CURRENT CLINICAL UROLOGY

ERIC A. KLEIN, MD, SERIES EDITOR

For other titles published in the series, go to
www.springer.com/series/7635

Robotic and Laparoscopic Reconstructive Surgery in Children and Adults

Edited by

Michael C. Ost, MD

Children's Hospital of Pittsburgh, Pittsburgh, PA

Humana Press

Editor
Michael C. Ost, MD
Pediatric Urology
Children's Hospital of Pittsburgh
Children's Hospital Drive
45th Street and Penn Avenue
4th Floor Faculty Building
Pittsburgh, PA 15201, USA
michael.ost@chp.edu

ISBN 978-1-4939-5783-5 ISBN 978-1-60327-914-7 (eBook)
DOI 10.1007/978-1-60327-914-7
Springer New York Dordrecht Heidelberg London

Printed on acid-free paper

Humana Press is part of Springer Science+Business Media (www.springer.com)

For my children, Lila, Jaitin, and Marcus.

Preface

I am thankful to have had the opportunity to work with Springer to create a unique textbook focusing on "Robotic and Laparoscopic Reconstructive Surgery in Children and Adults." The publication of this reference is timely and it is truly "one of a kind." It is not often that there is a union between adult and pediatric urologic surgical techniques. The breadth of this wonderful convergence is most clearly and consistently demonstrated when minimally invasive reconstructive techniques are utilized. I noted this observation from afar in my residency training, coveting a mastery of it in order to create a career and contribute toward the advancement of our very special field. In this regard, I pursued fellowship training in both minimally invasive urology (endourology–laparoscopy) and pediatric urology. I am grateful for having had the opportunity to learn from "the best in the business"; my time with Louis Kavoussi, MD, in New York and Steven Docimo in Pittsburgh was precious. Their teachings and mentorship are very much the embodiment of this book.

I am most appreciative of my colleagues and friends who have contributed to the authorship of this text. Michael Griffin, my developmental editor, certainly deserves special thanks. I am confident that pediatric urologists, adult urologists, fellows, and urology residents will find this textbook to be a comprehensive, yet concise, reference for all robotic and laparoscopic procedures that may be performed within our vast discipline.

Pittsburgh, PA — Michael C. Ost
March 2010

Contents

Part I Principles of Reconstructive Laparoscopy and Robotics in Urology

1 **Laparoscopic and Robotic Instrumentation for Urologic Reconstructive Surgery in Adults** 3
James F. Borin

2 **Instrumentation During Pediatric Robotic Anastomoses and Reconstruction** 17
Shahin Chandrasoma and Chester J. Koh

3 **Instrumentation During Pediatric Laparoscopic Anastomoses and Reconstruction** 29
Smart Zeidan and Alaa El-Ghoneimi

Part II Laparoscopic and Robotic Reconstructive Renal Surgery

4 **Adult Laparoscopic Partial Nephrectomy for Renal Cell Carcinoma** 43
Mohamed A. Atalla, Sero Andonian, and Manish A. Vira

5 **Adult Robotic-Assisted Partial Nephrectomy for Renal Cell Carcinoma** 55
Ronald S. Boris and Peter A. Pinto

6 **Pediatric Laparoscopic and Robotic Upper Pole Nephrectomy for Nonfunctioning Moieties** 73
Glenn M. Cannon and Richard S. Lee

Part III Laparoscopic and Robotic Reconstructive Renal Pelvis Surgery

7 **Adult Laparoscopic and Robotic-Assisted Pyeloplasty for Ureteropelvic Junction Obstruction** 85
Sarah P. Conley and Benjamin R. Lee

8 **Pediatric Laparoscopic (Infant, Pre-pubertal, and Teenager) Pyeloplasty for Ureteropelvic Junction Obstruction** **93**
Danielle D. Sweeney and Steven G. Docimo

9 **Pediatric Robotic (Infant, Pre-pubertal, and Teenager) Pyeloplasty for Ureteropelvic Junction Obstruction** **109**
Yoshiyuki Kojima and Pasquale Casale

Part IV Laparoscopic and Robotic Reconstructive Ureteral Surgery

10 **Laparoscopic Ureteroureterostomy and Correction of Ureteral Defects** **125**
Erica J. Traxel and Paul Noh

11 **Robotic Ureteroureterostomy and Correction of Ureteral Defects** **141**
Patricio C. Gargollo and Hiep T. Nguyen

Part V Laparoscopic and Robotic Reconstructive Bladder Surgery

12 **Robotic Radical Cystectomy and Use of Intestinal Segments for Reconstruction in the Adult Patient** **153**
Nikhil Waingankar, Mostafa A. Sadek, Michael J. Schwartz, Douglas S. Scherr, and Lee Richstone

13 **Laparoscopic Bladder Augmentation and Creation of Continent-Catheterizable Stomas in the Pediatric Patient** **167**
Kristin A. Kozakowski and Walid A. Farhat

14 **Laparoscopic Ureteral Reimplant Surgery to Correct Reflux Disease** **175**
Bekir Aras, Levent Gurkan, Ali Serdar Gözen, Dogu Teber, and Jens Rassweiler

15 **Robotic Ureteral Reimplant Surgery to Correct Reflux Disease** **185**
Craig A. Peters and Ryan P. Smith

Part VI Laparoscopic Orchiopexy in Children

16 **Laparoscopic and Robotic Orchiopexy for the Impalpable Undescended Testicle** **201**
Ahmad Z. Mohamed, Regina Norris, and Francis X. Schneck

Part VII Laparoscopic and Robotic Anastomoses for Radical Prostatectomy

17 Laparoscopic Anastomoses and Bladder Neck Reconstruction Following Radical Prostatectomy **221**
Ender Özden, Özcan Kılıç, Ali Serdar Gözen, Dogu Teber, and Jens Rassweiler

18 Robotic Anastomoses and Bladder Neck Reconstruction Following Radical Prostatectomy **235**
Marc C. Smaldone, Tina K. Schuster, and Stephen V. Jackman

Part VIII NOTES and LESS—Future Directions in MIS Reconstructive Surgery

19 The Role of NOTES and LESS in Minimally Invasive Reconstructive Urological Surgery **261**
Mark D. Sawyer and Lee Ponsky

Part IX Laparoscopy and Robotics in Incontinence and Pelvic Reconstructive Surgery

20 Laparoscopy and Robotics in Stress Urinary Incontinence and Pelvic Reconstructive Surgery **277**
Alvaro Lucioni and Kathleen C. Kobashi

Subject Index **293**

Contributors

Sero Andonian Department of Urology, McGill University Health Centre, Montreal, Canada, sero.andonian@muhc.mcgill.ca

Bekir Aras Department of Urology, Fatih Sultan Mehmet Training and Research Hospital, Istanbul, Turkey

Mohamed A. Atalla Laparoscopic and Robotic Urology, North Shore Long Island Jewish Health System, Arthur D. Smith Institute for Urology, Hofstra University School of Medicine, New Hyde Park, NY, USA, attala@att.net

James F. Borin Division of Urology, University of Maryland, Baltimore, MD, USA, jborin@smail.umaryland.edu

Ronald S. Boris Urologic Oncology Branch, National Cancer Institute, Bethesda, MD, USA, rboris@clarian.org

Glenn M. Cannon Department of Urology, Harvard Medical School, Children's Hospital Boston, Boston, MA, USA, cannongm2@upmc.edu

Pasquale Casale Division of Urology, The Children's Hospital of Philadelphia, Philadelphia, PA, USA, casale@email.chop.edu

Shahin Chandrasoma Division of Pediatric Urology, Keck School of Medicine, Children's Hospital Los Angeles, Institute of Urology, University of Southern California (USC), Los Angeles, CA, USA, schandrasoma@gmail.com

Sarah P. Conley Department of Urology, Tulane University School of Medicine, New Orleans, LA, USA, sconley2009@gmail.com

Steven G. Docimo Children's Hospital of Pittsburgh, Pittsburgh, PA 15232, USA, steven.docimo@chp.edu

Alaa El-Ghoneimi Faculty of Medicine, University of Paris VII, Paris, France; Department of Pediatric Surgery and Urology, Robert Debré Children University Hospital, Paris, France, alaa.elghoneimi@rdb.ap-hop-paris.fr

Walid A. Farhat Division of Urology, Department of Surgery, The Hospital for Sick Children, Toronto, ON, USA, walid.farhat@sickkids.ca

Patricio C. Gargollo Department of Pediatric Urology, Childrens Medical Center, UT Southwestern Medical Center, Dallas, TX, USA, patricio.gargollo@childrens.com

Ali Serdar Gözen Department of Urology, SLK-Klinikum Heilbronn, University of Heidelberg, Heilbronn, Germany, asgozen@yahoo.com

Levent Gurkan Department of Urology, SLK-Klinikum Heilbronn, University of Heidelberg, Heilbronn, Germany

Stephen V. Jackman Department of Urology, University of Pittsburgh Medical Center, 3471 Fifth Avenue, Suite 700, Pittsburgh, PA 15213, USA, jackmansv@upmc.edu

Özcan Kılıç SLK-Klinikum Heilbronn, University of Heidelberg, Heilbronn, Germany, drozcankilic@yahoo.com

Kathleen C. Kobashi Section of Urology and Renal Transplantation, Department of Urology, University of Washington, Virginia Mason Medical Center, Seattle, WA, USA, urokck@vmmc.org

Chester J. Koh Division of Pediatric Urology, Keck School of Medicine, Children's Hospital Los Angeles, Institute of Urology, University of Southern California (USC), Los Angeles, CA, USA, ckoh@chla.usc.edu

Yoshiyuki Kojima Division of Urology, The Children's Hospital of Philadelphia, University of Pennsylvania, Philadelphia, PA, USA; Department of Nephro-Urology, Nagoya City University Graduate School of Medical Sciences, Nagoya, Japan, ykojima0919@gmail.com

Kristin A. Kozakowski Urology, The Hospital for Sick Children, Toronto, ON, USA, kkoz99@gmail.com

Richard S. Lee Department of Urology, Harvard Medical School, Children's Hospital Boston, Boston, MA, USA, richard.lee@childrens.harvard.edu

Benjamin R. Lee Department of Urology, Tulane University School of Medicine, New Orleans, LA, USA, brlee@tulane.edu

Alvaro Lucioni The Continence Center at Virginia Mason Medical Center, Seattle, WA, USA, alvaro.lucioni@vmmc.org

Ahmad Z. Mohamed Department of Urology, Children's Hospital of Pittsburgh of UPMC, Pittsburgh, PA, USA, ahmad.mohamed@chp.edu

Hiep T. Nguyen Department of Urology, Children's Hospital Boston, Boston, MA, USA, hiep.nguyen@childrens.harvard.edu

Paul Noh Division of Pediatric Urology, Cincinnati Children's Hospital Medical Center, Cincinnati, OH, USA, paul.noh@cchmc.org

Regina Norris Division of Pediatric Urology, Children's Hospital of Pittsburgh of UPMC, Pittsburgh, PA, USA, regina.norris@chp.edu

Ender Özden SLK-Klinikum Heilbronn, University of Heidelberg, Heilbronn, Germany, eozden@omu-edu.tr

Craig A. Peters Division of Pediatric Urology, University of Virginia Children's Hospital, Charlottesville, VA, USA, cap9b@virginia.edu

Peter A. Pinto Urologic Oncology Branch, National Cancer Institute, Bethesda, MD, USA, pintop@mail.nih.gov

Lee Ponsky Division of Orologic Oncology, Department of Urology, Center of Urologic Oncology and Minimally Invasive Therapies, University Hospitals Case Medical Center, Cleveland, OH, USA, 3471 Fifth Avenue, Suite 700, Pittsburgh, PA 15213, USA, lee.ponsky@uhhospitals.org

Jens Rassweiler Department of Urology, SLK-Klinikum Heilbronn, University of Heidelberg, Heilbronn, Germany, jens.rassweiler@slk-kliniken.de

Lee Richstone North Shore-Long Island Jewish Health System, The Smith Institute for Urology, New Hyde Park, NY, USA

Mostafa A. Sadek Arthur D. Smith Institute for Urology, New Hyde Park, NY, USA

Mark D. Sawyer Division of Orologic Oncology, Department of Urology, Center of Urologic Oncology and Minimally Invasive Therapies, University Hospitals Case Medical Center, Cleveland, OH, USA, mark.sawyer@vanderbilt.edu

Douglas S. Scherr The New York Presbyterian Hospital, Weill Medical College of Cornell University, New York, NY, USA

Francis X. Schneck Division of Pediatric Urology, Children's Hospital of Pittsburgh of UPMC, Pittsburgh, PA, USA, schneckf@upmc.edu

Tina K. Schuster Department of Urology, University of Pittsburgh Medical Center, 3471 Fifth Avenue, Suite 700, Pittsburgh, PA 15213, USA, tschuster88@gmail.com

Michael J. Schwartz North Shore Long Island Jewish Health System, Arthur D. Smith Institute for Urology, Hofstra University School of Medicine, New Hyde Park, NY, USA

Marc C. Smaldone Department of Surgical Oncology, Fox Chase Cancer Center, 333 Cottman Avenue, Philadelphia, PA 19111, USA, smaldonemc@gmail.com

Ryan P. Smith Department of Urology, University of Virginia, Charlottesville, VA, USA, rps2k@virginia.edu

Danielle D. Sweeney Pediatric Urology, Dell Children's Hospital, Austin, TX, USA, danielledsweeney@gmail.com

Dogu Teber Department of Urology, SLK-Klinikum Heilbronn, University of Heidelberg, Heilbronn, Germany, doguteber@hotmail.com

Erica J. Traxel Division of Pediatric Urology, Department of Surgery, St. Louis Children's Hospital, Washington University School of Medicine, St. Louis, MO, USA, traxele@wudosis.wustl.edu

Manish A. Vira Department of Urology, North Shore Long Island Jewish Health System, Arthur D. Smith Institute for Urology, Hofstra University School of Medicine, New Hyde Park, NY, USA, mvira@nshs.edu

Nikhil Waingankar North Shore-Long Island Jewish Health System, Arthur D. Smith Institute for Urology, New Hyde Park, NY, USA, nwaingankar@nshs.edu

Smart Zeidan Department of Pediatric Surgery and Urology, Robert Debré Children University Hospital, Paris, France, smartzeidan@gmail.com

Part I
Principles of Reconstructive Laparoscopy and Robotics in Urology

Chapter 1

Laparoscopic and Robotic Instrumentation for Urologic Reconstructive Surgery in Adults

James F. Borin

Instruments employed in minimally invasive surgery often vary across different countries, regions, and institutions, often due to a matter of preference and training. Most procedures can be carried out quite effectively with a very basic set of tools: scissors, grasper, needle driver. However, more specific instruments will facilitate standard procedures and make challenging procedures feasible. The principles of open surgery are still paramount in the minimally invasive realm: adequate exposure, gentle dissection, minimal tissue manipulation, and watertight anastomoses. This chapter will highlight some, but not all, of the instruments commonly employed in laparoscopic and robotic-assisted reconstructive urologic surgery.

Laparoscopy vs. Robotics

Robot-assisted surgery is performed in a laparoscopic environment and therefore many of the standard laparoscopic instruments will be employed. Robotic surgery is at once both more versatile and yet more limiting than standard laparoscopy. The versatility comes in the form of the 30 EndoWrist® instruments available for the da Vinci surgical platform (Intuitive Surgical Inc., Sunnyvale, CA) [1]. While these instruments mirror their open or laparoscopic predecessors, the increased degrees of freedom inherent in the "wrist" provide for more functionality. However, of these 30 instruments, perhaps only 15 are commonly used, and most procedures will employ only 5 or 6. The limitation of robotic surgery, therefore, is the dearth of instruments available to the console surgeon. On the other hand, while the operating surgeon has command over a few basic instruments, essentially scissors, grasper, and needle drivers, the assistant can draw from the entire armamentarium of laparoscopic tools in order to provide retraction, dissection, or hemostasis. Thus, the skill and facility of the assistant will often dictate the complexity of reconstructive procedures which may be attempted.

This reliance on the assistant is one facet of robotic surgery which may make some skilled laparoscopic surgeons more reluctant to attempt complicated procedures. A case in point is partial nephrectomy. Using a pure laparoscopic approach, the surgeon is able to position the renal hilum occlusion device, whether Satinsky clamp or bulldogs, and may even provide his own suction during tumor excision and renorrhaphy. With a robotic approach, those tasks must be performed by an assistant. In order to partially compensate for this, some have advocated using an atraumatic grasper in the fourth arm to provide compression of the hilum, thereby removing this task from the assistant and obviating the need for bulldog clamps, which can be difficult to remove,

J.F. Borin (✉)
Division of Urology, University of Maryland, Baltimore, MD, USA
e-mail: jborin@smail.umaryland.edu

M.C. Ost (ed.), *Robotic and Laparoscopic Reconstructive Surgery in Children and Adults*, Current Clinical Urology, DOI 10.1007/978-1-60327-914-7_1, © Springer Science+Business Media, LLC 2011

or a Satinsky clamp, which could be inadvertently dislodged [2, 3]. There are also new instruments in development which will provide the console surgeon with the ability to suction/irrigate and even staple (personal communication; Intuitive Surgical, Inc., Sunnyvale, CA). Until such time, however, robotic surgery will continue to be a hybrid of a limited number of advanced wristed instruments and standard laparoscopic instruments controlled by an assistant. Although there is considerable overlap between standard laparoscopic and robotic instruments, this chapter will deal with them separately.

Standard Laparoscopic Instrumentation

Graspers and Dissectors

The main distinction between the various types of graspers and dissectors is the type of jaws they contain, whether traumatic or atraumatic. The latter are more versatile and can be used to handle any type of tissue, while the former are more specialized in their indications. Most instruments are 5 mm in width but can range from 3 to 12 mm; length ranges from 34 to 37 mm. The instrument jaws can be either curved or straight, single action (i.e., only one jaw moves, while the other remains stationary) or double action (both jaws move equally). The tip of the instrument can be blunt, tapered (dolphin), flat/rounded (duck-bill), curved (Maryland), or angled (Mixter) (Fig. 1.1).

Handles used for dissection generally have a mechanism that opens and closes freely, similar to a pair of scissors. Jaws may be smooth or serrated for atraumatic instruments, while traumatic instruments will contain a number of dull or sharp teeth in order to firmly grasp tissue. These may be used in conjunction with a ratcheted, locking handle.

Incision and Hemostasis

Instruments used to incise tissue are often coupled with an energy source, monopolar, bipolar, or harmonic. Cold scissors are an effective way to cut through thin areolar tissue in avascular

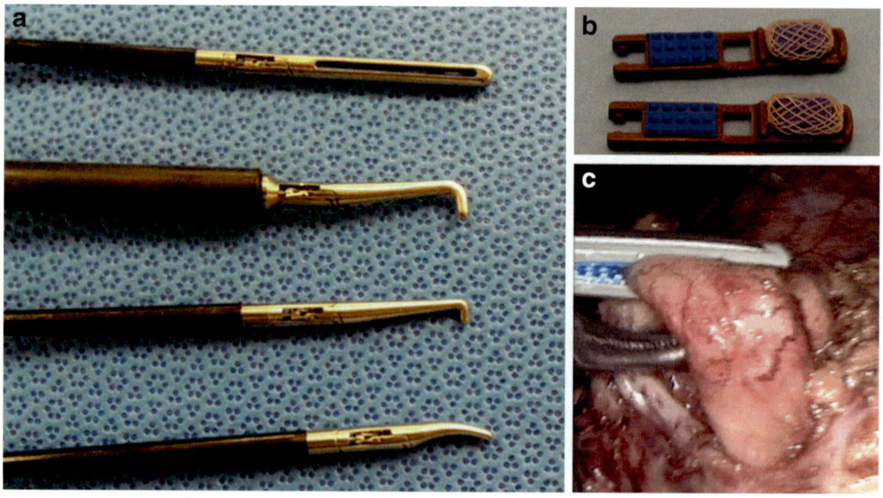

Fig. 1.1 Laparoscopic graspers. There is a diversity of jaw sizes and configurations. (**a**) (*top to bottom*) Fenestrated bowel grasper, 10 mm right angle (Mixter), 5 mm right angle, Maryland. (**b**) Disposable rubber and mesh inserts for Direct Drive atraumatic grasper (Applied Medical, Rancho Santa Margarita, CA). There is also an entire disposable instrument with similar grip. This is particularly useful for reconstruction involving the ureter as the soft jaws will not damage or devascularize this delicate structure (**c**)

planes; monopolar energy can be added in order to cauterize small vessels. There are a variety of scissor tips available: straight, hooked, curved, and microscissors, for example. The latter are similar to Potts scissors and may be helpful for ureteral spatulation during pyeloplasty or ureteroneocystostomy. While the majority of standard laparoscopic instruments are reusable and quite resistant to wear, scissors in particular can become dull over time. This is of particular importance during partial nephrectomy. Disposable scissors are one option, although they may be less robust and more difficult to maneuver than their reusable counterparts. Another option is a reusable shaft with disposable tip, which ensures a strong instrument and sharp blades with every use.

The monopolar hook electrode is useful for dissection, particularly around tubular structures, such as the renal hilum and ureter. Small vessels may be cauterized by placing them on stretch and applying short bursts of cautery. However, the hook cannot efficiently coagulate vessels larger than a few millimeters. Furthermore, monopolar energy is potentially more dangerous than bipolar or harmonic due to the pattern of current spread across the tissue as well as the possibility of current arcing through an insulation gap, which can result in unrecognized bowel injury [4].

In bipolar coagulation, energy flows from one jaw of the instrument to the other, which significantly reduces the flow of current into tissues and theoretically reduces thermal spread and capacitive coupling. Simple bipolar instruments use an electrosurgical unit (i.e., standard "Bovie"); the surgeon activates the bipolar energy with a foot pedal and uses visual cues, such as charring or cessation of bleeding, to determine when to discontinue the current. There are several so-called "smart" bipolar instruments which generally provide permanent sealing of vessels up to 7 mm in diameter, as well as lymphatics and tissue bundles. Their technology differs slightly, but overall performance in clinical testing has been similar among the various models [5]. One of the more popular models is the LigaSure™ vessel sealing system (Valleylab, Boulder, Colorado), which produces at least four times the current of a standard electrosurgery generator with one-fifth to one-twentieth the amount of voltage [6]. As opposed to a standard electrosurgical unit, the LigaSure™ uses TissueFect™ sensing technology to actively monitor changes in tissue impedance and provide a real-time adjustment of the energy output [7]. The LigaSure™ also has a cutting blade that is activated once the tissue has been coagulated or sealed. This allows for efficient, hemostatic dissection with a single instrument. It is available in a 5 or 10 mm diameter; the latter has larger jaws and can handle more tissue (Fig. 1.2).

Ultrasonic energy significantly limits thermal damage to adjacent tissue to $\leq$ 1 mm from the activation site [8]. The Harmonic ACE® (Ethicon Endo-Surgery, Cincinnati, OH) is an ultrasonic cutting and coagulating surgical device, also referred to as harmonic shears or harmonic scalpel. In this instrument, electrical energy is transformed into mechanical vibration within a handpiece that contains piezoelectric crystals. While the risk of local thermal damage and tissue charring is significantly reduced, the active blade does get quite hot due to ultrasonic vibrations and care must be taken to avoid inadvertently touching it to adjacent structures.

The above instruments are used for dissection as well as coagulating small vessels. However, for pure hemostasis, the argon beam coagulator (ABC) (Conmed, Utica, NY) is an exceedingly valuable tool. This is a non-contact monopolar energy device which delivers electric current generated by an electrosurgical unit via a stream of inert argon gas. The pressure of the gas helps to clear away a small amount of blood and debris, which facilitates coagulation of the bleeding point. The ABC has a depth of penetration of about 0.5 mm, causing extensive charring of the surface with minimal thermal damage (Fig. 1.2). It is especially useful in obtaining hemostasis in the partial nephrectomy bed after either clamped or unclamped tumor excision. The ABC can also be used to seal small avulsed vessels. Is it important to remember that ABC activation will release a stream of argon gas into the peritoneal cavity thereby increasing the pneumoperitoneal pressure. While the gas is rapidly absorbed and

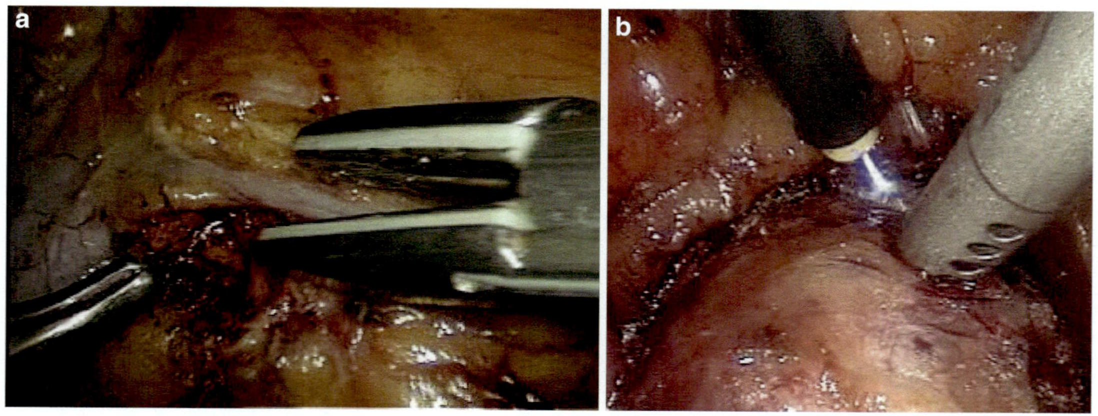

Fig. 1.2 Hemostatic devices: the 10-mm LigaSure^{TM} has large rounded, blunt jaws which are good for dissection and for fulguration of thick tissue. It may also be used to ligate larger vessels, such as the gonadal vein, shown here (**a**). The argon beam coagulator employs monopolar energy in a stream of argon gas to deliver a fine spray of cautery (**b**). A standard suction/irrigation tip with fenestrations is seen in the foreground

cleared from the body, prolonged activation must be coupled with either active suction or passive ventilation (i.e., opening one of the trocar side ports) in order to avoid prolonged elevation of pneumoperitoneum >20 mm Hg which can compromise venous return and/or cause air embolism.

Suturing

Needle drivers, like graspers, are available in several different configurations. The choice of instrument used is often due to personal preference; each type and style has its advantages and disadvantages. The jaws of the needle driver can be either serrated or smooth to allow for more or less play in the needle once locked in place. In addition, the tip can be straight or curved, solid or fenestrated (Fig. 1.3). The latter may be helpful in assuring the proper orientation of the needle. A heavy needle holder (i.e., Ethicon) may allow for easier passage of a needle through tissue, but prolonged suturing with heavy instruments may cause more shoulder strain. Conversely, lighter drivers (i.e., Storz, Snowden-Pencer) may be more comfortable to use over time at the potential expense of precision.

The locking mechanism is perhaps the most important quality of a needle driver and is most subject to personal preference. Mechanisms are generally either ratcheted or Castro-Viejo type (Fig. 1.3). The former allows for graduated pressure to be applied on the needle while still keeping it in place. With only a few clicks on

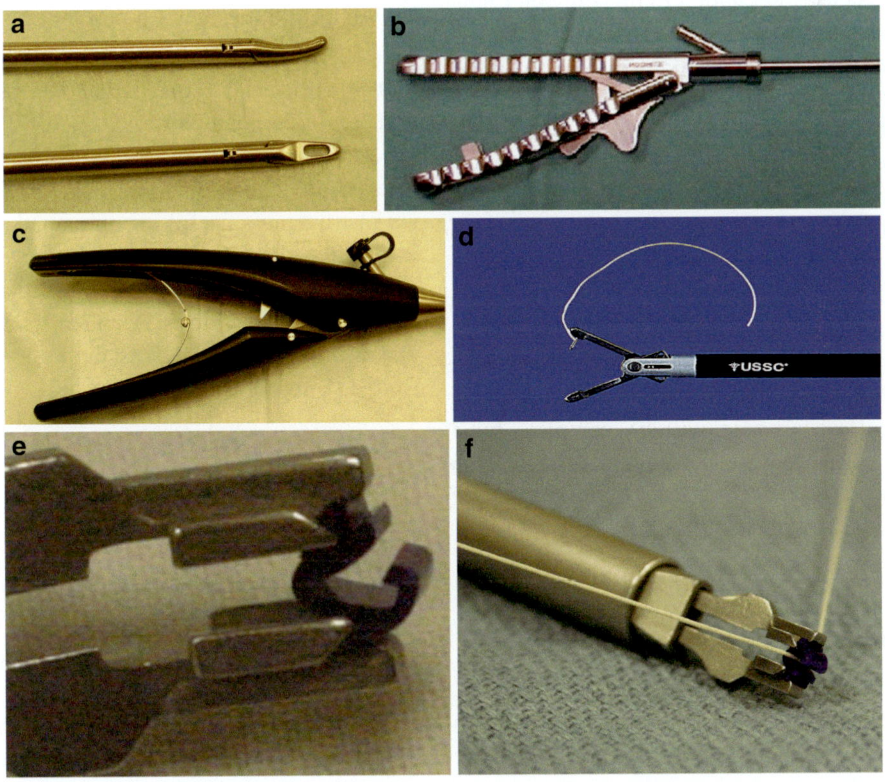

Fig. 1.3 Suturing instruments: laparoscopic needle driver jaws may be *curved* or *straight*, solid or fenestrated (**a**). Most manufacturers favor a ratchet mechanism for the handle (**b**), but Castro-Viejo style is another option (**c**). (**d**) Endo Stitch device with 9-mm straight needle. (**e**) The Lapra-Ty is a locking, absorbable clip delivered via a sturdy 10-mm laparoscopic applier. It is important to secure the suture within the deepest portion of the hinge in order to ensure maximum hold strength (**f**)

the ratchet mechanism, the angle of the needle may be easily adjusted before locking it firmly in place. Care must be taken when activating the release mechanism to avoid temporarily losing control of the needle. The Castro-Viejo-type mechanism is either locked or unlocked. The action is often a bit smoother than the ratchet type; however, once locked in place, it is more difficult to make fine adjustments to needle position.

Because laparoscopic suturing is a difficult skill to master, several adjuncts have been devised. The Endo Stitch device (Covidien/Autosuture, Mansfield, MA) is a 10-mm instrument that shuttles a 9-mm straight needle between two jaws, with tissue grasped in between (Fig. 1.3). It is particularly useful for pyeloplasty but not for renorrhaphy [9].

Perhaps one of the most versatile products in this category is the Lapra-Ty clip (Ethicon Endo-Surgery, Cincinnati, OH). It is placed on the end of piece of suture which is then used to secure two pieces of tissue. A laparoscopic applicator then delivers a second clip, thereby obviating the need for knot tying in many complex urologic laparoscopic procedures such as pyeloplasty, partial nephrectomy, and urethrovesical anastomosis (Fig. 1.3). The Lapra-Ty clip is composed of poly(*p*-dioxanone) (PDS) which breaks down via hydrolysis and, according to the manufacturer, can maintain a hold strength on a 3-0- or a 4-0-coated Vicryl suture for 10 days following placement; absorbance will be complete by 7 months. It has also been used successfully both experimentally and clinically on other types of suture (esp. Monocryl) [10].

Stapling/Clipping

These devices are a ubiquitous part of laparoscopic urologic surgery. The clips and staples are made of titanium which is MRI compatible and highly resistant to encrustation within the urinary tract [11]. The clip appliers hold a sheath of clips which can be fired repeatedly for vessel or ureter ligation. Applicators are either 5 or 10 mm in size, generally corresponding to the relative size of clips delivered. However, a newer version of the 5-mm instrument (Ligamax™ 5; Ethicon Endo-Surgery, Cincinnati, OH) will fire clips equivalent to a 10-mm device; this lower profile may facilitate control of vessels when there is little working room or visibility. Staplers deliver two triple-staggered rows of staples and simultaneously cut in between the rows. The type of material being divided will dictate the size of staples used. Generally, a 2.5-mm cartridge is used for vasculature and ≥3.5 mm for bowel or thick tissue. Non-absorbable polymer-ligating clips with a locking mechanism at the tip may provide more secure ligation of large vessels (Hem-o-lock clips; Teleflex Medical, Research Triangle Park, NC).

Suction/Irrigation

This device is available as an entirely disposable unit or a disposable unit which can be coupled with reusable cannulas of 5 or 10 mm diameter. The most common is a 5-mm cannula with a length of 32–36 cm (Fig. 1.2). A longer 45-cm instrument is useful for obese patients and is invaluable in robot-assisted procedures in order to allow the assistant more room to maneuver around the robotic arms. A battery-powered irrigation unit provides pressurized flow; suction is from a standard wall unit.

Retraction

Retraction can be provided by a variety of instruments depending on the structures surrounding the area to be exposed. An endo-peanut (Küttner) dissector is versatile and atraumatic; it can be used for bowel, liver, spleen, or even the vena cava or renal hilum. However, the surface area is small, only 5–10 mm, so for prolonged retraction of larger structures, a triangle, esophageal, PEER (Jarit/Integra Surgical, Plainsboro, NJ), or fan retractor may be more efficacious to prevent slippage (Fig. 1.4). If an additional assistant is not available to provide stationary retraction, an Endoholder® (Codman, Raynham, MA) is a

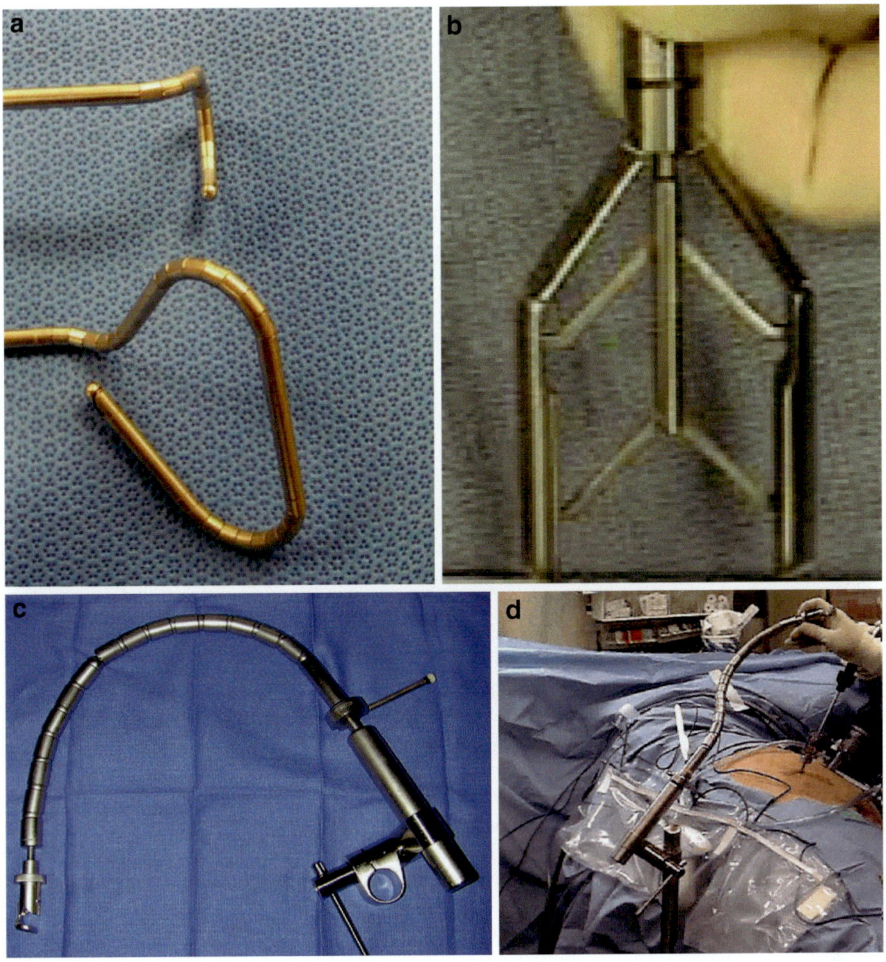

Fig. 1.4 Retractors: (**a**) several retractors contain a hinged mechanism which allows them to be delivered through a 5-mm port and then transformed into a round or a triangular configuration, particularly useful for retraction of spleen, liver, or pancreas (*top*: esophageal retractor, *bottom*: triangle or "snake" retractor). (**b**) The PEER retractor is available in 5 and 10 mm sizes and expands once delivered into the abdomen. It is helpful in retracting the kidney to expose the hilum for more efficient dissection of the renal vessels. (**c**) The Endoholder has a snake-like mechanism which allows it a great deal of flexibility. It is mounted to the side of the table and can be attached to any 5- or 10-mm instrument and then firmly locked in place to deliver consistent stable retraction (**d**). This obviates the need for a second assistant

useful device which can be attached to virtually any 5- or 10-mm instrument, holding it tightly in place (Fig. 1.4).

Vascular Clamps

Renal hilum occlusion during laparoscopic partial nephrectomy may be achieved via either a Satinsky or a bulldog clamp (Fig. 1.5). The Satinsky may occlude the hilum en bloc or just the artery alone. Bulldogs are generally placed across each individual vessel. The Satinsky is easier to place and requires less hilar dissection, although a separate, dedicated 12-mm port is necessary. Bulldogs (Klein Surgical, Bulverde, TX or Aesculap, Center Valley, PA) are placed with a laparoscopic applicator which is then removed from the field; they are later removed using the same applicator (Klein) or

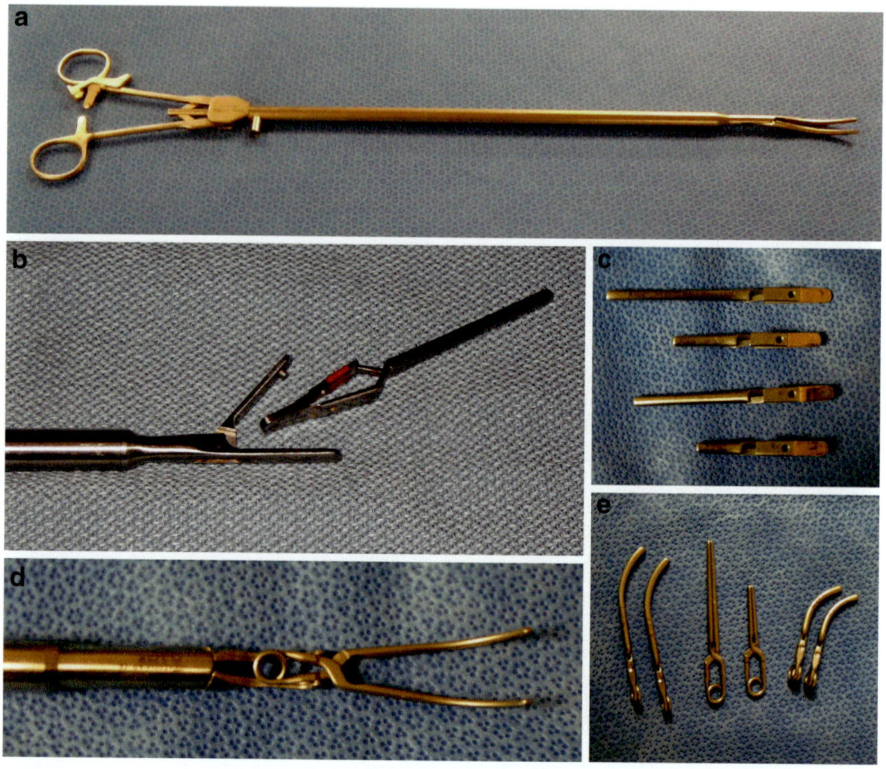

Fig. 1.5 Vascular clamps: (**a**) the Satinsky is a 10-mm instrument which can be used to occlude renal artery alone or artery and vein together; in the latter case, minimal hilar dissection is required. (**b**, **c**) Klein bulldogs require a single instrument for application or removal. (**d**, **e**) Aesculap bulldogs have a spring-like configuration and the jaws are thinner; application and removal are performed with separate devices

a special removal device (Aesculap) (Fig. 1.5). Occasionally, more than one bulldog must be placed on the renal artery to provide adequate occlusion.

Port-Site Closure

Lateral blunt-tipped trocar sites ≤10 mm may not require fascial closure [12]. However, for midline port sites > 5 mm, fascial closure is appropriate to decrease the incidence of hernias. Free-hand suturing is an option; however, closure with a Carter–Thomason device (Inlet Medical, Eden Prairie, MN) using Vicryl suture is fast and offers the most secure closure with few complications [13].

Robotic Instruments

The da Vinci Surgical System online catalog lists 39 instruments for use with 8-mm trocars [1]. The majority of these instruments have a limited life span of 10 uses; a computer chip housed in the instrument counts down each life. The da Vinci instruments are "wristed," that is, they contain a joint at the tip of the instrument which can articulate 90°. This provides greater maneuverability and dexterity than do straight instruments. A standard laparoscopic grasper or scissors has four degrees of freedom (dof): (1) in/out, (2) pitch (up/down), (3) yaw (left/right), (4) rotation (clockwise/counterclockwise). The da Vinci instrument, equipped with an EndoWrist®, has six dof: (1) in/out, (2) external yaw (left/right), (3) external pitch (up/down),

(4) rotation (clockwise/counterclockwise), (5) internal pitch (wristed portion up/down), (6) internal yaw (wristed portion left/right) [14]. Grip (open/close jaws) may also be considered an additional degree of freedom; thus da Vinci instruments are advertised to contain a total of seven dof. When a surgeon performs open suturing, his wrist is far removed from the needle; it is separated by the length of the needle driver, some 6 in. or so. When suturing with a da Vinci instrument, the "wrist" is only a few centimeters away from the needle. This design is thought to provide greater precision overall, and particularly for delicate maneuvers in confined spaces.

Of the available 8-mm instruments, only about half are commonly used by urologists (Table 1.1). For any given reconstructive case, generally five to six instruments will be employed: cautery/energy, bipolar forceps, large grasper, needle drivers (2), additional scissors (optional). The approximate robot-associated cost for a five-instrument procedure, including per use instrument cost, drapes, and disposables, is $1,425 (personal communication, Intuitive Surgical, Inc.). For some renal reconstructive procedures (pyeloplasty, ureteroureterostomy, pyelolithotomy), it may only be necessary to use two instrument arms of the robot instead of three. For maximum cost reduction, a total of three instruments can be employed for selected procedures: scissors (especially Hot Shears™), bipolar forceps, needle driver. Suturing can be performed effectively with a single needle driver in the dominant hand combined with bipolar forceps.

A combination of cost prohibition (approximately $200–320 each time a new instrument is used [15]) and inefficiency with exchanges may restrict the diversity of instruments employed during a single case. The current number and variety of da Vinci instruments is limited in comparison to the dozens available for standard laparoscopy by a variety of manufacturers. However, the versatility of the EndoWrist® design allows for instrument multifunctionality which obviates many of these concerns. For example, there is currently no robotic right-angle (Mixter) clamp. However, 90° angulation of a Maryland or PK® Dissecting Forceps produces a similar result and is quite useful to dissect out the renal vessels.

Monopolar Cautery

Monopolar instruments include the hook, spatula, and Hot Shears™. The hook and spatula represent the earliest iteration of instrumentation, combination of familiar tools from standard laparoscopy (L-hook) and open surgery (handheld bovie), respectively. The hook is quite useful for blunt and fine dissection as well as targeted cautery. The spatula is excellent for blunt dissection with less risk of accidental perforation of underlying vessels due to its blunt tip. The Hot Shears™ is a curved scissors which mimics its laparoscopic counterpart (Fig. 1.6). This instrument has the most versatility as it can be used for fine, blunt, and sharp dissections. Many surgeons who previously used the hook or the spatula now

Table 1.1 Eight-millimeter da Vinci instruments commonly used in urologic surgery

Energy-based	
Monopolar	Hot Shears™ (Curved), hook, spatula
Bipolar forceps	Maryland, PK® Dissecting, PreCise™, fenestrated
Ultrasonic	Harmonic® Curved Shears
Needle drivers	Large, Large SutureCut™, Mega, Mega SutureCut™
Forceps	ProGrasp™, Cadiere, Tenaculum, DeBakey
Graspers	Cobra, Thoracic, Graptor™
Cold scissors	Curved, round tip, Potts
Clip appliers	Small (titanium clip), large Hem-o-Lok®

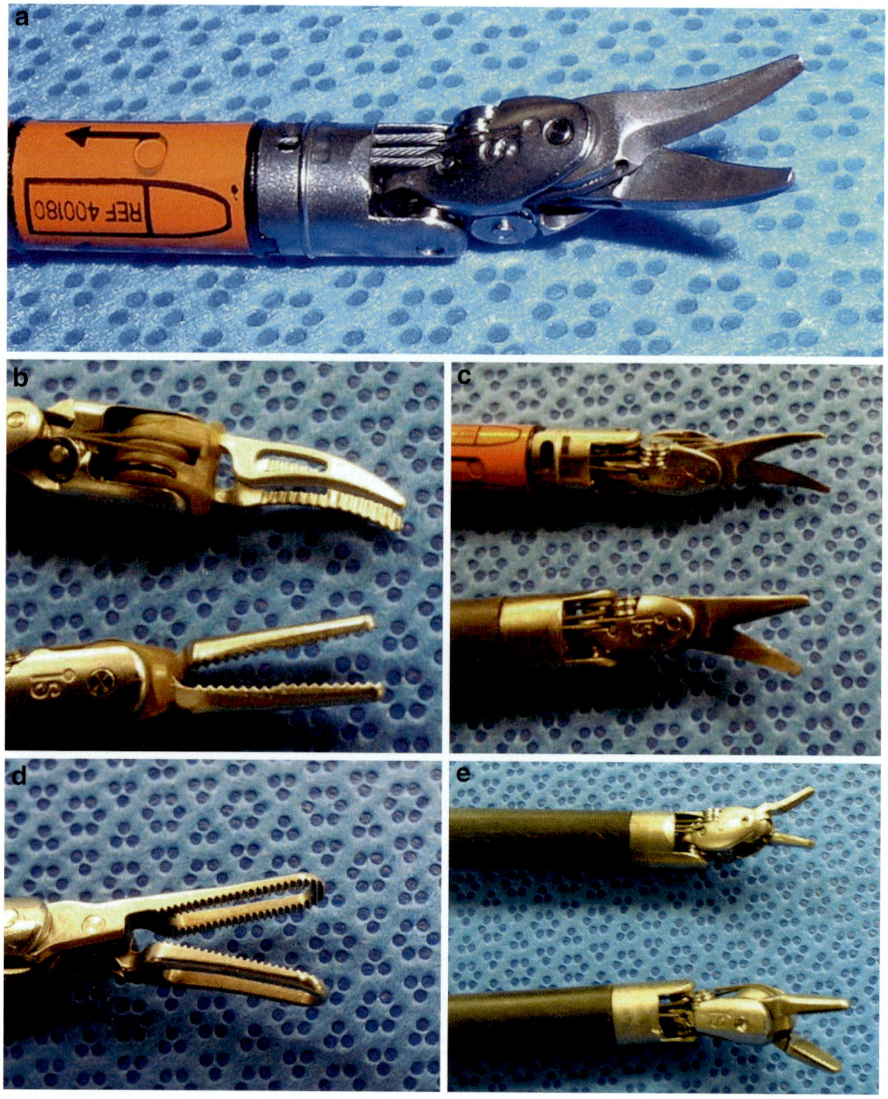

Fig. 1.6 Robotic instruments: (**a**) Hot Shears™—note the thick metal cables which provide articulation at the "wristed" joint. (**b**) Bipolar forceps: Maryland (*top*), PK (*bottom*). (**c**) Hot Shears™ (*top*) and cold scissors (*bottom*) are very similar in size and shape. (**d**) The ProGrasp™ has large oval, fenestrated jaws with small teeth for a firm grip. (**e**) The most popular size of needle driver is large (*top*). The mega (*bottom*) is shown in comparison

exclusively employ Hot Shears™. There is also potentially a cost savings of $80/case in this strategy. While Hot Shears™ are more expensive on a per use basis compared to the other two instruments ($320 vs. $200), they do obviate the requirement of an additional scissors ($200/use), which would almost certainly need to be employed in conjunction with hook or spatula during a reconstructive procedure. However, although rated for 10 uses, the Hot Shears™ can become dull prematurely which may necessitate employing an additional scissor for sharp dissection; this shortcoming may nullify their cost advantage.

Bipolar Cautery

The Maryland and PreCise™ bipolar forceps perform well as dissectors, graspers, and retractors. Their jaws are curved and triangle shaped, respectively, and surgeon's preference will dictate which one is used, although the Maryland is generally a more familiar design due to its laparoscopic predecessor (Fig. 1.6). The narrow tips of each allow for targeted delivery of bipolar energy, although thick tissue (especially fat) may be grasped within the entire jaw for quick and thorough coagulation. There is no sensor mechanism associated with either of these; similar to monopolar cautery, the surgeon uses visual cues to determine when sufficient coagulation has occurred. They have medium grip strength and thus may be used to grasp and retract tissue as well as to suture, although they function better in "catching" rather than "throwing" a needle because of the potential for slippage. In comparison, the da Vinci large needle driver has very high grip strength.

A newer bipolar option is the PK® Dissecting Forceps, which is a so-called "smart" instrument. It will sound an unpleasant warning when too much tissue has been grasped or when the jaws are touching; the generator will not deliver any energy until the proper adjustment is made. A satisfying tone will sound to signify that coagulation or vessel sealing has been achieved. The jaws are similar to a laparoscopic Maryland and longer and narrower than the da Vinci Maryland, which is more like a curved triangle (Fig. 1.6). The tips are rounded which makes them very useful for blunt dissection. The cost of these instruments is similar ($270 vs. $290/use); however, the PK requires a proprietary "smart" generator, whereas the others can use a standard electrosurgical unit. Furthermore, the PK has a weak (low) grip strength which may allow for more efficient coagulation—less risk of grasping the tissue too tightly causing the jaws to touch—however, this difference can be noticeable during grasping as tissue is more prone to slippage. Similar to the other bipolar instruments, the PK may be used to assist in suturing as the low-profile weak jaws are less damaging to tissue than is a standard needle driver.

Ultrasonic Energy

The da Vinci is capable of supporting a Harmonic® Curved Shears. This is a two-piece instrument; a shaft with a harmonic insert. The shaft has 20 lives while each insert is disposable. The total cost is about $430 per use [15]. In order to ensure efficient energy transfer, the "active" vibrating blade of the ultrasonic shears must be continuous from the piezoelectric crystal to the tip of the instrument. Therefore, it does not have any wristed articulation, so the maneuverability is limited, similar to its standard laparoscopic counterpart.

Scissors

While the cautery shears have more versatility than cold scissors, they are more prone to early dullness; therefore it is essential to have more than one type of scissors available. The three types offered are round tip, curved, and Potts. The round tip are perhaps the least useful because they have a straight blade with a blunted tip, possibly valuable for cutting through thick scar tissue as they have a strong closing force. The curved scissors are very similar in design to the hot scissors; both have narrow tips good for dissecting and a jaw length of 1.3 cm (Fig. 1.6). The former were an earlier iteration and were designed with a medium closing force and strong opening force; the hot scissors have a strong closing force and a medium opening force. Finally, Potts scissors recreate the standard open instrument; they have very narrow jaws designed for fine work. Some have employed them during nerve dissection in radical prostatectomy but they may be most useful for ureteral spatulation in a pyeloplasty or ureteroneocystostomy.

Graspers

Intuitive Surgical offers 13 graspers or forceps, but some are specialized for cardiac or thoracic procedures and would not have much use in urological surgery. By far the most popular and versatile is the ProGrasp™. The jaws are oval shaped, 2.8 cm in length, with a large fenestration and fine, atraumatic teeth (Fig. 1.6). They have high grip strength, so there is little risk of tissue slippage. The most common use of this device is via the fourth arm as an adjunct to retraction. Cadiere forceps, a precursor to the ProGrasp™, also contain an ovoid fenestrated jaw; the length is shorter at 2.0 cm and the atraumatic teeth are significantly more prominent, although grip strength is weak. The Cobra grasper has a solid rectangular jaw, 2.0 cm in length, with prominent serrations and four interlocking teeth at the tip. Although it also has weak grip strength, the teeth may make it impractical for grasping some tissues (i.e., bowel).

Needle Drivers

The most popular suturing instrument is the large needle driver (Fig. 1.6); with a jaw length of 1.0 cm and very high closing strength, it is ideal for the majority of urologic suturing, most of which involve SH, RB-1, or CT-1 needles and suture ranging from 0 to 5-0. The large SutureCut™ driver is another option. This is a modification of the large needle driver wherein a sharpened edge at the base of each jaw functions as a scissors which can be used to cut sutures. This obviates the need for an assistant to cut sutures and improves on the practice of using two needle drivers to tear the needle off the end of the suture. One caveat is that inexperience with this device can result in inadvertent suture transection; therefore practice is important prior to using it in a live case. The other two needle drivers available, Mega and Black Diamond Micro, are either too large or too small, respectively, to be utility instruments in urologic reconstructive surgery. The latter may be useful for very fine sutures with small needles in specific situations, but needle slippage can be problematic even with RB-1 needles.

Clip Appliers

There are two clip appliers, both of which have wristed articulation and are engineered to be discarded after 100 clips are applied. The small clip applier delivers an individual small titanium clip, while the large one applies a large Hem-o-Lok® clip, a non-absorbable polymer-ligating clip with a locking mechanism. In both cases, the instrument must be removed, reloaded manually, and then replaced if a second clip is to be deployed. With a skilled assistant, this process can be fairly rapid; on the other hand, a skilled assistant is generally able to deliver titanium or Hem-o-Lok® clips with tremendous accuracy and economy using a standard laparoscopic applier. The da Vinci clip appliers may be advantageous for use when a skilled assistant is unavailable; however, the process of reloading may be slower.

Five-Millimeter Instruments

There are 10 5-mm instruments available which duplicate their 8-mm counterparts (Table 1.2).

Table 1.2 Five-millimeter da Vinci instruments

Energy-based	
Monopolar	Hook, spatula
Ultrasonic	Harmonic® Curved Shears
Needle drivers	5-mm needle driver
Forceps	Maryland, DeBakey
Graspers	Schertel, bowel
Cold scissors	Curved, round tip

These were initially designed for pediatric use but may also be valuable for reconstruction in adults. While they do articulate, there is not a single wrist joint but rather a series of three joints providing a snake-like curvature. Energy-based instruments include a hook and a spatula as well as a (non-articulating) harmonic scalpel. There are no bipolar instruments, so a Maryland grasper is most commonly employed. Each 5-mm instrument is rated for 20 uses with an approximate cost of $230/use. In order to use the 5-mm instruments, 5-mm da Vinci cannulas must be employed, for an upfront cost of about $2,400 for two trocars and an obturator [15].

References

1. EndoWrist® Instrument and Accessory Catalog. June 2009. http://www.intuitivesurgical.com/products/endowrist_instruments/871145_I_I&A_Catalog_2009_Public_Screen.pdf. Accessed Sep 1, 2009.
2. Bhayani SB, Das N. Robotic assisted laparoscopic partial nephrectomy for suspected renal cell carcinoma: retrospective review of surgical outcomes of 35 cases. BMC Surg. 2008;8:16.
3. Figenshau R, Bhayani S, Venkatesh R, Wang A. Robotic renal hilar control and robotic clip placement for partial nephrectomy. J Endourol. 2008;22:2657–9.
4. Tulikangas PK, Smith T, Falcone T, et al. Gross and histologic characteristics of laparoscopic injuries with four different energy sources. Fertil Steril. 2001;75:806–10.
5. Newcomb WL, Hope WW, Schmelzer TM, et al. Comparison of blood vessel sealing among new electrosurgical and ultrasonic devices. Surg Endosc. 2009;23:90–6.
6. Biyani CS, Murphy M. Instruments used in laparoscopic reconstructive urology. In: Ramalingam M, Patel VR, editors. Operative atlas of laparoscopic reconstructive urology. London: Springer; 2009. pp. 27–36.
7. TissueFect™ Sensing Technology: Precisely Managing Energy Delivery. http://www.ligasure.com/ligasure/pages.aspx?page=Technology/TissueFect. Accessed Dec 27, 2009.
8. Bishoff JT, Allaf ME, Kirkels W, et al. Laparoscopic bowel injuries: incidence and clinical presentation. J Urol. 1999;161:887–90.
9. Jarrett TW, Chan DY, Charambura TC, et al. Laparoscopic pyeloplasty: the first 100 cases. J Urol. 2002;167:1253–6.
10. Abdelshehid CA, Borin JF, Sala LG, et al. In vitro analysis of Lapra-Ty clip strength. J Endourol. 2006;20:A79.
11. Grubb RL 3rd, Sundaram CP, Yan Y, et al. Use of titanium staples during upper tract laparoscopic reconstructive surgery: initial experience. J Urol. 2002;168:1366–9.
12. Shalhav AL, Barret E, Lifshitz DA, et al. Transperitoneal laparoscopic renal surgery using blunt 12 mm trocar without fascial closure. J Endourol. 2002;16:43–6.
13. Elashry OM, Nakada SY, Wolf JS Jr, et al. Comparative clinical study of port-closure techniques following laparoscopic surgery. J Am Coll Surg. 1996;183:335–44.
14. Eichel L, Ahlering TA, Clayman RV. Robotics in urologic surgery: risks and benefits. AUA Update Series. 2005;24:106–11.
15. Instrument & Accessory Price List. EndoWrist® USA; April 2009.

Chapter 2

Instrumentation During Pediatric Robotic Anastomoses and Reconstruction

Shahin Chandrasoma and Chester J. Koh

Introduction

For the past four decades, patients have increasingly chosen the minimally invasive option for their urologic surgical needs to avoid the morbidity of large incisions, and this generally has led to shorter hospital stays, less pain medication requirements, and earlier return to normal activity levels in adult patients. This is especially true for adult patients who have undergone ablative urologic procedures such as nephrectomy or adrenalectomy by conventional laparoscopic techniques. The advantages of minimally invasive surgery also apply to pediatric patients and especially for those who have undergone ablative pediatric urology procedures with similar benefits seen in these patients. Of note, the first reported use of laparoscopy in pediatric urology was for patients with nonpalpable undescended testes in the 1960s [1], and diagnostic laparoscopy in this setting has gained widespread acceptance among pediatric urologists. Over the last two decades, laparoscopic surgical techniques have improved significantly in the adult and pediatric patient populations since the first reported laparoscopic pyeloplasty in the adult population in 1993 [2] and the first pediatric laparoscopic pyeloplasty in 1995 [3], both by the use of conventional laparoscopy. In children, this has led to a reliably safe and effective approach to the kidney for reconstructive urological procedures that require extensive suturing with similar success rates and potential benefits with regard to cosmesis, intraoperative blood loss, postoperative stay, and the length of the overall hospital stay.

However, for pediatric urology cases, the limitations of conventional laparoscopic equipment and the steep learning curve associated with its use in pediatric reconstructive procedures have led to only a modest adoption among pediatric urologists for these types of procedures. The da Vinci Surgical System from Intuitive Surgical (Sunnyvale, CA) has introduced the benefits of an intuitive interface, three-dimensional visualization, and greater degrees of instrument articulation and control that allow for robotic-assisted laparoscopic procedures. The increased precision of and facility with instrumentation offered by robotic assistance is readily seen in pediatric procedures, specifically those that are reconstructive in nature, and thus require extensive dissection and suturing. This has helped to increase the utilization of minimally invasive techniques for pediatric reconstructive procedures.

The most commonly performed robotic procedures in the pediatric population to date are pyeloplasty and extravesical ureteral reimplantation [4]. As technology has advanced, with finer degrees of control and ever-improving visualization through smaller and smaller cameras, the use of robotic-assisted laparoscopic surgery in pediatric urology should continue to rapidly

C.J. Koh (✉)
Division of Pediatric Urology, Keck School of Medicine, Children's Hospital Los Angeles, Institute of Urology, University of Southern California (USC), Los Angeles, CA, USA
e-mail: ckoh@chla.usc.edu

M.C. Ost (ed.), *Robotic and Laparoscopic Reconstructive Surgery in Children and Adults*, Current Clinical Urology, DOI 10.1007/978-1-60327-914-7_2, © Springer Science+Business Media, LLC 2011

increase, as more surgical techniques are adapted to the robotic-assisted laparoscopic option. The close approximation of these techniques to their open counterparts facilitates the transition to the minimally invasive option. In this chapter, we will describe the robotic instrumentation available for use with the Da Vinci surgical robot and discuss its advantages in various procedures in the field of pediatric urology.

The Da Vinci Surgical System

The Da Vinci Surgical System from Intuitive Surgical (Sunnyvale, CA) consists of a surgeon console, a patient-side cart with the interactive robotic arms (the "robot"), a vision cart (the "video tower"), and the proprietary *EndoWrist* robotic instruments. Since its approval for clinical use by the US Food and Drug Administration in 2000, the Da Vinci surgical robot has greatly expanded the field of minimally invasive surgery in the field of urology, and most notably in the surgical management of prostate cancer. For men diagnosed with localized prostate cancer, robotic-assisted laparoscopic prostatectomy has become a widely performed procedure in the USA as both patients and surgeons have rapidly adopted this minimally invasive surgical alternative to open surgery. In addition, the Da Vinci surgical robot has gained acceptance for pediatric urology procedures as the technological advances appear to be particularly useful for the reconstructive nature of most pediatric urologic procedures.

The patient-side cart with the robotic arms consists of up to four working arms, although the fourth arm is seldom used in the pediatric population because of the smaller working spaces in pediatric patients. In addition, avoiding the fourth arm can reduce the initial capital investment required for the system. The three main robotic arms consist of the camera arm and two instrument arms, where each arm is attached to their respective laparoscopic ports. The middle camera arm is specifically designed to hold the system's camera telescope, while the two side arms control the robotic instruments, which are inserted and removed by the bedside assistant.

The camera arm consists of two cameras in a single metallic sheath and is designed to mimic the binocular function of a surgeon's eyes. The signal from each of the two cameras is delivered to the surgeon console, which processes the two images to provide the surgeon with a single three-dimensional image. This provides the surgeon with superior surgical visualization during the procedure due to the 10-fold magnification and the sense of depth perception that is not seen with conventional laparoscopy.

The surgeon console is a distinct unit at which the surgeon is comfortably seated while handling the robotic controls. The degree of control includes arm position, focus, zoom, camera position, and instrument movement, with a relatively short learning curve before one becomes comfortable with the controls. The motion control is enhanced by the console system, which can translate the surgeon's precise movements and imbuing fluidity of action to the surgical field, while dampening any potential hand or arm tremors. This novel control system has the potential for future ergonomic benefits for surgeons, which most likely will be shown as robotic experience among surgeons grows.

The robotic instruments have proprietary "EndoWrist" articulation that allows for more precise control and improved manipulation of tissue than is offered with standard laparoscopic instruments. It mimics the seven degrees of freedom present in human wrist articulation and therefore gives the console surgeon the ability to perform precise finite movements with the robotic instruments. This close approximation to a surgeon's movements during open surgery has the potential for shorter learning curves with this minimally invasive modality as opposed to previous minimally invasive options.

In summary, the Da Vinci Surgical System's combination of robotic technological advances, magnified visualization, and precise operator control has led to a transformation of standard open surgical techniques in children for pediatric urology procedures to their minimally invasive counterparts, where these procedures can now be performed via small laparoscopic incisions instead of a large open incision.

Instruments

A wide range of instruments are available for the Da Vinci robotic surgical system which approximate those used in both open surgery and traditional laparoscopy. Common instruments in open surgery and laparoscopy, such as needle drivers and Maryland dissectors, have robotic counterparts that were created for use with the Da Vinci system. The most obvious advantage of these newly adapted instruments over their laparoscopic predecessors is the presence of the articulating EndoWrist technology as previously described, which increases the flexibility of the instrument tips and thus augments the instrument's utility by making it possible to approach and grasp tissue from many different directions, as opposed to the plane directly accessibly by the port. This in turn allows for more effective traction and tissue exposure, as the instrument's movement is similar to the surgeon's hand and wrist movements, as opposed to traditional laparoscopy where a surgeon's movements are opposite to those of the internal instruments.

The camera telescope with three-dimensional visualization is available in two sizes: 12 and 8.5 mm. A 5-mm camera telescope is also available but is limited to two-dimensional visualization as seen in conventional laparoscopy since this telescope contains a single camera. For the robotic instruments, a wide range of instruments are currently available in both 8 and 5 mm sizes. However, certain instruments are currently not available in the 5 mm size, and this includes the electrocautery-capable monopolar curved scissors (Hot Shears). Despite this limitation, with the goals of improved cosmesis and smaller skin incisions in mind, we utilize the 8.5-mm telescope and the 5-mm instruments for the majority of our pediatric robotic procedures, where the 12-mm telescope and the 8-mm instruments are reserved for adolescent patients. In general, the 5-mm instruments have a longer articulating tip than the 8-mm instruments; however, we have not experienced any negative sequelae with the use of the 5-mm instruments during robotic procedures in children.

A number of instruments in particular are useful for the pediatric surgical specialist. The initial dissection during a typical procedure is dependent on a combination of blunt dissection and dissection with cautery; this is especially apparent in the exposure of the kidney and the renal pelvis, as tissue planes are well defined and often can be bluntly developed initially. We recommend the use of a cautery instrument in the right hand and a grasping instrument in the left hand.

The most commonly used monopolar cautery device in the 5 mm size is the monopolar cautery instrument with either a hook or a spatula tip (Fig. 2.1), since the monopolar curved scissors (Hot Shears) are available only in the 8 mm size. Advantages of the monopolar cautery hook include its capability for blunt dissection near potentially delicate posterior structures prior to the initiation of cautery, as well as its small contact focus of cautery, which allows for precise incision and exposure of tissue planes with the blunt tip of the instrument. The monopolar curved scissors (Hot Shears) can provide sharp dissection with a smaller contact focus of cautery as compared to the monopolar cautery hook; however, its capability for blunt dissection may be limited due to the sharp edges at the scissors' distal tip, as well as to its sole availability in the 8 mm size. Another alternative for a cautery

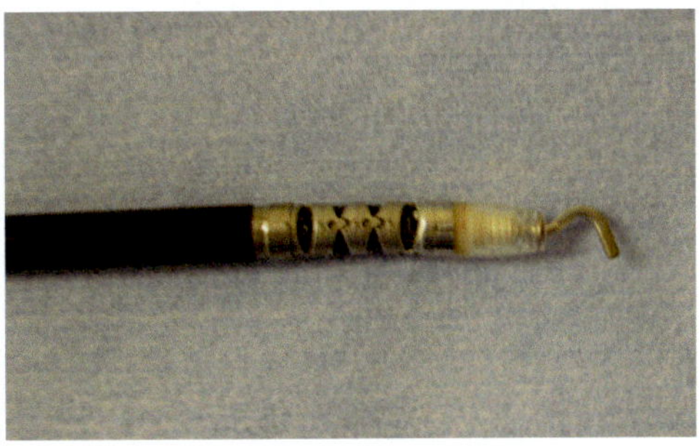

Fig. 2.1 Monopolar cautery hook—5 mm

instrument are the harmonic curved shears, which are available in 5 and 8 mm sizes. As with the laparoscopic harmonic instruments, the cautery energy is transmitted between the jaws of the device, and this containment of energy may help to avoid inadvertent cautery injury to surrounding structures.

A variety of grasping instruments are available for the Da Vinci robot for pediatric procedures. Routine forceps and graspers in the 5 mm sizes include the Maryland dissectors (Fig. 2.2) and the DeBakey forceps (Fig. 2.3). If a larger grasper is required, the atraumatic bowel graspers (Fig. 2.4) and the sharp-toothed Schertel graspers are available in the 5 mm sizes for creating and maintaining surgical exposure. As with the cautery instruments, other graspers and forceps are available that can provide more forceful traction, such as the ProGrasp forceps. But they are available only in the 8 mm sizes and thus may have limited utility for pediatric procedures. Unfortunately, the bipolar Maryland forceps are also available only in the 8 mm size, and this may be one instrument that, if available in the 5 mm size, could help to increase surgeon's efficiency and reduce operative times in pediatric procedures, as many robotic surgeons use the bipolar Maryland forceps as their grasping instrument. This allows the use of bipolar cautery in the grasping instrument without the need for an instrument change. The combination of finite movements with the Maryland forceps with the added ability to deliver hemostasis with the use of bipolar energy would be beneficial in pediatric cases.

For cutting purposes, only two types of scissors are currently available in the 5 mm size:

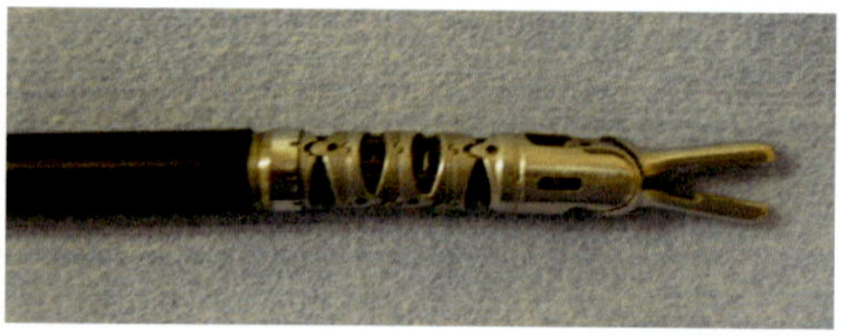

Fig. 2.3 DeBakey forceps—5 mm

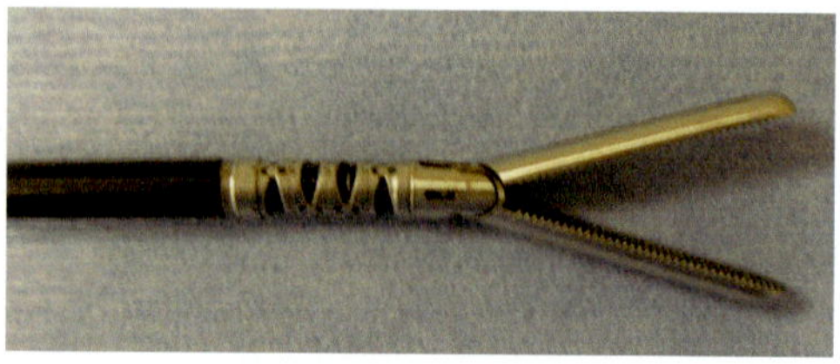

Fig. 2.4 Bowel graspers—5 mm

curved scissors (Fig. 2.5) and round-tip scissors. In most instances, the curved scissors are useful for general dissection and cutting. However, certain procedural steps, such as the spatulation of a ureter prior to a dismembered pyeloplasty anastomosis, may necessitate a straight incision with the round-tip scissors. The relatively wide distal tips of the round-tip scissors may limit its usefulness for small-caliber ureteral spatulations. For fine-cutting purposes, Potts scissors with sharp pinpoint tips are available, but only in the 8 mm size.

For pediatric procedures, the needle driver (Fig. 2.6) and the 5-mm grasping instruments listed above are usually sufficient for suture placement and knot tying in an instrument-tie manner. In general, one is advised to handle reuseable portions of the suture with the needle driver as opposed to the grasping instruments, since the needle driver tends to better preserve

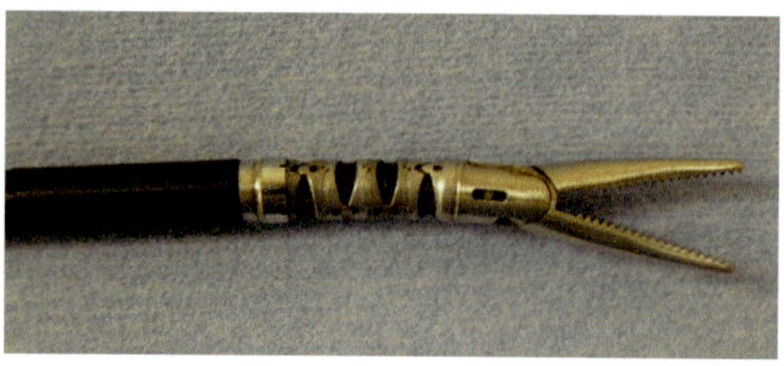

Fig. 2.2 Maryland dissector—5 mm

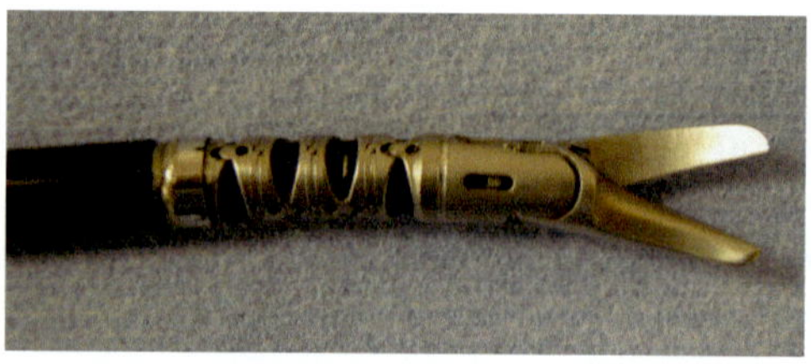

Fig. 2.5 Curved scissors—5 mm

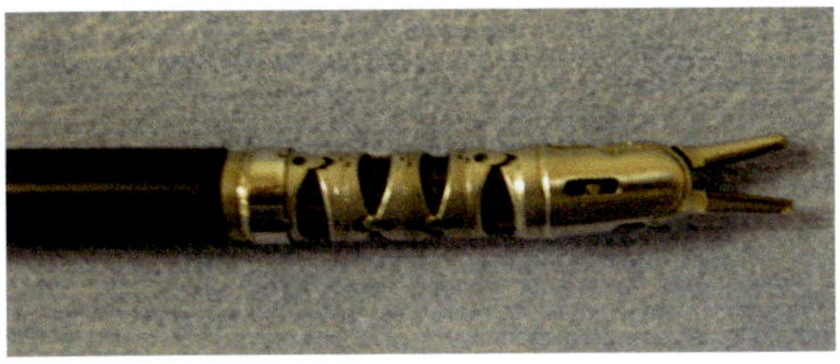

Fig. 2.6 Needle driver—5 mm

the suture integrity when handling a suture. A larger variety of other instruments are also available, but only in the 8 mm size. Instrument ties with the Black Diamond microforceps may be facilitated by the instrument's narrow tips, as it is easier to wrap the suture around the narrow tips of these forceps. Another instrument available only in the 8 mm size is the SutureCut needle driver, which has a small scissor blade in the base of the instrument's tips that can be used for cutting suture without the need for an instrument change or an assistant. One must take care not to prematurely cut one's suture. Future technological advances may allow for these instruments to become available in the 5 mm sizes.

In addition to the wide variety of robotic instruments available with the proprietary "EndoWrist" articulation, the pediatric robotic surgeon also has the ability to use traditional laparoscopic instruments either through one of the robotic instrument ports or through an accessory 5-mm laparoscopic port. We generally encourage the use of a 5-mm accessory port to potentially increase surgeon's efficiency and to reduce operative times. Attaching the CO_2 gas inflow to the accessory port may also decrease the incidence of poor camera visualization due to fogging. In addition, the accessory port can also provide the capability for the bedside assistant to assist with retraction, suture placement and removal, as well as suction and irrigation without the need for an instrument change. Furthermore, the entire gamut of laparoscopic instruments such as clip appliers and scissors can be utilized during the robotic procedure. And the accessory port can serve as the conduit in which to place ureteral wires and stents into the ureter without the need for a separate incision or puncture.

As robotic technology continues to evolve, the list of robotic instruments is expected to grow with miniaturization of the instruments and improved surgeon's capabilities in the robotic setting. This should be especially beneficial for the pediatric urologic patient where an increasing number of pediatric reconstructive procedures can be performed in a minimally invasive fashion with the potential for clinical benefits such as improved cosmesis, decreased hospital length of stays, and reduced pain medication requirements. In the next paragraphs, several robotic procedures in pediatric urology are described with respect to their instrumentation needs.

Robotic-Assisted Laparoscopic Pyeloplasty

Pyeloplasty for the surgical management of ureteropelvic junction (UPJ) obstruction is one of the most common uses for the Da Vinci robot in the pediatric urology field. UPJ obstruction is more commonly being diagnosed in the perinatal period due to early detection with antenatal ultrasound imaging, as opposed to later in childhood or even adulthood for symptomatic manifestation [5]. Accompanying this trend is the rising concern that prenatal diagnosis of UPJ obstruction can lead to anxiety in expecting parents with worries that their newborn will require surgical intervention early in life [6]. For this reason, minimally invasive modalities for the surgical management of UPJ obstruction in infants and children may help to alleviate the concerns of parents by giving them a less invasive surgical option rather than open surgery.

Primary UPJ obstruction can be due to intrinsic obstruction with an aperistaltic segment of ureter at the level of the renal pelvis with an interruption of ureteral muscular development leading to contractile discontinuity and functional obstruction [7]; due to high insertion of the ureter into the pelvis; or due to extrinsic compression from a crossing lower pole renal vessel that crosses anterior to the UPJ. Other potential causes of UPJ obstruction include persistent congenital valvular mucosal folds [8] and upper ureteral polyps [9]. Secondary UPJ obstruction can be seen secondary to severe vesicoureteral reflux when the dilated tortuous ureter kinks and impedes urine flow. Initial repair of the UPJ obstruction is generally recommended in these cases [10].

Surgical repair of UPJ obstruction is commonly performed using a dismembered pyeloplasty technique as described by Anderson and Hynes [11]. This technique via an open incision has become the gold standard for UPJ reconstruction as it allows for extensive flexibility in the excision of abnormal ureteral segments, as well as the preservation of aberrant crossing vessels. The laparoscopic adaptation of this technique was first reported in adults in 1993 [2], and subsequently in children in 1995 [3]. With the laparoscopic technique with peritoneal insufflation and direct endoscopic visualization, rapid identification of the obstructed UPJ, as well as the rapid detection of a crossing vessel, if present, is possible. However, one of the limitations of the laparoscopic technique was the steep learning curve for the ureteral reconstruction, which involves extensive laparoscopic suturing and hence has resulted in only a modest adoption by pediatric urologists.

The EndoWrist articulation of the Da Vinci system allows a surgeon to mimic actual hand and wrist movements to help overcome the technical demands of intracorporeal suturing. Robotic-assisted laparoscopic pyeloplasty has been described as a cutting-edge improvement over laparoscopic pyeloplasty [12], with comparable results to open surgery [13]. The 10-fold magnification and three-dimensional visualization appear to shorten the learning curve for surgeons with limited experience in minimally invasive reconstruction [14]. However, the benefit to experienced laparoscopic surgeons may be limited.

Robotic-assisted laparoscopic pyeloplasty has also been shown to be safe and successful in infants [15] and in reoperative cases [16]. When directly compared to open surgery, robotic-assisted laparoscopic pyeloplasty has led to decreased lengths of hospital stays and reduced pain medication requirements, as well as similar operative times when compared to open surgery once a surgeon has gained sufficient experience [17].

Robotic-assisted laparoscopic techniques have also been described for difficult intrarenal collecting systems or for failed pyeloplasties for which successful robotic ureterocalicostomies were performed [18]. In addition, for patients with lower ureteral obstruction, robotic-assisted laparoscopic ureteroureterostomy has been successfully performed in both single and duplicated collecting systems [19].

Useful 5-mm Instruments

Exposure/initial dissection of the renal pelvis in the retroperitoneal space can be accomplished with the *monopolar cautery hook* in the right hand and the *Maryland dissector or DeBakey forceps* in the left hand. The use of *curved scissors* is limited by the lack of cautery in the 5-mm version of this instrument.

Transection of the renal pelvis and the ureter can be performed with *curved scissors or round-tip scissors. Spatulation* may be facilitated by the straight tips of the *round-tip scissors*; however, the wider tips of these scissors as compared to the *curved scissors* may limit this advantage in small ureters.

Anastomosis may be performed with two *needle drivers* or the use of one *needle driver* and one grasping instrument such as the *DeBakey forceps*, with the caveat that one should preferentially handle reusable portions of the suture with the *needle driver* as opposed to the grasping instruments.

Robotic-Assisted Laparoscopic Renal Surgery

The Da Vinci robot has been used for other types of renal surgeries such as complete and partial nephrectomy, pyelolithotomy, calyceal diverticulectomy, and adrenalectomy in the pediatric population [20]. This should not be surprising given the access to and visualization of the kidney demonstrated in reconstructive procedures such as the dismembered pyeloplasty. The 10-fold magnification and three-dimensional visualization allow for careful identification of key structures in these procedures, which can be difficult to identify in the typical pediatric patient. However, the benefits of robotic surgery over conventional laparoscopy have yet to be demonstrated for pediatric urology procedures that are primarily extirpative in nature.

While robotic-assisted laparoscopic partial nephrectomies in adult patients are common for the removal of small kidney tumors [21], robotic-assisted laparoscopic partial nephrectomies in children are often performed for the removal of benign nonfunctioning upper pole segments. In the small working space of a pediatric patient, the Da Vinci system's optics and fine articulation and instrument control may allow for precise movements and potentially safer procedures. Often, these nonfunctioning upper pole segments have their own vascular supply, which necessitates identification and control of the upper pole blood supply without the need for clamping of the lower pole vascular supply. Hence warm ischemia time is usually not necessary when this procedure is applied to children because of their duplicated vascular anatomy. As with laparoscopic partial nephrectomies, the distinction between the poles is often clearly demarcated, and extensive mobilization of the duplex kidney is usually unnecessary [22].

The surgical procedure for a robotic-assisted laparoscopic partial nephrectomy closely resembles that of the conventional laparoscopic technique. The arterial supply to the nonfunctioning upper pole segment, if located, is clamped to allow ischemic delineation of the borders of the upper pole on the cortex of the kidney. Once the borders are delineated, the ischemic upper pole can be removed with electrocautery or harmonic curved shears similar to the conventional laparoscopic technique [23].

Robotic-assisted laparoscopic partial nephrectomy has been described in the adult population [24], with the adaptation of the robotic procedure to utilize a single laparoscopic port [25]. Robotic-assisted laparoscopic partial nephrectomy has also been reported as a safe option for use in children, with a relatively short learning curve and the potential for enhanced safety and efficiency for this minimally invasive option because of the magnified visualization and fine dexterity of the robotic instruments [26].

Useful 5-mm Instruments

Exposure/initial dissection of the kidney in the retroperitoneal space can be accomplished with the *monopolar cautery hook* in the right hand and the *Maryland dissector or DeBakey forceps* in the left hand. The use of *curved scissors* is limited by the lack of cautery in the 5-mm version of this instrument.

Partial nephrectomy of a nonfunctioning upper pole can be performed using *monopolar cautery hook* or *harmonic curved shears*. If significant upper pole vessels are encountered, laparoscopic clipping or robotic suture ligation may be necessary. Yet in many instances, due to the atretic nature of the upper pole vessels, simple cautery or the use of the harmonic instrument may be sufficient for vascular control.

Hemostasis with mattress sutures, if necessary, may be performed with two *needle drivers*, or the use of one *needle driver* and one grasping instrument such as the *DeBakey forceps*, with the caveat that one should preferentially handle reusable portions of the suture with the *needle driver* as opposed to the grasping instruments.

Robotic-Assisted Laparoscopic Ureteral Reimplantation

Vesicoureteral reflux is commonly due to a primary defect at the level of the ureterovesical junction (UVJ) or may occur secondarily when the normal UVJ is overwhelmed by increased intravesical pressure. Primary reflux is usually related to an inadequate length of the intramural ureter, with a tunnel length that is shorter than the optimal tunnel length-to-diameter ratio of 5:1 reported by Paquin [27].

There are numerous techniques for ureteral reimplantation described in the urologic literature, all of which are associated with excellent success rates. Some are performed with intravesical ureteral dissection and tunnel creation [27, 28], while others are performed extravesically, without violation of the bladder mucosa [29, 30]. One of the most difficult steps in these procedures is accessing the native ureter, especially if an extravesical approach is chosen.

Utilization of the Da Vinci robot provides clear unobstructed views of the posterior pelvis from a cephalad point of view, as similarly seen in established robotic procedures such as the robotic-assisted radical prostatectomy. A transperitoneal approach to the distal ureter is feasible once the overlying peritoneum is safely incised and the ureter is identified. We prefer the extravesical Lich-Gregoir technique where the robotic instruments allow for precise placement of interrupted sutures on the newly created bladder muscle flaps to create a new submucosal tunnel for the reimplanted ureter.

Intravesical approaches are also possible using the Da Vinci surgical system. Olsen noted that the transvesical technique was effective in a porcine model where eight pigs with induced vesicoureteral reflux underwent transvesical placement of the robotic camera and the ports into the bladder after induction of pneumovesicum, with successful Cohen cross-trigonal reimplantations in all specimens [31]. The robotic approach was preceded by conventional laparoscopic transvesical reimplantation in children with subsequent high success rates, but it was noted that smaller bladder capacities were associated with higher rates of complication, namely urinary leakage [32]. More recently, robotic-assisted laparoscopic intravesical ureteral reimplantation has been safely and successfully performed in children at several pediatric centers [20, 33]. And successful tapering and reimplantation of megaureters have also been reported [20]. Given the advantages of magnified visualization of the distal ureter and bladder, fine instrument control, and facilitated suturing capabilities, robotic-assisted laparoscopic reimplantation may find greater acceptance in the near future among pediatric urologists.

Useful 5-mm Instruments

Exposure/initial dissection of the distal ureter in the perivesical space can be accomplished with the *monopolar cautery hook* in the right hand and the *Maryland dissector or DeBakey forceps* in the left hand. The use of the *monopolar cautery hook* is especially advantageous as the ureter can be retracted with the hook instrument with minimal risk of ureteral injury. The use of *curved scissors* is limited by the lack of cautery in the 5-mm version of this instrument.

Creation of the bladder muscle flaps may best be accomplished with the use of the *monopolar cautery hook* due to the lack of cautery with the 5-mm *curved scissors*. Bladder distension via the Foley catheter may assist with this dissection and may help prevent bladder mucosal perforation.

Closure of the muscle flaps over the ureter to complete the extravesical reimplantation may be performed with two *needle drivers*, or the use of one *needle driver* and one grasping instrument such as the *DeBakey forceps*, with the caveat that one should preferentially handle reusable portions of the suture with the *needle driver* as opposed to the grasping instruments.

Robotic-Assisted Laparoscopic Bladder Surgeries

Other procedures in the field of pediatric urology to which robotic assistance has been applied involve the urinary bladder, with the greatest benefits seen in procedures requiring extensive laparoscopic suturing. In the pediatric population, children with neurogenic bladder related

Table 2.1 Common instruments in pediatric robotic urologic surgery

- Monopolar cautery hook or spatula (5 mm; 8 mm) (Fig. 2.1)
- Maryland dissector (5 mm; 8 mm with bipolar) (Fig. 2.2)
- DeBakey forceps (5 mm; 8 mm) (Fig. 2.3)
- Bowel grasper (5 mm; 8 mm) (Fig. 2.4)
- Round-tip scissors (5 mm; 8 mm)
- Curved scissors (5 mm—without cautery) (Fig. 2.5)
- Needle driver (5 mm; 8 mm) (Fig. 2.6)
- ProGrasp forceps (8 mm only)
- Harmonic curved shears (5 mm; 8 mm)
- Monopolar curved scissors (Hot Shears) (8 mm only)

to their myelomeningocele represent a group of patients that may require bladder augmentation with lifelong catheterization, either through their native urethra or through a catheterizable appendicovesicostomy [34]. Limited application of minimally invasive techniques to these types of procedures may be in part due to the extensive suturing required for these types of reconstruction. Previous reports of laparoscopic reconstructions include the extracorporeal creation of a neobladder after laparoscopic radical cystectomy [35], although intracorporeal diversions have also been successfully performed with conventional laparoscopy in the porcine model [36].

With the goal of pediatric applications in mind, complete intracorporeal robotic-assisted bladder augmentation was successfully performed in a porcine model [37]. Furthermore, clinical applications of the Da Vinci robot for reconstructive bladder procedures have been described including intracorporeal augmentation with Mitrofanoff appendicovesicostomy [38], antegrade cutaneous colon tube creation [39], and urachal cyst excision with bladder reconstruction [40].

Another potential benefit of robotic-assisted laparoscopic surgery is the potential for combined surgical procedures to be performed in children in a single anesthetic session. Simultaneous robotic-assisted laparoscopic appendicovesicostomy with nephrectomy and orchiopexy was previously reported [41]. This provides new possibilities for patients with multiple urinary tract abnormalities, where robotic-assisted laparoscopic surgery can lead to complete surgical repair of all abnormalities in a single session.

The Future

As robotic technology evolves with improvements and miniaturization of the robotic instruments, more reconstructive procedures in pediatric urology most likely will be performed in a minimally invasive fashion. This should benefit most pediatric urology patients with expected reductions in length of hospital stays, reductions in pain medication requirements, earlier return to normal activity, and improved cosmesis. In addition, one can foresee possible applications of robotic technology to emerging modalities of minimally invasive surgery, such as natural orifice translumenal endoscopic surgery (NOTES), as shown in animal studies using the robotic system [42]. As advocates for pediatric health, pediatric robotic surgeons should strive to be at the forefront of these emerging technologies to ensure that they are properly applied to the pediatric patient.

References

1. Timchenko A. Methods of laparoscopy in children. Klin Khir. May 1969;5:10–4.
2. Kavoussi LR, Peters CA. Laparoscopic pyeloplasty. J Urol. 1993;150:1891.
3. Peters CA, Schlussel RN, Retik AB. Pediatric laparoscopic dismembered pyeloplasty. J Urol. 1995;153:1962–5.
4. Casale P. Robotic pyeloplasty in the pediatric population. Curr Urol Rep. Jan 2009;10(1):55–9.
5. Brown T, Mandell J, Lebowitz RL. Neonatal hydronephrosis in the era of sonography. AJR. May 1987;148(5):959–63.

6. Harding LJ, Malone PS, Wellesley DG. Antenatal minimal hydronephrosis: is its follow-up an unnecessary cause of concern? Prenat Diagn. Aug 1999;19(8):701–5.
7. Hanna MK. Antenatal hydronephrosis and ureteropelvic junction obstruction: the case for early intervention. Urology. May 2000;55(5):612–5.
8. Maizels M, Stephens FD. Valves of the ureter as a cause of primary obstruction of the ureter: anatomic, embryologic and clinical aspects. J Urol. May 1980;123(5):742–7.
9. Thorup J, Pedersen PV, Clausen N. Benign ureteral polyp as a cause of intermittent hydronephrosis in a child. J Urol. Dec 1981;126(6):796–7.
10. Lebowitz RL, Blickman JG. The coexistence of ureteropelvic junction obstruction and reflux. AJR. Feb 1983;140(2):231–8.
11. Anderson JC, Hynes W. Retrocaval ureter; a case diagnosed pre-operatively and treated successfully by a plastic operation. Br J Urol. Sep 1949;21(3):209–14.
12. Peters CA. Robotically assisted paediatric pyeloplasty: cutting edge or expensive toy? BJU Int. Dec 2004;94(9):1214–5.
13. Atug F, Woods M, Burgess SV, Castle EP, Thomas R. Robotic-assisted laparoscopic pyeloplasty in children. J Urol. 2005;174:1440–2.
14. Passerotti C, Peters CA. Pediatric robotic-assisted laparoscopy: a description of the principle procedures. Sci World J. 20 Jun 2006;6:2581–8.
15. Kutikov A, Nguyen M, Guzzo T, Canter D, Casale P. Robot-assisted pyeloplasty in the infant – lessons learned. J Urol. 2006;176:2237–40.
16. Passerotti CC, Nguyen HT, Eisner BH, Lee RS, Peters CA. Laparoscopic reoperative pediatric pyeloplasty with robotic assistance. J Endourol. 2007;21:1137–9.
17. Lee RS, Retik AB, Borer JG, Peters CA. Pediatric robot assisted laparoscopic dismembered pyeloplasty: comparison with a cohort of open surgery. J Urol. Feb 2006;175(2):683–7.
18. Casale P, Mucksavage P, Resnick M, Kim SS. Robotic ureterocalicostomy in the pediatric population. J Urol. Dec 2008;180(6):2643–8.
19. Passerotti CC, Nguyen HT, Lais A, Dunning P, Harrell B, Estrada C, Lee R, Retik AB, Peters CA. Robot-assisted laparoscopic ileal bladder augmentation: defining techniques and potential pitfalls. J Endourol. Feb 2008;22(2):355–60.
20. Estrada CR, Passerotti CC. Robotic surgery in pediatric urology. Arch Esp Urol. May 2007;60(4):471–9.
21. Aron M, Koenig P, Kaouk JH, Nguyen MM, Desai MM, Gill IS. Robotic and laparoscopic partial nephrectomy: a matched-pair comparison from a high-volume centre. BJU Int. Jul 2008;102(1):86–92.
22. Janetschek G, Seibold J, Radmayr C, Bartsch G. Laparoscopic heminephroureterectomy in pediatric patients. J Urol. Nov 1997;158(5):1928–30.
23. Jackman SV, Cadeddu JA, Chen RN, Micali S, Bishoff JT, Lee BR, Moore RG, Kavoussi LR. Utility of the harmonic scalpel for laparoscopic partial nephrectomy. J Endourol. Oct 1998;12(5):441–4.
24. Patel MN, Bhandari M, Menon M, Rogers CG. Robotic-assisted partial nephrectomy. BJU Int. May 2009;103(9):1296–311.
25. Kaouk JH, Goel RK. Single-port laparoscopic and robotic partial nephrectomy. Eur Urol. May 2009;55(5):1163–9.
26. Lee RS, Sethi AS, Passerotti CC, Retik AB, Borer JG, Nguyen HT, Peters CA. Robot assisted laparoscopic partial nephrectomy: a viable and safe option in children. J Urol. Feb 2009;181(2):823–8.
27. Paquin AJ Jr. Ureterovesical anastomosis: the description and evaluation of a technique. J Urol. Nov 1959;82:573–83.
28. Politano VA, Leadbetter WF. An operative technique for the correction of vesicoureteral reflux. J Urol. Jun 1958;79(6):932–41.
29. Lich R Jr. Obstructive diseases of the urinary tract in children. J Ark Med Soc. Sep 1961;58:127–30.
30. Gregoir W. The surgical treatment of congenital vesico-ureteral reflux. Acta Chir Belg. Apr 1964;63:431–9.
31. Olsen LH, Deding D, Yeung CK, Jørgensen TM. Computer assisted laparoscopic pneumovesical ureter reimplantation a.m. Cohen: initial experience in a pig model. APMIS Suppl. 2003;109:23–5.
32. Kutikov A, Guzzo TJ, Canter DJ, Casale P. Initial experience with laparoscopic transvesical ureteral reimplantation at the Children's Hospital of Philadelphia. J Urol. Nov 2006;176(5):2222–5.
33. Lendvay TS. Robotic-Assisted Laparoscopic Management of Vesicoureteral Reflux. Adv Urol. 2008;Vol. 2008:Article ID 732942, 4 pages. doi:10.1155/2008/732942.
34. Mitrofanoff P. Trans-appendicular continent cystostomy in the management of the neurogenic bladder. Chir Pediatr. 1980;21(4):297–305.
35. Huang J, Lin T, Xu K, Huang H, Jiang C, Han J, Yao Y, Guo Z, Xie W, Yin X, Zhang C. Laparoscopic radical cystectomy with orthotopic ileal neobladder: a report of 85 cases. J Endourol. May 2008;22(5):939–46.
36. Wagner A, Munter M, Makarov D, Nielsen M, Scorpio D, Kavoussi LR. Totally laparoscopic creation of a novel stapled orthotopic neobladder in the porcine model. J Endourol. Jan 2008;22(1):151–6.
37. Passerotti CC, Diamond DA, Borer JG, Eisner BH, Barrisford G, Nguyen HT. Robot-assisted laparoscopic ureteroureterostomy: description of technique. J Endourol. Apr 2008;22(4):581–4.
38. Gundeti MS, Eng MK, Reynolds WS, Zagaja GP. Pediatric robotic-assisted laparoscopic augmentation ileocystoplasty and Mitrofanoff appendicovesicostomy: complete intracorporeal – initial case report. Urology. Nov 2008;72(5):1144–7.

39. Lendvay TS, Shnorhavorian M, Grady RW. Robotic-assisted laparoscopic Mitrofanoff appendicovesicostomy and antegrade continent enema colon tube creation in a pediatric spina bifida patient. J Laparoendosc Adv Surg Tech A. Apr 2008;18(2):310–2.
40. Yamzon J, Kokorowski P, De Filippo RE, Chang AY, Hardy BE, Koh CJ. Pediatric robot-assisted laparoscopic excision of urachal cyst and bladder cuff. J Endourol. Oct 2008;22(10):2385–8.
41. Rosito T, Andreoni CR, Iizuca F, Ortiz V, Macedo A Jr. Combined laparoscopic appendicovesicostomy (Mitrofanoff) with nephrectomy and orchidopexy in an 8-year-old boy. J Pediatr Urol. Aug 2008;4(4):317–8.
42. Haber GP, Crouzet S, Kamoi K, Berger A, Aron M, Goel R, Canes D, Desai M, Gill IS, Kaouk JH. Robotic NOTES (Natural Orifice Translumenal Endoscopic Surgery) in reconstructive urology: initial laboratory experience. Urology. Jun 2008;71(6):996–1000.

Chapter 3

Instrumentation During Pediatric Laparoscopic Anastomoses and Reconstruction

Smart Zeidan and Alaa El-Ghoneimi

Instrumentation for open surgery has seen relatively little change over the last several decades. Laparoscopic surgery is equipment intensive. Each surgical specialty has different requirements for instruments, and laparoscopic urology involves gaining access, visualization, placement of instruments, dissection and hemostasis of target tissues, extraction of specimens, and wound closure. Adaptations of adult laparoscopic instruments continue to be made for appropriate application and improvement of the safety of laparoscopic procedures in infants and children. This chapter gives an overview of the basic equipment and instruments that should be available.

Instrumentation for Visualization

Four components are required to create a laparoscopic image: *laparoscope, light source, camera*, and *monitor*.

Laparoscopes that are most commonly used are rigid and have 0° or 30° lenses (range 0–70° lenses) and a size of 10 mm (range 1.9–12 mm). They contain a rod lens system as optical system and glass fibers for the transmission of light. The quality of the laparoscopes in terms of visualization and light transmission is inversely related to its diameter. To start with endoscopic surgery in children, it is advisable to start with 5-mm-diameter laparoscope as these laparoscopes give good view and allow for sufficient light transmission for most operations in children. Moreover, as it is also advised to start with 5-mm-diameter instruments, the laparoscope can be moved to different port sites. After gaining experience, the surgeon can decide whether smaller laparoscopes give a sufficient view. It is advisable to use 30° laparoscopes for most operations that allow for looking behind structures, except for retroperitoneal approach where the 0° laparoscope facilitates the orientation in the retroperitoneal space [1].

Light sources use high-intensity halogen, mercury, or xenon vapor bulbs with an output of 250–300 W. In addition to manual control of the brightness, some units also have automatic adjustment capabilities to prevent too much illumination that may result in a "washed-out" image. Any breakage of fibers in the fiber optic cable, which may occur during sterilization and/or improper handling, will result in decreased light transfer from the light source to the laparoscope. Appropriate adapters must be purchased when the cable and the endoscope are from different manufacturers than the light source. Recent advances in laparoscopic technology have combined the light source and camera capabilities into a single working instrument. This integrated laparoscope is available in 5 and 10 mm sizes. Cold light does not exist: the temperature at the end of the light cable rises up

A. El-Ghoneimi (✉)
Faculty of Medicine; Department of Pediatric Surgery and Urology, Robert Debré Children University Hospital, University of Paris VII, Paris, France
e-mail: alaa.elghoneimi@rdb.ap-hop-paris.fr

M.C. Ost (ed.), *Robotic and Laparoscopic Reconstructive Surgery in Children and Adults*, Current Clinical Urology, DOI 10.1007/978-1-60327-914-7_3, © Springer Science+Business Media, LLC 2011

to 225°C within seconds and at the end of the laparoscope up to 95°C within 15 min [2]. The cable should therefore always be attached to the laparoscope and wiping the lens clean against surrounding tissues should not be done especially in children because the bowel is more fragile than in adults.

The camera system consists of a camera and a video monitor. The camera is attached directly to the end of the laparoscope and transfers the view of the surgical field through a cable to the camera box unit. After reconstruction of the optical information, it is displayed on one or two video monitors. All currently made cameras can be gas or soak sterilized. The quality of the cameras has been greatly improved over the years [3]. A wide variety of cameras are currently available: single-chip, single-chip/digitized, three-chip, three-chip/digitized, interchangeable fixed focus lenses, zoom lenses, beam splitter, and direct coupler. Digitized images are preferable to analog as their recorded fidelity is preserved. The digital signal prevents image quality degradation and improves color, contrast, sharpness, and depth of field when compared to conventional systems [4]. Video advances such as high-definition television produce an extremely high-resolution image in a wide screen format, which provides superior image quality and visualization during endoscopy. In order to obtain a "true" upright image of the surgical field on the monitor, the camera's orientation mark must be placed at the 12 o'clock position. With 0° laparoscopes, the camera is locked to the eyepiece in the "true" position; the system is maintained in this orientation throughout the procedure. If the assistant inadvertently rotates the laparoscope, the image will also rotate which can be very disorienting. In contrast, with the 30° laparoscope, the camera is loosely attached to the eyepiece of the laparoscope so that the laparoscope can be rotated. Accordingly, the assistant must hold the camera in the upright, "true," position with one hand while rotating the laparoscope through a 360° arc in order to peer over and around vascular and other intra-abdominal structures; the 30° lens thus provides the surgeon with a more complete view of the surgical field than does a 0° lens. The most vexing problem with regard to the laparoscope is "fogging" of the lens. To prevent fogging of the laparoscope after insertion into the warm intraperitoneal cavity, it is advisable to initially warm the laparoscope in a container holding warm saline prior to its passage into the abdomen. In addition, wiping of the tip with a commercial defogging fluid or with povidone iodine solution (Betadine®) is also recommended. Should the image remain poor, the laparoscopist should check for moisture build-up occurring between the eyepiece and the camera; both components need to be disconnected and carefully cleansed with a dry gauze pad. All these measures should be used to have clear images. This problem is frequently seen in children because of the limited working space and of the fact that the surrounding structures are close to the laparoscope. In the retroperitoneal approach, the retroperitoneal fat should be kept away from the field to avoid any contact with the laparoscope [5]. The role of the assistant is crucial in maintaining the laparoscope away from the target organ and surrounding structures. A self-retaining instrument to hold the camera stable is of great advantage in reconstructive surgery.

Instrumentation for Insufflation/Insufflators

Laparoscopic insufflation is accomplished with CO_2. It allows the surgeon to obtain and maintain the pneumoperitoneum at a specific abdominal pressure. Current insufflation machines are automated and allow manual settings to regulate intra-abdominal pressure and CO_2 flow rates. In addition, most machines monitor the total volume of CO_2 infused. Intra-abdominal pressure should be kept below 15 mmHg in the pediatric patient to avoid potentially severe physiologic consequences [6, 7]. Most operations in children can be well performed using a pressure not higher than 10 mmHg. To be able to obtain a good working space with a low intra-abdominal pressure, optimal muscle relaxation is required. As far as flow is concerned, a low flow, e.g., 2 l/min, is sufficient when trocars do not leak. In children, major gas leaks should be prevented as this will lead to hypothermia [8].

Instrumentation for Access

Trocars

Trocars enable the laparoscopist to introduce working instruments into the gas-filled abdomen. They also maintain or re-establish a pneumoperitoneum by conveying the insufflant and may serve as pathways for delivering dissected tissue from the surgical area to the outside of the abdomen. Typically, a trocar consists of an *outer hollow sheath* (also called cannula or port) and an *inner obturator*, which is removed as soon as the outer sheath has entered the peritoneal cavity. A variety of trocars, both *disposable and reusable*, are available. Standard models range from 3 to 20 mm in diameter and from 5 to 15 cm in length.

There are *ports* with and without a stopcock for CO_2 insufflations and with and without a valve (Fig. 3.1a). Some ports (e.g., 3 mm diameter) have a partial membrane as a valve (Fig. 3.1b). When no instrument is inside, they leak CO_2. To prevent leakage when no instrument is present, a blunt obliterator should be inserted. It is advisable to start building up experience in endoscopic surgery with ports and corresponding laparoscope and instruments of the same diameter, which allows for changing laparoscope

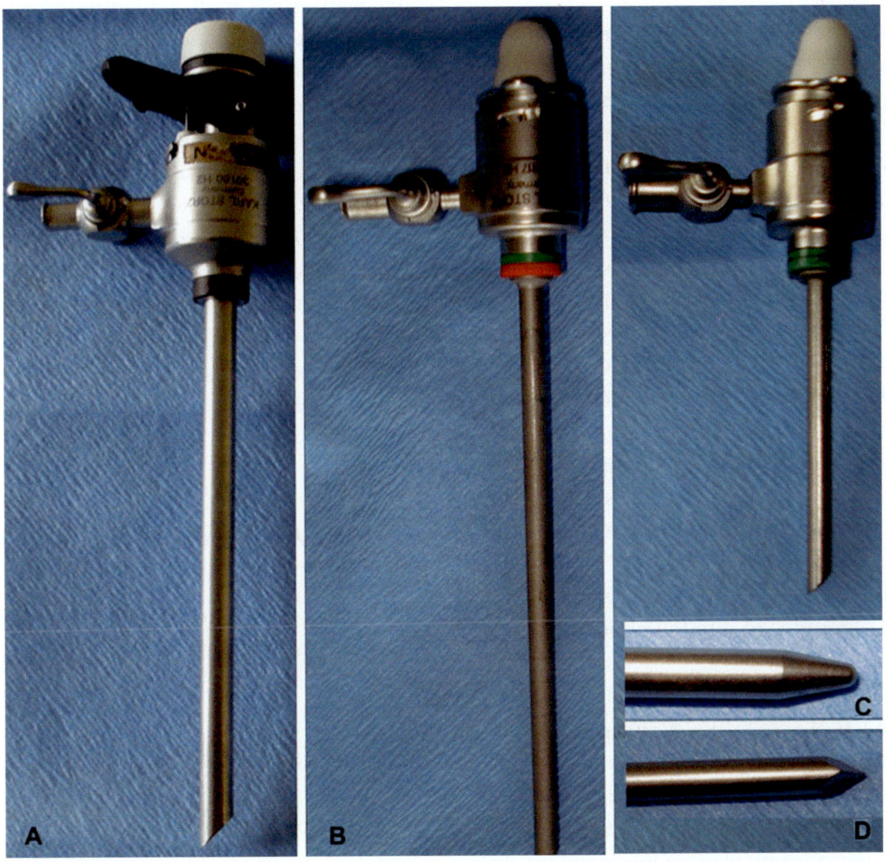

Fig. 3.1 Trocar. (**a**) Standard 5-mm reusable port with stopcock and valve. (**b**) Three-millimeter reusable ports with stopcock and without valve (two different lengths). (**c**) Blunt conical obturator's tip. (**d**) Sharp pyramidal obturator's tip

and instruments to all available port sites. Two- and three-millimeter instruments are available. The 2-mm instruments are fragile and bend easily. Moreover the beaks of these instruments are so narrow that accidental perforation may easily occur and firm grasping will cause tissue damage. In contrast, 3-mm instruments to be used in concert with 3.3-mm port are quite strong and are less likely to cause accidental perforation. Most 3-mm instruments are now available in an insulated form and most of the operations in children can be done with 3-mm instruments. The total 3-mm arsenal however is much more limited than the 5-mm arsenal. The length of the port should depend on the thickness of the body wall to be pierced. In general, ports for use in children may be shorter, not only because of the thinner body wall but also because of the limited working space.

The obturator's tip may be sharp pyramidal, sharp conical, eccentric, needle-like and blunt conical (Fig. 3.1c, d). The purpose is to facilitate the introduction of a port through the various layers of tissue or to obliterate the port if only a ring-like valve is present. A plastic *safety shield* covers the sharp tip of most disposable trocars. It retracts as the tip of the obturator traverses the abdominal wall but springs forward and locks in its deployed position as soon as the trocar enters the peritoneal cavity, thereby protecting intraperitoneal contents from injury. When inserted in an open way, it is advisable to insert the port together with a blunt conical obturator to prevent damage of tissues caused by the edge of the port and to allow a smaller hole for insertion.

Several *innovative trocar systems* and *devices* have been introduced into the clinical practice of laparoscopy:

The *EndoTip*™ *system* (Karl Storz, Culver City, CA) is a screw-like nondisposable device which has no sharp points or cutting edges. A small fascial incision is made after which the port is screwed in clockwise direction. This process can be supervised by using a telescope inside the port at the same time. By doing so the tissues are not cut but pouched away. The port is removed by screwing in counter clock direction.

The disposable *One-Step*™ *port* (InnerDyne, Inc., Sunnyvale, CA) has an adjustable seal which allows introduction of laparoscopic instruments within a range of 4.4–12 mm in diameter. Siloxane™ coating provides smooth passage of instruments and a removable cap facilitates removal of tissues. The initial passage of this port is facilitated by its narrow profile: 2.1 mm at the distal tip and 3.8 mm along the main body; next a blunt-tipped obturator is introduced in order to expand it to a 5, 10, or 12 mm size, dependent upon the surgeon's needs. As such, the tissues of the abdominal wall are stretched rather than incised, thereby precluding the need for placement of fascia sutures at the end of the procedure.

Blunt trocars have no safety shields and are nonbladed. They are passed through the abdominal wall either with a rotating or with a side-to-side forward action. Because they dilate and stretch the abdominal wall tissues, rather than cutting the tissue, no fascia sutures are used to close these port sites, especially if they are off the midline.

Reducers allow downsizing of working channels in $\geq$10 mm trocars to accommodate smaller 5-mm working instruments without any leakage of CO_2; however the development of multi-port technology has resulted in valves that can accommodate 5–12-mm instruments without the need for a reducer.

Primary Access and Port Placement

The kidney can be accessed by retroperitoneal or transperitoneal approach.

Retroperitoneal Access

Lateral Approach

The patient is placed laterally, with sufficient flexion of the operating table so as to expose the area of trocar placement, between the last rib and

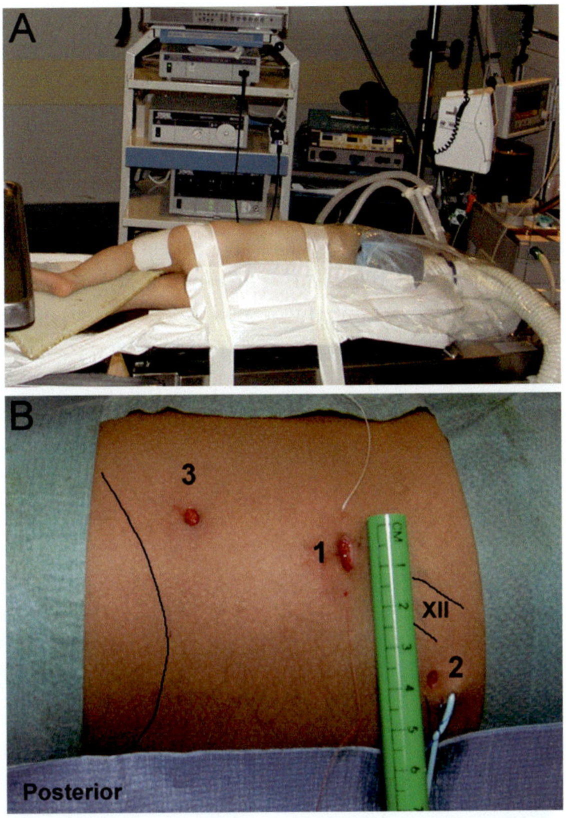

Fig. 3.2 (**a**) Patient positioning for left retroperitoneal laparoscopic renal surgery. The patient is placed laterally, with sufficient flexion of the operating table so as to expose the area of trocar placement, between the last rib and the ileac crest; for younger children as shown, a lumbar support is sufficient for the exposure. The child is rapped by two adhesive bands, one on the greater trochanter level and a second on the chest to keep the child on perpendicular angle with the table. The surgeon, assistant, and scrub nurse are all on the back side of the child. The front side of the child is left free for the monitor. (**b**) Port placement and landmarks for left retroperitoneal laparoscopic pyeloplasty. Retroperitoneal access is achieved via the first incision (*1*), at the tip of the 12th rib, and is used for the laparoscope. Second port (*2*), placed in the costovertebral angle, is used for the needle holder and scissors and to place the double J stent. Third port (*3*) is placed near to the iliac crest at the anterior axillary line and is used for the grasping forceps. The first port is 3 or 5 mm n diameter and the other ports are 3 mm. In this case a transanastomotic pyelostomy stent was used

the ileac crest (Fig. 3.2). In infants and young children (under 6 years), our preference is to put a lumber padding to laterally flex the patient without flexing the operating table. Retroperitoneal access is achieved through the first incision, 15–20 mm in length and one finger width from the lower border of the tip of the 12th rib. The use of narrow retractors with long blades allows a deep dissection with short incision. The Gerota's fascia is approached by a muscle-splitting blunt dissection, then it is opened under direct vision and the first blunt trocar (3 or 5 mm diameter) is introduced directly inside the opened Gerota's fascia [9–13]. A working space is created by gas insufflation dissection, and the first trocar is fixed with a purse-string suture that is applied around the deep fascia to ensure an airtight seal and to allow traction on the main trocar if needed to increase the working space. This type of fixation is preferable to the single used self-retaining trocar, because in children this type of trocars has relatively big size that interferes with the mobility of instruments. Second trocar (3 mm diameter) is inserted posteriorly in the costovertebral angle, in front of the lumbosacral muscle. Third trocar (3 mm diameter) is inserted in the anterior axillary line, a finger width from the top of the iliac crest [14]. To avoid transperitoneal insertion of this trocar, the working space is fully developed and the deep surface of the anterior wall muscles is identified before the trocar insertion. Insufflation pressure does not exceed 10 mmHg, and the CO_2 flow rate is progressively increased from 1 to 3 l/min. Age is not a limiting factor for this approach. Young children have less fat and the access is easier; we have used this access in other indications as nephrectomy for children as young as 3 weeks [15].

Prone Posterior Approach

The access begins with an incision in the costovertebral angle at the edge of the paraspinous muscles. The secondary trocars are placed just above the iliac crest, one medially at the edge of the paraspinous muscles and one laterally at the posterior clavicular line [16].

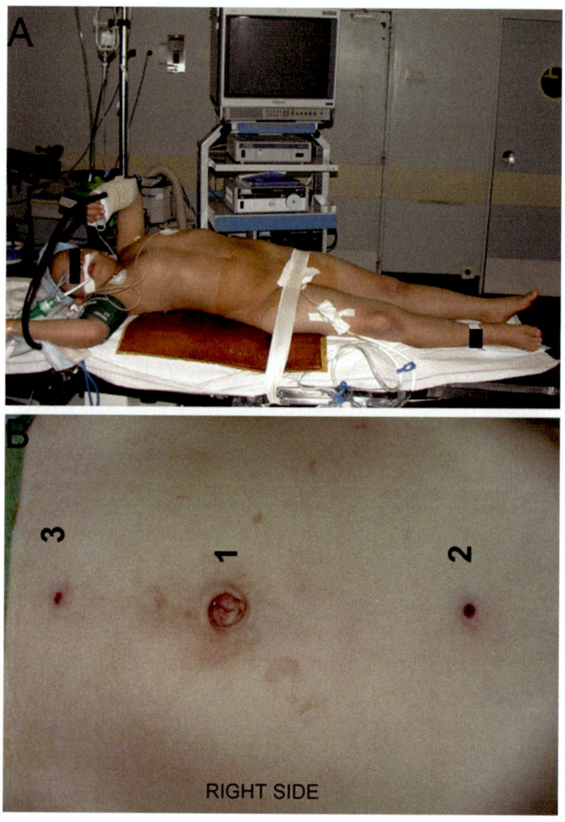

Fig. 3.3 (**a**) Patient positioning and trocar placement for left transperitoneal laparoscopic renal surgery. The child is positioned on semiflank position with the surgeon standing in front of the abdomen (opposite side of pyeloplasty). (**b**) Port placement and landmarks for left transperitoneal laparoscopic pyeloplasty. First port (*1*) is inserted under vision through a midline trans-umbilical incision and is used for the laparoscope. Second port (*2*) is inserted midway between the umbilicus and the symphysis pubis and is used for the needle holder and scissors. Third port (*3*) is placed midway between the umbilicus and the xiphoid, and is used for the grasping forceps. The same configuration can be used for the opposite side after modification of the child's position

Other Techniques to Access the Retroperitoneal Space

Since the description by Gaur in 1992 [17], the balloon dissection has been the method applied by most of the urologists. Disadvantages of the balloon are the cost of the disposable material and the possible complications with rupture of the balloon [18]. On the other hand, the balloon dissection allows creating a working space without opening the Gerota's fascia, which is important for radical nephrectomy of malignant tumors in adults.

Capolicchio et al. [19] described a modification of the lateral access. They recommend the insertion of the first trocar through the costovertebral angle. This modification helped the authors to avoid the accidental peritoneal tear during the access through the first lateral incision and also allowed a smaller incision for the laparoscope.

Micali et al. [20] reported the use of the Visiport visual trocar to access directly to the retroperitoneal space. The advantage of this method is the possibility to use a small incision for the first trocar, which is interesting in the reconstructive surgery.

Transperitoneal Access

Several options exist in terms of patient positioning. The most frequently described is the flank position [21]. Most pediatric surgeons use an open method for the introduction of the first trocar in order to prevent the rare but often life-threatening complications of vascular or hollow viscous perforation by the Veress needle or the blind insertion of the first port [22]. The pneumoperitoneum is created through an open umbilical approach. The child is positioned with the surgeon standing in front of the abdomen (opposite side of pyeloplasty). The most frequent configuration has been with the umbilical port and two ipsilateral ports in the mid-clavicular line above and below the umbilicus. A fourth trocar may be placed in the mid-axillary line if needed for exposure to retract the liver or the spleen if needed. The kidney is exposed by medial mobilization of the colon. In our experience, we insert the laparoscope through the umbilicus, and the operating trocars are inserted midway between the umbilicus and the symphysis pubis and between the umbilicus and the xiphoid process (Fig. 3.3). This configuration is available for both sides and we have used it successfully in cases of horseshoe kidney [23].

Instrumentation for Grasping and Blunt Dissection

The variety of manipulative instruments for laparoscopic surgery is increasing all the time. Each instrument has a handle, a shaft, and an end. Most instruments have a grip handle. Handles can have an electrocautery connection and/or a locking mechanism. Most graspers and dissectors are used in the 5 mm size but are available in a range from 3 to 12 mm, in both disposable and reusable forms. Grasping instruments have either a single-action or a double-action tip design. Wide variations exist with regard to configuration of tip, surface characteristics of the jaws, handle design, and possible electrosurgical properties. Various tip designs include blunt-coarse, pointed, straight, curved, and angled. The surface of the jaws may be atraumatic or traumatic. Indeed in children, instrument with a traumatic end has limited use. Instrument may be reasonably atraumatic when used in adults but are traumatic when used in children.

Instrumentation for Incising and Hemostasis

Laparoscopic scissors are available in disposable and non-disposable forms. As in open surgery, two types of scissors are used: dissecting scissors and scissors to cut ligatures or sutures. The blades of laparoscopic scissors are shorter than their open surgical counterparts. The configuration of the tip may be useful for selective situations: serrated tips for cutting fascia, hooked tips for cutting sutures, microscissors for spatulating the ureter during a pyeloplasty, and curved tips for dissection. Incision of the tissue is achieved using either an electrosurgical or a mechanical approach.

Electrosurgical instrument. Different electrodes are available: needle electrodes (Corson-type) produce fine cuts, spatula electrodes are utilized in blunt dissection and cutting, hook electrodes (J and L configurations) are of particular value during dissection of vessels, as tissue can be pulled away from delicate structures before activating the cutting current. Most of these instruments require the use of monopolar high-frequency electrosurgery (MHFE). MHFE has the potential hazards of collateral damage caused by insulation failure, inadvertent contact with other metal instruments, or capacitive coupling. If nondisposable MHFE instruments are used, they should be checked after each operation for insulation failure. The probe, if coagulating current is being used, should not be activated unless it is in direct contact with the tissue to be incised; if cutting current is being used, it is helpful to activate the probe <1 mm from the tissue and then initiate contact. In our current practice in children, the limited working space makes the use of MHFE more dangerous. In the retroperitoneal approach, MHFE should be avoided to prevent collateral damage especially of the intraperitoneal structures that could be hurt accidentally through the peritoneum.

Hemostasis is most safely achieved by utilizing bipolar devices which require less energy for performance. Bipolar high-frequency electrocautery (BHFE) coagulates between the beak of the instrument and decreases likelihood of injury to surrounding tissue. It has the great disadvantage of being basically a non-cutting instrument, which means that after coagulation, another instrument has to be brought in for cutting. A variation on bipolar electrosurgery is the LigaSure vessel sealing system (Valleylab, Inc., Boulder, CO). The system consists of a 5-mm Maryland-style grasper/dissector or a 10-mm grasping device, with a cutting blade to transect the coagulated vascular structure, and both are connected to a bipolar radio frequency generator. When the vascular structure is grasped by the instrument, the tissue is evaluated by a feedback-response system which subsequently delivers the optimal energy required to seal the vessel effectively. Due to the high-current and low-voltage output, the vascular structure enclosed by the jaws of the instrument degrades quickly and a protein-based seal is created; this mechanism of electrical current delivery to the tissues results in less charring and less collateral thermal damage [24]. Vessels up to 7 mm appear to be effectively occluded with this device.

Ultrasonic device provides another option for dissection in endoscopic surgery. Ultrasonic energy can be used for sealing vessels and for cutting tissue. The end of the instrument may have different shapes, but the shear is most often used because it can dissect, coagulate, and transect at the same time. For use in children, 5-mm-diameter shears are available. In ultrasonic surgery, electrical energy is transformed into mechanical energy by the use of a piezoelectric crystal system. Rapid mechanical vibrations, produced by this system, are capable of creating the following effects on tissue: cavitation, coaptation/coagulation, and cutting. Multifunctionality (grasping, cutting, dissecting, and coagulation) is provided when a scissor-type tip is utilized [25]. In addition to the low risk of local thermal damage and tissue charring due to its working temperature of <80°C, the depth of penetration is limited to the targeted tissue and a 1 mm area on either side of the point of application [26]. This device has two blades; only one of them is nonheat conductor. In order to prevent collateral thermal damage, the metallic blade should be carefully watched. As ultrasonic coagulation blanches the tissues, in contrast to HFE coagulation, which blackens the tissues, collateral damage may be harder to see. A disadvantage of the use of ultrasonic energy is the high cost of the shears, which at present are available only in a disposable version. We frequently use this device during nephrectomy in children but with care to watch carefully the metallic blade not to be in contact with surrounding structures as renal vein when coagulating the renal artery; this can

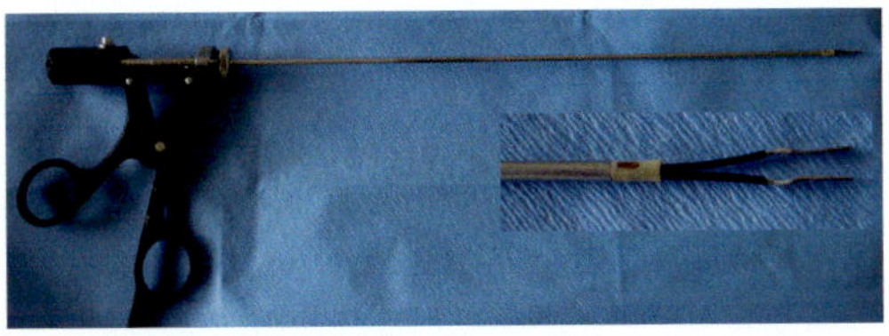

Fig. 3.4 A 3-mm bipolar electrosurgery with thin blades: the perfect device for delicate dissection of the pelviureteral junction in children

severely damage the wall of the vessels resulting in bleeding. Our preference in delicate dissection in children (e.g., dissection of the pelviureteric junction) is the BHFE (Fig. 3.4). This exists in 3-mm instruments with thin blades to help precise hemostasis [27].

Instrumentation for Suturing and Tissue Anastomosis

The ability to ligate and to suture tissues in endoscopic surgery is very important. A significant amount of practice is needed in order to achieve a sufficient level of proficiency.

Laparoscopic needle holders have one fixed jaw and one jaw that opens by squeezing the spring-loaded handle of the instrument. Due to the length and narrow shaft of the needle holders, they all have a locking mechanism to secure the needle in the jaw of the needle holder. This is done with a ratchet, spring-loaded, or a Castro-Viejo-type mechanism. Some needle holders also possess a valuable feature, which allows the jaws to rotate around the main axis, relative to the handle. Again for use in children in whom the manipulation angle is often smaller than 60°, it is advantageous to have a needle holder with curved beak so that the tip can be well visualized. For internal tying, the pieces of thread to be used should be short, e.g., 10 cm; in our practice, the suture material for laparoscopic pyeloplasty in children is a 6-0 absorbable suture with a tapered three-eighth of circle needle, used in conjunction with a 3-mm needle holder (Fig. 3.5), placed from the most dependant portion of the pelvis to the most inferior point or the vertex of the ureteral spatulation. The suture is tied using the intracorporeal technique with the knots placed outside the lumen. The same stitch is used to run the anterior wall of the anastomosis (Fig. 3.6).

Knot pushers are utilized during extracorporeal knot-tying techniques. Knot pushers which work independent of the suture material either slide (Clarke-Reich) or cinch (Gazayerli) the knot into place. Integral knot pushers are part of a system that contains a preformed ligature loop. As soon as the loop of the pre-knotted suture is passed over the tissue to be secured, the knot is delivered and secured around the target tissue with the integral pusher. The suture is then cut and the plastic knot pusher is removed and discarded. We do not recommend extracorporeal knotting when using fine sutures. In pyeloplasty procedure, the 6-0 sutures are too fragile to resist the extracorporeal tension.

The *Endo Stitch* (US Surgical Corp., Norwalk, CT) device is an innovative disposable 10-mm instrument that facilitates laparoscopic suture placement and knot tying. The suture is secured to the center of a straight needle which has a pointed end on both sides, thereby allowing for tissue penetration in either direction. By shuttling the needle back and forth between the jaws of the

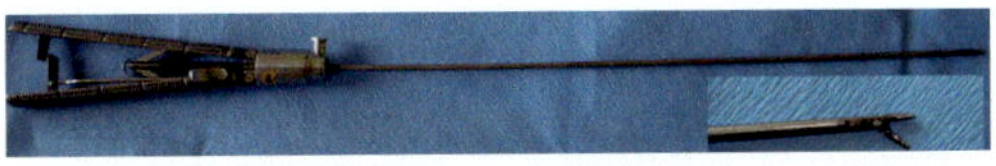

Fig. 3.5 A 3-mm needle holder: the indispensable device for suturing with 6-0 absorbable suture

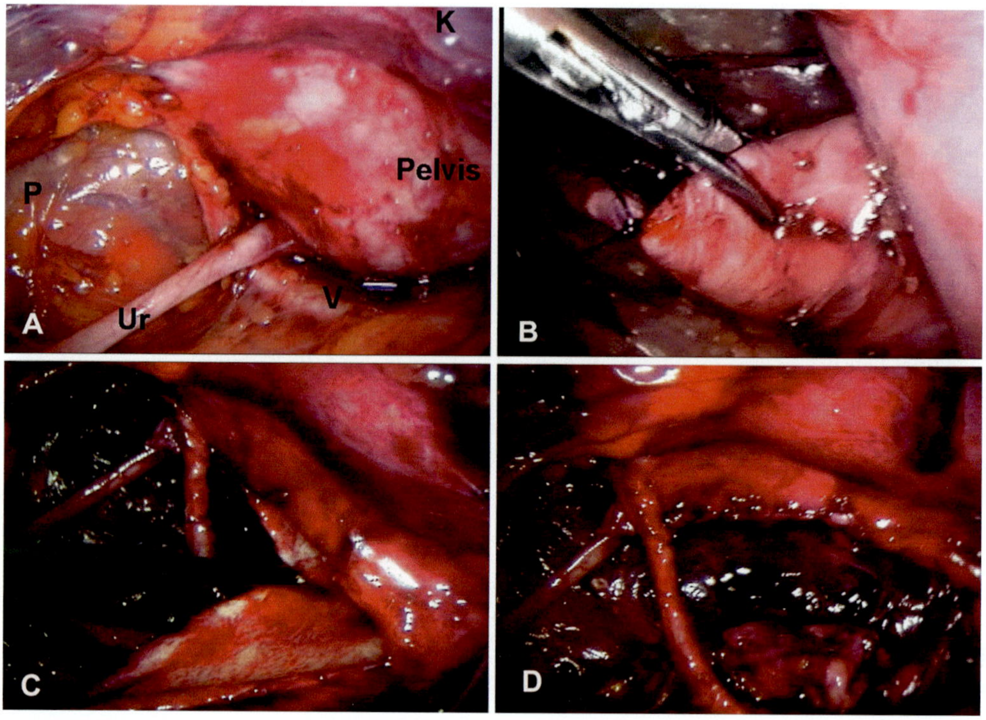

Fig. 3.6 Left retroperitoneal laparoscopic pyeloplasty for hydronephrosis secondary to aberrant crossing vessels. (**a**) The kidney is approached posteriorly and the renal pelvis is first identified. Aberrant crossing vessels are identified anteriorly to the PUJ. (**b**) A stay suture is placed at the PUJ for traction and the renal pelvis partly divided by scissors at the most dependant part and gentle traction on the stay suture helps to define this point. The traction suture also helps to mobilize the ureter so that the scissors can be in the axis of the ureter. (**c**) After placement of the stay suture, the ureter is completely divided and the UPJ and the pelvis are delivered anterior to the vessels with the help of the stay suture. Then the anastomosis is performed. A reduction of the renal pelvis is done when needed. (**d**) The final aspect at the end of the pyeloplasty. V, crossing vessels; Ur, ureter; P, peritoneum; K, kidney

instrument after each passage through the tissue, it applies a long known principle used in sewing machines. As such, passing the needle through the tissue and regrasping the needle after it has traversed the tissue becomes a simple task, as it is all done by a one-handed squeeze of the handle and a flip of the needle-securing lever, respectively. This device is rarely applicable in children, as most of the surgery is done with 3- and 5-mm trocars and instruments.

Instrumentation for Aspiration and Irrigation

In contrast to open surgery in which a swab with gauze can immediately restore vision during bleeding or can immediately clean leakage from the bowel, endoscopic surgery largely depends on suction and irrigation for these matters. Moreover as the amount of light that can be brought in endoscopic surgery is limited and blood absorbs light, blood even in areas remote from the direct area to be operated upon has to be removed in endoscopic surgery. These are available as either a disposable or a non-disposable device; a combination of aspiration and irrigation in one instrument is most practical. The aspirator, which is connected to a suction system, consists of a 3–10-mm metal tube with suction being controlled by either a one-way stopcock or a spring-controlled trumpet valve. The irrigation channel is also operated either by a one-way stopcock or by a trumpet valve. The irrigation fluid is pressurized within a range of 250–700 mmHg to allow for effective delivery of the irrigant and flushing of any bleeding site to allow for accurate hemostasis.

Conclusions

The specificity of working with children limits the use of most of the adult laparoscopic devices. Surgeons should be aware of the specific instrumentation in children. The main difficulties are the limited working space, the limited area of trocar insertion, and the relative fine structures to deal with compared to adults. If the surgeon is willing to reproduce the excellent open surgery functional results in children, a careful adaptation of instruments, sutures, and techniques should be applied and modified continuously. To achieve such goals, small and short instruments should be used. Aggressive monopolar diathermy dissection should be avoided. Reconstructive surgery such as pyeloplasty requires specific pediatric instrumentation and sutures to be comparable with open surgery instruments.

Although great improvement has been achieved in pediatric instrumentation, suturing devices are not yet optimal and still time consuming and the main limit for surgeons is to practice the laparoscopic approach for reconstructive surgery.

Critical Operative Steps

- Access to the retroperitoneum and creation of the working space are the keys of success in the retroperitoneal renal surgery.
- First trocar should be placed inside the Gerota's fascia behind the kidney.
- In retroperitoneal surgery, orientation is paramount. Landmarks, i.e., psoas, kidney, peritoneum, inferior vena cava, should be frequently checked.
- A stay stitch placed at the pyeloureteral junction helps to mobilize the ureter in the axis of the scissors and to keep traction by fixing it to the psoas muscle to give stability and to facilitate the suturing.
- Transperitoneal approach is more adapted for pelvic kidney and horseshoe kidneys.

Critical Instruments and Supplies

- A purse-string suture applied around the deep fascia to fix the first trocar and to ensure an airtight seal and to allow traction to increase the working space
- For pelviureteral anastomosis, a 6-0 absorbable suture with a tapered three-eighth of the circle needle is used in conjunction with 3-mm needle holder.
- MHFE should be avoided to prevent collateral damage.
- A 3-mm BHFE with thin blades is the perfect device in delicate dissection of the pelviureteral junction in children.
- Suturing device is rarely applicable in children, as most of the surgeries are done with 3- and 5-mm trocars and instruments.

References

1. El-Ghoneimi A. Retroperitoneal laparoscopic pyeloplasty in children. In: Esposito C, Settimi A, editors. Handbook of pediatric laparoscopic surgery. Naples: Litho Car; 2006. pp. 175–88.
2. Georgeson KE. Instrumentation. In: Bax NMA, Georgeson KE, Najmaldin A, et al., editors. Endoscopic surgery in children. Berlin: Springer; 1999. pp. 8–13.
3. Kourambas J, Preminger GM. Advances in camera, video, and imaging technology in laparoscopy. Urol Clin North Am. 2001;28:5–14.
4. Aslan P, Kuo RL, Hazel K, et al. Advances in digital imaging during endoscopic surgery. J Endourol. 1999;13:251.
5. El-Ghoneimi A. Laparoscopic nephrectomy and pyeloplasty. In: Docimo SG, Canning DA, Khoury AE, editors. The Kelalis–King–Belman textbook of clinical pediatric urology. London: Informa Healthcare; 2007. pp. 487–96.
6. Halachmi S, El-Ghoneimi A, Bissonnette B, et al. Hemodynamic and respiratory effect of pediatric urological laparoscopic surgery: a retrospective study. J Urol. 2003;170:1651–4.
7. Pennant JH. Anesthesia for laparoscopy in the pediatric patient. Anesthesiol Clin North Am. 2001;19:69–88.
8. Ott DE. Laparoscopic hypothermia. J Laparoendosc Surg. 1991;3:127–31.
9. El-Ghoneimi A, Valla JS, Steyaert H, et al. Laparoscopic renal surgery via a retroperitoneal approach in children. J Urol. 1998;160:1138–41.

10. El-Ghoneimi A, Farhat W, Bolduc S, et al. Laparoscopic dismembered pyeloplasty by a retroperitoneal approach in children. BJU Int. 2003;92:104–8.
11. El-Ghoneimi A. Pediatric laparoscopic surgery. Curr Opin Urol. 2003;13:329–35.
12. El-Ghoneimi A, Abou-Hashim H, Bonnard A, et al. Retroperitoneal laparoscopic nephrectomy in children: at last the gold standard? J Pediatr Urol. 2006;2(4):357–63.
13. Carr M, El-Ghoneimi A. Anomalies and surgery of the ureteropelvic junction in children. In: Wein AJ, Kavoussi LR, Novick AC, Partin AW, Peters CA, editors. Campbell–Walsh urology. Philadelphia, PA: Saunders Elsevier; 2006. pp. 3359–82.
14. El-Ghoneimi A. Laparoscopic renal surgery. In: Smith AD, Badlani GH, Bagley DH, Clayman RV, et al., editors. Smith's textbook of endourology. Hamilton, ON: BC Decker; 2007. pp. 857–64.
15. El-Ghoneimi A. Renal dysplasia and cystic disease options. In: Dociomo SG, editor. Minimally invasive approaches to pediatric urology. London: Taylor & Francis; 2005. pp. 105–18.
16. Peters C. Laparoendoscopic renal surgery in children. J Endourol. 2000;14:841–7.
17. Gaur D. Laparoscopic operative retroperitoneoscopy: use of a new device. J Urol. 1992;148:1137–9.
18. Adams JB, Micali S, Moore RG, et al. Complications of extraperitoneal balloon dilation. J Endourol. 1996;10:375–8.
19. Capolicchio JP, Jednak RJ, Anidjar M, et al. A modified access technique for retroperitoneoscopic renal surgery in children. J Urol. 2003;170: 204–6.
20. Micali S, Caione P, Virgili G, et al. Retroperitoneal laparoscopic access in children using a direct vision technique. J Urol. 2001;165:229–32.
21. Peters C. Laparoendoscopic renal surgery in children. J Endourol. 2000;14:841–7.
22. Esposito C, Ascione G, Garipoli V, et al. Complications of pediatric laparoscopic surgery. Surg Endosc. 1997;11:655.
23. Carr M, El-Ghoneimi A. Anomalies and surgery of the ureteropelvic junction in children. In: Wein AJ, Kavoussi LR, Novick AC, Partin AW, Peters CA, editors. Campbell–Walsh urology. Philadelphia, PA: Saunders Elsevier; 2006. pp. 3359–82.
24. Kennedy JS, Buysse SP, Lawes KR, et al. Recent innovations in bipolar electrosurgery. Minim Invasive Ther Allied Technol. 1999;8:95–9.
25. Strate T, Bloechle C, Broering D, et al. Hemostasis with the ultrasonically activated scalpel. Surg Endosc. 1999;13:727.
26. Bishoff JT, Allaf ME, et al. Laparoscopic bowel injuries: incidence and clinical presentation. J Urol. 1999;161(3):887–90.
27. El-Ghoneimi A. Pediatric laparoscopy. In: Kumar U, Gill IS, editors. Tips and tricks in laparoscopic urology. London: Springer; 2006. pp. 201–10.

Part II
Laparoscopic and Robotic Reconstructive Renal Surgery

Chapter 4

Adult Laparoscopic Partial Nephrectomy for Renal Cell Carcinoma

Mohamed A. Atalla, Sero Andonian, and Manish A. Vira

This chapter contains a video segment which can be found at the URL: http://www.springerimages.com/ost

Abbreviations

CKD	chronic kidney disease
LPN	laparoscopic partial nephrectomy
LRN	laparoscopic radical nephrectomy
NSS	nephron-sparing surgery
OPN	open partial nephrectomy
PSM	positive surgical margin
RCC	renal cell carcinoma
WIT	warm ischemia time

Epidemiology

Renal cell carcinoma (RCC) is the most common malignancy of the kidney and accounts for approximately 3% of adult cancers [1]. The incidence rate has steadily increased over the last three decades, particularly among African-Americans [2]. During 2009, it is estimated that approximately 57,760 new cases of kidney cancer will be diagnosed and 12,980 people will die of the disease in the United States [3]. With a 35% 5-year mortality, RCC is the most lethal urological malignancy [4]. The improvement in and increased application of cross-sectional imaging modalities have led to an increase in the incidental detection of renal masses. Historically, radical nephrectomy has been described as the standard surgical therapy for renal masses. With a better understanding of the heterogeneity of tumor biology and advancement of surgical technique, treatment options have evolved to include surveillance, ablation, and minimally invasive nephron-sparing techniques.

Indications

In 2009, motivated by the divergence in current clinical practice, the American Urological Association commissioned a panel to develop guidelines for the management of stage 1 renal cancer [5]. The guideline thoroughly outlined the factors surrounding the decision-making process that clinicians and patients face when confronted with the myriad of treatment options. Several studies have now concluded that partial nephrectomy provides cancer control similar to radical nephrectomy [6]. Furthermore, partial nephrectomy has been shown to decrease risk of end-stage renal failure requiring renal replacement therapy when compared to radical nephrectomy [7–9]. Laparoscopic partial nephrectomy (LPN) was first reported in 1993 [10, 11]. With subsequent improvement in instrumentation and technology, the technique has evolved and now can be considered a laparoscopic replication of the classic partial nephrectomy technique [12].

M.A. Vira (✉)
Department of Urology, North Shore Long Island Jewish Health System, Arthur D. Smith Institute for Urology, Hofstra University School of Medicine, New Hyde Park, NY, USA
e-mail: mvira@nshs.edu

M.C. Ost (ed.), *Robotic and Laparoscopic Reconstructive Surgery in Children and Adults*, Current Clinical Urology, DOI 10.1007/978-1-60327-914-7_4, © Springer Science+Business Media, LLC 2011

Classically, absolute indications for nephron-sparing surgery (NSS) were localized renal mass in a solitary kidney [13], bilateral synchronous renal masses, or a renal mass in a patient with chronic renal insufficiency [6, 14]. Relative indications for partial nephrectomy included hereditary forms of RCC such as von Hippel–Lindau disease and hereditary papillary renal cell carcinoma in which there is increased risk of metachronous renal malignancies [1]. Relative indications for partial nephrectomy also included patients at increased risk for chronic kidney disease (CKD) secondary to hypertension or diabetes mellitus [15]. These criteria have largely been supplanted with a generalized recommendation that NSS should be attempted, laparoscopically or open, for all small renal masses unless contraindicated even with a normal contralateral kidney.

Contraindications to partial nephrectomy include masses with renal vein or inferior vena cava tumor thrombus, locally advanced masses, masses with associated lymphadenopathy, and masses in patients with bleeding diathesis. Previously used size limitations for NSS gradually have been abolished with more reports of oncologic efficacy [16]. Specifically, recent reports have expanded the indications for NSS to include tumors larger than 4 cm in carefully selected patients [17, 18]. Simmons et al. evaluated LPN for tumors between 4 and 7 cm in size and showed equivalent oncological outcomes when compared to a similar cohort that underwent laparoscopic radical nephrectomy (LRN) [19]. Patients with tumor thrombus, lymphadenopathy, metastatic disease, or stage V CKD at surgery were excluded from the study. Overall mortality, cancer-specific mortality, and recurrence rates were similar after a median follow-up of 57 months. Interestingly, there was a significantly higher incidence of CKD in the LRN group. These findings underscore not only the oncologic efficacy of the treatment of localized RCC but also the importance of NSS in the avoidance of future CKD.

In patients with a normal contralateral kidney, the disadvantages of partial nephrectomy including increased risk of perioperative complications, local recurrence, and tumor multifocality have to be weighed against the risk of future CKD in deciding between partial and radical nephrectomy [7–9]. In a review of 878 open partial nephrectomy (OPN) patients, the rate of operative mortality was 1%, urine leak 7%, abscess 1%, bleeding 2%, and re-operation 2% [15]. Regarding local recurrence, the incidence in partial nephrectomy series has been reported to be 0–10% depending on tumor size, histology, and stage. In tumors 4 cm or less, the local recurrence rate is even lower at 0–3% [6]. Histologic subtype, i.e., papillary type 1, rather than tumor size has proven to be the most reliable predictor of multicentricity [20, 21].

In early studies of LPN, as the technique was being refined, patient and tumor selection was fairly stringent and included patients with unifocal, small, polar, and exophytic tumors. As the technique advanced and experience increased, larger, hilar, endophytic, and collecting system-abutting lesions were successfully resected laparoscopically [22]. LPN became a viable alternative to OPN for the majority of patients with small renal tumors. As LPN became more widespread, several studies directly compared LPN to OPN. LPN repeatedly was associated with measures of lower morbidity. These include decreased narcotic requirements, improved cosmesis, earlier resumption of diet, shorter hospitalization, earlier return to work, and lower expense [23, 24]. However, several studies have reported increased complications with LPN. In a large series from the Cleveland Clinic, LPN was associated with a shorter surgical time and lower blood loss but longer warm ischemia (27.8 min versus 17.5 min) and higher rate of intraoperative complications (5% versus 0%) when compared to OPN [25]. Similarly, in a multi-center comparison of 771 LPN to 1028 OPN, LPN was associated with longer ischemic time and increased postoperative complications (especially urological) while again demonstrating its benefits of shorter operative time, decreased blood loss, and shorter hospital stays [26]. These retrospective studies are undoubtedly affected by a certain element of selection bias in that the early experience with LPN (i.e., learning curve) is included in the comparison. Nevertheless, the advantages of lower blood loss, shorter hospitalization, and earlier convalescence are evident. Prospective randomized trials are lacking and understandingly difficult to conduct.

Ultimately, a well-informed decision about the treatment choice is based on a good understanding of the risks and benefits of the treatment alternatives. In most stage 1 renal tumors, alternatives to LPN include OPN, laparoscopic or open radical nephrectomy, percutaneous or laparoscopic thermal ablation, and observation [5]. For each of these options, surgeon and center experience and patient selection have a significant effect on short-term and long-term outcomes.

Preoperative Preparation

Adequate preoperative imaging is crucial to map out a successful approach for every LPN. A contrast-enhanced CT or MRI is essential for planning. Three-dimensional rendering is optional with some reports of additional benefit [27]. Metastases, lymphadenopathy, tumor thrombus, and metachronous lesions should be excluded. Tumor size, location, and relationship to the collecting system dictate the actual resection, while body habitus and vascular and collecting system anatomy dictate the approach and port placement. In addition to preoperative imaging, intraoperative ultrasound should always be utilized in confirming the location of the tumor and delineation of the extent of endophytic lesion resection.

Given that at least 20% of incidentally discovered small renal masses represent benign lesions, a renewed interest in percutaneous biopsy has been expressed in recent years. Traditionally, high rate of false-negative and nondiagnostic results rendered the biopsy powerless in preventing surgical resection for small renal masses [28]. However, improvement in biopsy accuracy and diagnostic methods have popularized percutaneous renal biopsy, particularly in patients contemplating active surveillance or suspected of harboring metastases from other organs or lymphoma [29].

Technique

The authors prefer a magnesium citrate bowel prep 1 day prior to surgery. Preoperative antibiotics are administered intravenously. Sequential lower extremity compression boots and an orogastric tube are used. Placement of a ureteral catheter for intraoperative retrograde injection of dyed saline to identify collecting system entry is rarely needed and reserved for central deep tumors. The patient is secured to the operating table at a 45° angle over a gel chest roll with the ipsilateral arm padded and flexed over the chest (Fig. 4.1). Once the patient is adequately secured,

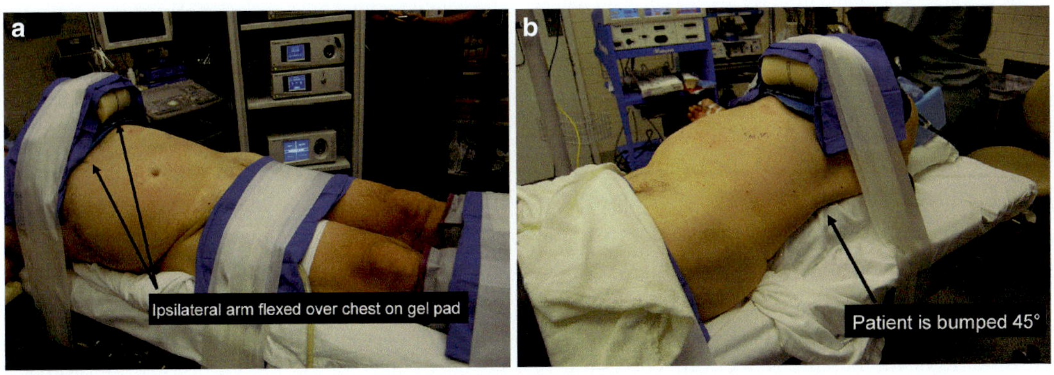

Fig. 4.1 (**a**, **b**) Patient Position. The patient is secured to the operating table at a 45° angle over a gel chest roll with the ipsilateral arm padded and flexed over the chest

the operating room table can be rotated to full tilt on the contralateral side to maximize exposure to the renal fossa.

A transperitoneal approach is preferred. While some centers advocate a retroperitoneoscopic approach for posterior or posterolateral tumors [30], we reserve this approach for patients who have had multiple prior abdominal surgeries. Abdominal insufflation is achieved with a Veress needle puncture through the umbilicus or in the ipsilateral upper quadrant (two finger breadths below costal margin). Most procedures are completed using three trocars. A 10-mm laparoscope port is placed periumbilically. Working ports are placed in the sub-xiphoid space and in the ipsilateral mid-axillary line at the level of the umbilicus. Port placement can be shifted cephalad and lateral for upper pole or posterior tumors and for overweight and obese patients. Regardless of the location, ports should be at least 8–10 cm apart with an angle of at least 90° (Fig. 4.2).

lateral splenic ligaments are divided to medially reflect the spleen, splenic flexure, and pancreas en bloc. On the right side, the duodenum is sharply released from the renal hilum and inferior vena cava with care taken to avoid the use of thermal dissection.

The ureter is then isolated medial to the lower pole and the gonadal vein is identified. The mass is localized and exposed by correlating with preoperative imaging and with the aid of intraoperative ultrasonography using a laparoscopic flexible 7-MHz probe. The renal capsule overlying the resection site is circumscribed using monopolar cautery while preserving the perirenal fat overlying the tumor. If the renal hilum is to be clamped, the vascular anatomy is delineated and the vessels are dissected carefully. A bulldog clamp is applied to each vessel separately, or a laparoscopic Satinsky clamp is applied through a separate stab incision, so as not to occupy a working port (Fig. 4.3).

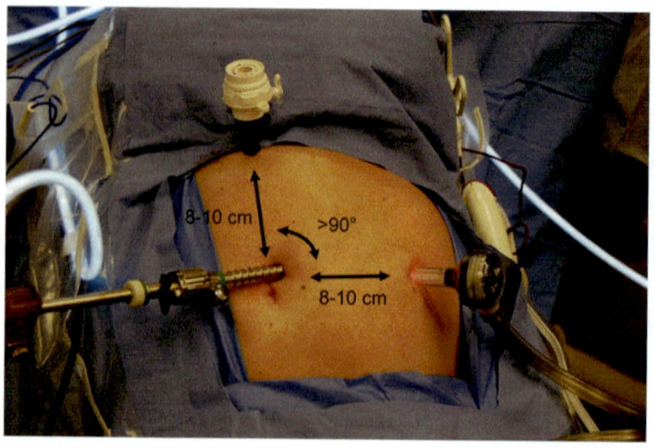

Fig. 4.2 Trocar Positioning. Regardless of exact position of the trocars, they should be at least 8–10 cm apart and at an angle of $\geq 90°$

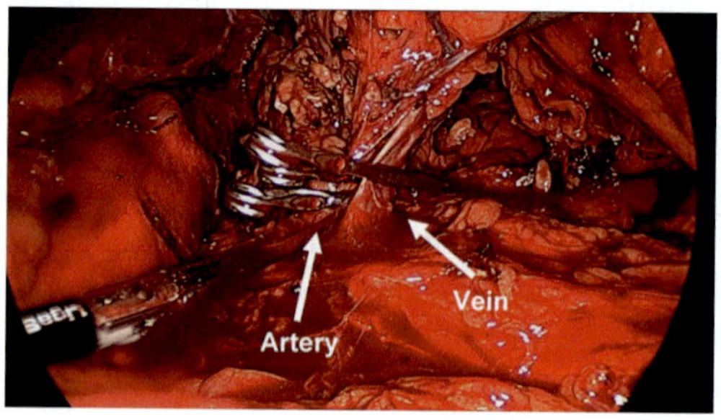

Fig. 4.3 Bulldog clamps are applied to the artery and vein separately for total hilar occlusion during resection of the tumor

A combination of monopolar hot shears, atraumatic grasper, suction irrigator, and the LigaSure Atlas sealer/divider (ValleyLab, Boulder, CO) is used for dissection. After inspecting the bowel for inadvertent injury during trocar placement, the small bowel is mobilized medially to expose the white line of Toldt. The white line is then incised from the inferior margin of the kidney around the splenic or the hepatic reflection. The colon is reflected medially to expose Gerota's fascia and the renal hilum. On the left side, lienorenal and

A combination of sharp and thermal dissection is used to excise the tumor with a small margin of normal parenchyma. Visualized perforating vessels can be ligated with a clip applier during the dissection. Collecting system entry is repaired using a polyglactin suture, although in the authors' experience, this step may not be necessary for minor violations. A biopsy of the base of the cortical defect is sent for frozen section to ensure complete resection. The defect is then fulgurated using an argon beam coagulator (Conmed, Utica, NY). The renorrhaphy is performed using 2-0 polyglactin suture on a CT-1 (GS-21) needle with a Lapra-Ty (Ethicon Endo-Surgery, Cincinnati, OH) knotted at the end. This can be performed in a running fashion, but several sutures might be needed depending on the defect size. The use of a Surgicel (Johnson and Johnson; New Brunswick, NJ) bolster and hemostatic sealants is optional but may not be necessary (Fig. 4.4) [31].

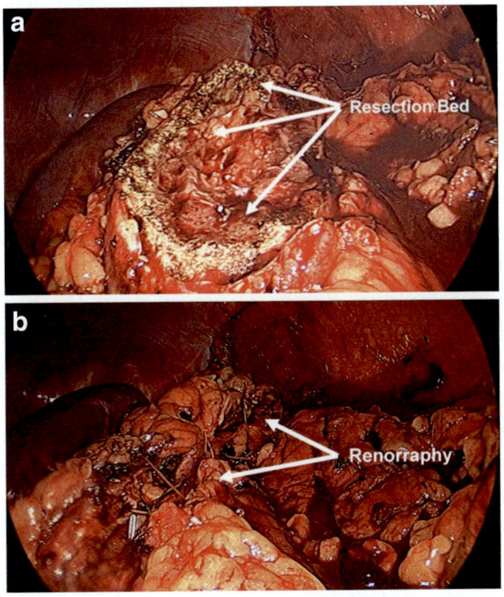

Fig. 4.4 (a) Renal defect after resection of 4.5 cm renal mass. (b) Renorraphy using suture ligation and reapproximation of capsular edges. Lapra-Ty adapters are used to secure sutures

After hilar unclamping, hemostasis is confirmed by lowering the intraperitoneal pressure to less than 10 mmHg. The tumor is placed in an entrapment bag and extracted via an extension of the periumbilical incision or a separate lower midline incision. Fascial defects of port sites that are 10 mm or larger should be closed using a wound closure device and a polyglactin suture. An external drain is left posterior to the kidney if collecting system entry is suspected. If a ureteral catheter is placed, it is removed at the conclusion of the procedure.

Special Considerations

Hilar Control

To perform an adequate resection during LPN, hilar control is often necessary to achieve a bloodless operative field. The primary concern with hilar occlusion is renal injury secondary to warm ischemia. In the largest comparative study to date, renal functional outcomes at 3 months postoperatively were similar in LPN and OPN, with 97.9 and 99.6% of operated upon renal units retaining function [26]. Hilar dissection and clamping (and resultant warm ischemia) can be safely avoided for smaller, exophytic, polar lesions [32]. Recently, an alternative to hilar clamping has been reported. The renal parenchyma can be clamped directly using a Satinsky clamp or other device with regional ischemia resulting in similar success rates [33, 34]. These alternatives, however, are not feasible for hilar or central lesions.

While the potentially harmful effects of vascular occlusion, including reperfusion injury after unclamping, are best avoided by resection under full perfusion, to approach larger, deeper, and more central tumors, hilar control is necessary. Intraoperative hemorrhage is decreased facilitating a more accurate dissection and deliberate reconstruction [35]. Laparoscopic bulldog clamps (Aesculap, Center Valley, PA) are the most widely used instruments to temporarily occlude the renal vessels. Bulldog clamps allow selective clamping of the main renal artery or, if preferred, individual polar branches (thereby reducing the effect of warm ischemia to the remainder of the kidney). Unlike the laparoscopic Satinsky clamp, after being applied, the clamps no longer occupy a working port. Care must be taken to avoid dislodgement from the applicator during removal of the clamps, as they can be easily lost in the peritoneal cavity, especially given the angled position of the patient. Another option of clamping the renal vessels laparoscopically is the use of a laparoscopic Satinsky clamp (Aesculap, Center Valley, PA), which allows en bloc clamping of the entire renal hilum. Use of a Satinsky obviates the need for unnecessary dissection of individual hilar vessels but can occupy an additional port or require a separate stab incision.

The deleterious effects of warm ischemia have been well documented [36]. Prolonged periods of ischemia result in acute tubular necrosis and renal failure. Intravenous mannitol (12.5 gm) is often administered prior to clamping for its protective effects. Mannitol is a free radical scavenger that decreases intracellular edema, decreases intra-renal vascular resistance, increases blood flow and glomerular filtration rate of superficial nephrons, and causes an osmotic diuresis [37, 38]. In addition, furosemide can be administered after unclamping to promote diuresis.

One approach to minimizing ischemic injury is to decrease warm ischemia time (WIT). Several surgeons have reported early unclamping of the vessels prior to a bolstering renorrhaphy with significant improvement in WIT over traditional techniques [39, 40]. WIT can also be reduced using on-demand clamping. This technique involves a full dissection of the hilum but involves clamping only if excessive bleeding occurs during the tumor resection [41]. This technique, however, is associated with a higher transfusion rate and higher potential for intraoperative complications. Another approach to reducing ischemic injury is to clamp only the artery. Early animal models of open partial nephrectomy did demonstrate a favorable effect with artery-only clamping, but this benefit has not been replicated in LPN [42]. The lack of benefit may be due to the passive venous occlusion as a result of the pneumoperitoneum.

Thirty minutes of warm ischemia has been arbitrarily designated as the safe WIT in LPN. While there is no absolute cutoff for WIT, it is generally accepted that length of WIT correlates with an increased risk and severity of renal dysfunction. Bhayani et al. [36] compared WIT less than and more than 30 min in a cohort of patients who underwent LPN. Median postoperative serum creatinine showed no significant change, and none of the 118 patients developed renal insufficiency. Porpiglia et al. reported similar results [43]. In their study, glomerular filtration rate (GFR) was not significantly different 3 months after LPN with warm ischemia of more than 30 min in 18 patients. Notably, in both studies, the vast majority of patients had a normal contralateral kidney. Patients with renal insufficiency, hypertension, or diabetes mellitus do not tolerate warm ischemia well and may be more susceptible to ischemic injury when WIT exceeds 30 min.

While the effects of WIT seem transient, the long-term effects are still uncertain. Efforts to minimize warm ischemia are important but should not jeopardize cancer control, hemostasis, or collecting system closure. In particular, when more complex renal lesions are approached and the surgeon feels that the ischemic time to resect and reconstruct the kidney will be longer than 30 min, cold ischemia techniques should be contemplated. Gill et al. described a laparoscopic ice slush technique that replicates techniques used in OPN. Slush is introduced through a separate trocar into a 12-mm entrapment bag into which the mobilized kidney is placed after the renal hilum is clamped using a laparoscopic Satinsky clamp [44]. Alternatively, cold saline irrigation through a 7-Fr ureteral catheter was described by Guillonneau et al. [45]. This technique also identified the open collecting system by visualization of saline outflow. Postoperative creatinine was higher in the cold ischemia group when compared to the control group (1.45 versus 1.26 mg/dl), but this was not statistically significant. A more invasive method of cold ischemia was described by Janetschek et al. [46]. An angiocatheter inserted through a percutaneous femoral puncture was advanced under fluoroscopic guidance to the renal artery. Following a mannitol infusion, the renal artery was clamped. The angiocatheter was then infused with a cold Ringer's lactate and mannitol solution during the resection. While this technique may have a renal protective effect, it is not without its risks [47].

Hemostasis

Several techniques have been described to achieve hemostasis in the nephrotomy defect. The first is by using a bipolar coagulation forceps

[48]. This technique allows simultaneous dissection and hemostasis. The argon beam coagulator is also a favored device for fulguration of the nephrotomy defect, albeit with a very shallow depth of penetration. In addition to the cost and non-availability in some centers, one disadvantage is a sudden rise of peritoneal pressure, which can lead to pneumothorax. This risk can be mostly avoided by passive venting of insufflation gas during coagulation [48].

A wide variety of hemostatic agents and tissue sealants have been used in LPN to aid in hemostasis and help reduce urine leakage [49]. These agents include fibrin gel or *Tisseel* (Baxter, Deerfield, IL), thrombin gelatin matrix or *FloSeal* (Baxter, Deerfield, IL), bovine serum albumin or *BioGlue* (Cryolife, Kennesaw, GA), and oxidized regenerated methylcellulose or *Surgicel* (Johnson and Johnson, New Brunswick, NJ). No single agent has proved superior, but each complements a sutured renorrhaphy; therefore, the choice of hemostatic agent depends on surgeon's preference. A retrospective survey of 18 centers with 1,347 cases of LPN found that 16 centers used hemostatic agents in addition to performing concomitant suturing of the nephrotomy bed [31]. While these hemostatic agents are useful, the key to successful hemostasis is an adequate suture renorrhaphy. Johnston et al. [32] compared fibrin glue alone to sutured bolster repair of the collecting system and reported a 41% incidence of postoperative hemorrhage or urinary leakage after fibrin glue compared to 11% when sutured bolsters were used. Overall rates of hemorrhage and urine leakage after LPN are low with a suture renorraphy and the use of hemostatic agents and tissue sealants has not been proven to reduce these rates.

Dissectors

The choice of dissecting instrument has been governed largely by surgeon's preference. Tumor resection has traditionally been performed using a combination of sharp and blunt non-thermal dissection. While it was widely accepted that a non-thermal dissection is required for accurate assessment of tumor margin status, this notion was challenged by Phillips et al. [50]. Despite some degree of cellular damage, pathologic evaluation of margin status was unhindered after dissection using bipolar and ultrasonic instruments. In light of these findings, portions, if not the entire dissection, can be performed using a Harmonic Scalpel (Ethicon Endo-Surgery; Cincinnati, OH) or a LigaSure device.

A device used with success in liver resections, the Habib probe (AngioDynamics; Queensbury, NY) was evaluated for safety in LPN by Andonian et al. [51] in a pilot study. This four-pronged bipolar radio frequency device ablates a hemostatic plane around the planned dissection plane. The TissueLink (TissueLink Medical; Dover, NH), a saline-coupled radio frequency tool was evaluated by several authors in LPN [52–54]. This device transmits energy from a standard electrosurgical generator through conductive fluid to produce a virtually bloodless dissection. The device likely has not enjoyed widespread use because of its cost and higher depth of penetration (4–7 mm) with potential for excessive damage to remaining normal renal parenchyma.

Outcomes

Positive Margins

Margin status at the time of surgery is an important early surrogate for adequacy of resection during LPN. As compared to OPN with cold ischemia, the luxury of awaiting the result of a frozen section prior to renorrhaphy and hilar unclamping is not afforded by the constraints of WIT. A positive surgical margin (PSM) often requires taking down the renorrhaphy and likely either re-clamping of the vessels or an open conversion to accomplish a deeper resection. In cases of extensive PSM, a completion nephrectomy may be considered.

In the current experience of LPN, the overall incidence of PSM is low. In a retrospective multi-institutional survey of 17 centers in the United States and Europe, the PSM rate on frozen section was 2.4% [55]. Out of 21 cases of PSM, 14 underwent immediate radical nephrectomy and the rest were followed. In a multi-center study of 511 patients who underwent LPN, 9 patients (1.8%) were found to have a PSM [56]. Two underwent complete radical nephrectomy revealing no residual tumor. Of the seven patients followed conservatively, one patient with VHL died of metastatic RCC 10 months postoperatively and the remaining six patients were disease-free at a median follow-up of 32 months. Similarly, other surgeons have advocated that patients found to have a microscopic PSM following resection can be followed with vigilant observation and frequently spaced axial imaging to help detect early evidence of recurrence [57].

Tumor Spillage and Port Site Metastasis

Laparoscopic port site metastasis is defined as recurrent malignant lesions developing at trocar sites, without evidence of peritoneal carcinomatosis [58]. In a retrospective review of over 1,000 laparoscopic cases, only two cases (0.18%) of port site metastases were reported, suggesting that it is a rare event [59]. There are five reported cases of port site metastasis after LRN [60]. The first case of port site metastasis after LPN was reported recently [58]. Schneider et al. [61] evaluated surgical measures to reduce port site metastasis in a porcine model. These measures included making smaller skin incisions, securing trocars to prevent dislodgement and gas leak, using sterile water or heparin-supplemented irrigant to irrigate the field and wounds, and using entrapment bags for specimen retrieval. In this animal model, these measures reduced recurrence from 63.8 to 13.8%.

Recurrence and Survival

Overall cancer-specific survival rates in patients with localized RCC are 91% at 5 years and 80% at 10 and 20 years. In an aggregate review of 1,800 patients who had undergone LPN, cancer-specific survival exceeded 90% after a mean follow-up of 3 years (range of 2–6 years) [26]. The risk of local recurrence was found to be 0–10% and was lowest for patients who underwent nephron-sparing surgery for lesions of ≤ 4 cm [6]. Negative predictors of survival include high tumor grade, high tumor stage, bilateral disease, and tumors greater than 4 cm [62]. Location of the tumor (central versus peripheral; endophytic versus exophytic) is a significant technical consideration for nephron-sparing surgery but is not a significant prognosticator of cancer-specific outcomes [63].

Complications

In addition to general complications that are possible with laparoscopic abdominal surgery, LPN has an added risk of complications in the short and intermediate postoperative period [64]. Complications most notable to LPN are hemorrhage and urinary fistula development. In a review of 878 patients, the rate of operative mortality was 1%, urinary fistula 7%, abscess 1%, bleeding 2%, and re-operation 2% [15]. Simmons and Gill [22] found an overall complication rate of 19%, of which 71% were minor. The complications included a 4.5% rate of bleeding and 2% rate of urinary fistula development. An international survey of 1,347 LPNs revealed a 2.7% incidence of hemorrhage requiring a blood transfusion and a 1.9% incidence of urinary fistula [31].

Rates of urinary fistula development vary across the literature, but intuitively, the incidence correlates with depth of tumor involvement and resection [65]. Urinary fistula is initially managed conservatively with external drainage. If leakage persists, a ureteral stent or nephrostomy tube can be placed to allow for urinary diversion. Rarely are other interventions necessary for persistent urinary leaks [66]. Investigating techniques for prevention of urinary leaks have not yielded unequivocal results. While deep cortical suturing of collecting system entry points can help accelerate closure, they risk excluding calyces and damaging interstitial vessels that can lead to arteriovenous malformations [67, 68].

Intraoperative conversion to an open procedure can be as high as 4.32% [69]. Common causes for conversion include vascular injuries and concerns about margins. Certain tumor characteristics strongly correlate with the risk of technical complications in some series. Patients with a functionally solitary kidney, bilateral lesions, and large or centrally located tumors posed an increased risk for complications [70]. A shift in the management of postoperative hemorrhage in the absence of hemodynamic instability has been observed toward percutaneous angioembolization.

Future Directions

As more centers adopt minimally invasive techniques for renal surgery, the volume of data available for meaningful analyses grows and matures. Critical analysis, with emphasis on prospective and balanced data, is critical for continued improvement in care. The recently published AUA Guideline will help drive the push for NSS for localized tumors and help reduce the incidence of CKD due to surgery for RCC. As new techniques are developed, we expect the emphasis on reducing invasiveness to parallel the emphasis on oncological outcomes in the next few years. Robotic and laparoendoscopic single-site techniques have been described and explored by various centers, and time will tell whether they will have a place in the treatment armamentarium [71].

Summary

LPN is a technically challenging procedure that is feasible and safe. Short and intermediate outcomes are excellent and comparable to classical approaches. Having equivalent outcomes and improved recovery will aid in further spread and development of LPN techniques. Research into techniques to further preserve precious renal function is needed as an aging population with prevalent risk factors continues to have a rising incidence of RCC.

Critical Operative Steps

1. Adequately pad and secure patient to the operating table.
2. Place ports at least 8 cm apart and shift cephalad and lateral if necessary.
3. Expose ureter, renal hilum, and tumor while preserving fat overlying tumor.
4. Circumscribe resection line after intraoperative ultrasound.
5. Clamp hilum using individual bulldogs or laparoscopic Satinsky.
6. Resect tumor with sharp and blunt dissection.
7. Biopsy base of tumor for frozen section.
8. Perform renorrhaphy with or without bolster and sealants.
9. Place drain posterior to the kidney or resection site.
10. Extract tumor in entrapment sac.

Critical Instruments and Supplies

1. Ligasure Atlas (ValleyLab, LS1037)
2. Ultrasound unit with laparoscopic 7-MHz probe
3. Laparoscopic Satinsky (e.g., Aesculap, PM177R)
4. Laparoscopic bulldog clamps and applicator (e.g., Aesculap, PL526R)
5. Argon beam coagulator (e.g., Conmed, E2520H)
6. Needle drivers (e.g., Karl Storz, 26173 KL)
7. Lapra-Ty and applier (Ethicon, ESXC200, and KA200)
8. Surgicel (Johnson & Johnson, ET1951)
9. Entrapment sac (e.g., Covidien, 173050G)

References

1. Linehan WM, Rini BI, Yang JC. Cancer of the kidney. In: DeVita VT, Lawrence TS, Rosenberg SA, editors. DeVita, Hellman, and Rosenberg's cancer: principles and practice of oncology. Vol I. 8th ed. Philadelphia, PA: Wolters Kluwer/Lippincott Williams & Wilkins; 2008. pp. 1331–7.
2. Chow WH, Devesa SS, Warren JL, Fraumeni JF, Jr. Rising incidence of renal cell cancer in the United States. JAMA. 5 May 1999;281(17): 1628–31.
3. Jemal A, Siegel R, Ward E, Hao Y, Xu J, Thun MJ. Cancer statistics, 2009. CA Cancer J Clin. Jul–Aug 2009;59(4):225–49.
4. Lipworth L, Tarone RE, McLaughlin JK. The epidemiology of renal cell carcinoma. J Urol. Dec 2006;176(6 Pt 1):2353–8.
5. Novick AC, Campbell SC, Belldegrun A, et al. Guideline for management of the clinical stage 1 renal mass; 2009. Located at: American Urological Association Education and Research, Inc.
6. Uzzo RG, Novick AC. Nephron sparing surgery for renal tumors: indications, techniques and outcomes. J Urol. Jul 2001;166(1):6–18.
7. Lau WK, Blute ML, Weaver AL, Torres VE, Zincke H Matched comparison of radical nephrectomy vs nephron-sparing surgery in patients with unilateral renal cell carcinoma and a normal contralateral kidney. Mayo Clin Proc. Dec 2000;75(12):1236–42.
8. McKiernan J, Simmons R, Katz J, Russo P Natural history of chronic renal insufficiency after partial and radical nephrectomy. Urology. Jun 2002;59(6): 816–20.
9. Sorbellini M, Kattan MW, Snyder ME, Hakimi AA, Sarasohn DM, Russo P Prognostic nomogram for renal insufficiency after radical or partial nephrectomy. J Urol. Aug 2006;176(2):472–6; discussion 476.
10. McDougall EM, Clayman RV, Anderson K Laparoscopic wedge resection of a renal tumor: initial experience. J Laparoendosc Surg. Dec 1993;3(6):577–81.
11. Winfield HN, Donovan JF, Godet AS, Clayman RV Laparoscopic partial nephrectomy: initial case report for benign disease. J Endourol. Dec 1993;7(6): 521–6.
12. Gill IS, Desai MM, Kaouk JH, et al. Laparoscopic partial nephrectomy for renal tumor: duplicating open surgical techniques. J Urol. Feb 2002;167(2 Pt 1):469–76; discussion 475–6.
13. Fergany AF, Saad IR, Woo L, Novick AC Open partial nephrectomy for tumor in a solitary kidney: experience with 400 cases. J Urol. May 2006;175(5):1630–3; discussion 1633.
14. Novick AC Renal-sparing surgery for renal cell carcinoma. Urol Clin North Am. May 1993; 20(2):277–82.
15. Oakley NE, Hegarty NJ, McNeill A, Gill IS Minimally invasive nephron-sparing surgery for renal cell cancer. BJU Int. Aug 2006;98(2): 278–84.
16. Hafez KS, Fergany AF, Novick AC Nephron sparing surgery for localized renal cell carcinoma: impact of tumor size on patient survival, tumor recurrence and TNM staging. J Urol. Dec 1999;162(6):1930–3.
17. Simmons MN, Chung BI, Gill IS. Perioperative efficacy of laparoscopic partial nephrectomy for tumors larger than 4 cm. Eur Urol. Jan 2009;55(1):199–207. Epub 26 Jul 2008.
18. Mitchell RE, Gilbert SM, Murphy AM, Olsson CA, Benson MC, McKiernan JM Partial nephrectomy and radical nephrectomy offer similar cancer outcomes in renal cortical tumors 4 cm or larger. Urology. Feb 2006;67(2):260–4.
19. Simmons MN, Weight CJ, Gill IS Laparoscopic radical versus partial nephrectomy for tumors >4 cm: intermediate-term oncologic and functional outcomes. Urology. May 2009;73(5):1077–82.
20. Kletscher BA, Qian J, Bostwick DG, Andrews PE, Zincke H Prospective analysis of multifocality in renal cell carcinoma: influence of histological pattern, grade, number, size, volume and deoxyribonucleic acid ploidy. J Urol. Mar 1995;153(3 Pt 2): 904–6.
21. Ornstein DK, Lubensky IA, Venzon D, Zbar B, Linehan WM, Walther MM Prevalence of microscopic tumors in normal appearing renal parenchyma of patients with hereditary papillary renal cancer. J Urol. Feb 2000;163(2):431–3.
22. Simmons MN, Gill IS Decreased complications of contemporary laparoscopic partial nephrectomy: use of a standardized reporting system. J Urol. Jun 2007;177(6):2067–73; discussion 2073.
23. Beasley KA, Al Omar M, Shaikh A, et al. Laparoscopic versus open partial nephrectomy. Urology. Sep 2004;64(3):458–61.
24. Schiff JD, Palese M, Vaughan ED, Jr., Sosa RE, Coll D, Del Pizzo JJ Laparoscopic vs open partial nephrectomy in consecutive patients: the Cornell experience. BJU Int. Oct 2005;96(6):811–4.
25. Gill IS, Matin SF, Desai MM, et al. Comparative analysis of laparoscopic versus open partial nephrectomy for renal tumors in 200 patients. J Urol. Jul 2003;170(1):64–8.
26. Gill IS, Kavoussi LR, Lane BR, et al. Comparison of 1,800 laparoscopic and open partial nephrectomies for single renal tumors. J Urol. Jul 2007;178(1):41–6.
27. Coll DM, Uzzo RG, Herts BR, Davros WJ, Wirth SL, Novick AC 3-dimensional volume rendered computerized tomography for preoperative evaluation and intraoperative treatment of patients undergoing nephron sparing surgery. J Urol. Apr 1999;161(4):1097–102.
28. Lane BR, Samplaski MK, Herts BR, Zhou M, Novick AC, Campbell SC Renal mass biopsy—a renaissance? J Urol. Jan 2008;179(1):20–7.

29. Richter F, Kasabian NG, Irwin RJ, Jr., Watson RA, Lang EK Accuracy of diagnosis by guided biopsy of renal mass lesions classified indeterminate by imaging studies. Urology. Mar 2000;55(3):348–52.
30. Haber GP, Gill IS Laparoscopic partial nephrectomy: contemporary technique and outcomes. Eur Urol. Apr 2006;49(4):660–5.
31. Breda A, Stepanian SV, Lam JS, et al. Use of haemostatic agents and glues during laparoscopic partial nephrectomy: a multi-institutional survey from the United States and Europe of 1347 cases. Eur Urol. Sep 2007;52(3):798–803.
32. Johnston WK, 3rd, Montgomery JS, Seifman BD, Hollenbeck BK, Wolf JS, Jr. Fibrin glue v sutured bolster: lessons learned during 100 laparoscopic partial nephrectomies. J Urol. Jul 2005;174(1):47–52.
33. Simon J, Bartsch G, Jr., Finter F, Hautmann R, de Petriconi R Laparoscopic partial nephrectomy with selective control of the renal parenchyma: initial experience with a novel laparoscopic clamp. BJU Int. Mar 2009;103(6):805–8.
34. Verhoest G, Manunta A, Bensalah K, et al. Laparoscopic partial nephrectomy with clamping of the renal parenchyma: initial experience. Eur Urol. Nov 2007;52(5):1340–6.
35. Novick AC Renal hypothermia: in vivo and ex vivo. Urol Clin North Am. Nov 1983;10(4):637–44.
36. Bhayani SB, Rha KH, Pinto PA, et al. Laparoscopic partial nephrectomy: effect of warm ischemia on serum creatinine. J Urol. Oct 2004;172(4 Pt 1): 1264–6.
37. Lang F Osmotic diuresis. Ren Physiol. 1987; 10(3–4):160–73.
38. Nosowsky EE, Kaufman JJ The protective action of mannitol in renal artery occlusion. J Urol. Mar 1963;89:295–9.
39. Baumert H, Ballaro A, Shah N, et al. Reducing warm ischaemia time during laparoscopic partial nephrectomy: a prospective comparison of two renal closure techniques. Eur Urol. Oct 2007;52(4):1164–9.
40. Nguyen MM, Gill IS Halving ischemia time during laparoscopic partial nephrectomy. J Urol. Feb 2008;179(2):627–32; discussion 632.
41. Bollens R, Rosenblatt A, Espinoza BP, et al. Laparoscopic partial nephrectomy with "on-demand" clamping reduces warm ischemia time. Eur Urol. Sep 2007;52(3):804–9.
42. Orvieto MA, Zorn KC, Mendiola F, et al. Recovery of renal function after complete renal hilar versus artery alone clamping during open and laparoscopic surgery. J Urol. Jun 2007;177(6):2371–4.
43. Porpiglia F, Renard J, Billia M, et al. Is renal warm ischemia over 30 minutes during laparoscopic partial nephrectomy possible? One-year results of a prospective study. Eur Urol. Oct 2007;52(4): 1170–8.
44. Gill IS, Abreu SC, Desai MM, et al. Laparoscopic ice slush renal hypothermia for partial nephrectomy: the initial experience. J Urol. Jul 2003;170(1):52–6.
45. Guillonneau B, Bermudez H, Gholami S, et al. Laparoscopic partial nephrectomy for renal tumor: single center experience comparing clamping and no clamping techniques of the renal vasculature. J Urol. Feb 2003;169(2):483–6.
46. Janetschek G, Abdelmaksoud A, Bagheri F, Al-Zahrani H, Leeb K, Gschwendtner M Laparoscopic partial nephrectomy in cold ischemia: renal artery perfusion. J Urol. Jan 2004;171(1):68–71.
47. Beri A, Lattouf JB, Deambros O, et al. Partial nephrectomy using renal artery perfusion for cold ischemia: functional and oncologic outcomes. J Endourol. Jun 2008;22(6):1285–90.
48. Janetschek G, Jeschke K, Peschel R, Strohmeyer D, Henning K, Bartsch G Laparoscopic surgery for stage T1 renal cell carcinoma: radical nephrectomy and wedge resection. Eur Urol. Aug 2000; 38(2):131–8.
49. Msezane LP, Katz MH, Gofrit ON, Shalhav AL, Zorn KC Hemostatic agents and instruments in laparoscopic renal surgery. J Endourol. Mar 2008;22(3):403–8.
50. Phillips JM, Narula N, Deane LA, et al. Histological evaluation of cold versus hot cutting: clinical impact on margin status for laparoscopic partial nephrectomy. J Urol. Dec 2008;180(6):2348–52.
51. Andonian S, Adebayo A, Okeke Z, Lee BR Habib laparoscopic bipolar radiofrequency device: a novel way of creating an avascular resection margin in laparoscopic partial nephrectomy. J Laparoendosc Adv Surg Tech A. Dec 2008;18(6):853–6.
52. Coleman J, Singh A, Pinto P, et al. Radiofrequency-assisted laparoscopic partial nephrectomy: clinical and histologic results. J Endourol. Jun 2007;21(6):600–5.
53. Tan YH, Young MD, L'Esperance JO, Preminger GM, Albala DM Hand-assisted laparoscopic partial nephrectomy without hilar vascular clamping using a saline-cooled, high-density monopolar radiofrequency device. J Endourol. Nov 2004; 18(9):883–7.
54. Urena R, Mendez F, Woods M, Thomas R, Davis R Laparoscopic partial nephrectomy of solid renal masses without hilar clamping using a monopolar radio frequency device. J Urol. Mar 2004;171(3):1054–6.
55. Breda A, Stepanian SV, Liao J, et al. Positive margins in laparoscopic partial nephrectomy in 855 cases: a multi-institutional survey from the United States and Europe. J Urol. Jul 2007;178(1):47–50; discussion 50.
56. Permpongkosol S, Colombo JR, Jr., Gill IS, Kavoussi LR Positive surgical parenchymal margin after laparoscopic partial nephrectomy for renal cell carcinoma: oncological outcomes. J Urol. Dec 2006;176(6 Pt 1):2401–4.
57. Yossepowitch O, Thompson RH, Leibovich BC, et al. Positive surgical margins at partial

nephrectomy: predictors and oncological outcomes. J Urol. Jun 2008;179(6):2158–63.

58. Castillo OA, Vitagliano G, Diaz M, Sanchez-Salas R Port-site metastasis after laparoscopic partial nephrectomy: case report and literature review. J Endourol. Apr 2007;21(4):404–7.
59. Rassweiler J, Tsivian A, Kumar AV, et al. Oncological safety of laparoscopic surgery for urological malignancy: experience with more than 1,000 operations. J Urol. Jun 2003;169(6):2072–5.
60. Lee BR, Tan BJ, Smith AD Laparoscopic port site metastases: incidence, risk factors, and potential preventive measures. Urology. Apr 2005;65(4): 639–44.
61. Schneider C, Jung A, Reymond MA, et al. Efficacy of surgical measures in preventing port-site recurrences in a porcine model. Surg Endosc. Feb 2001;15(2):121–5.
62. Bostwick DG, Murphy GP Diagnosis and prognosis of renal cell carcinoma: highlights from an international consensus workshop. Semin Urol Oncol. Feb 1998;16(1):46–52.
63. Black P, Filipas D, Fichtner J, Hohenfellner R, Thuroff JW Nephron sparing surgery for central renal tumors: experience with 33 cases. J Urol. Mar 2000;163(3):737–43.
64. Breda A, Finelli A, Janetschek G, Porpiglia F, Montorsi F. Complications of laparoscopic surgery for renal masses: prevention, management, and comparison with the open experience. Eur Urol. Apr 2009;55(4):836–50. Epub 20 Jan 2009.
65. Zorn KC, Gong EM, Orvieto MA, Gofrit ON, Mikhail AA, Shalhav AL Impact of collecting-system repair during laparoscopic partial nephrectomy. J Endourol. Mar 2007;21(3):315–20.
66. Meeks JJ, Zhao LC, Navai N, Perry KT, Jr., Nadler RB, Smith ND Risk factors and management of urine leaks after partial nephrectomy. J Urol. Dec 2008;180(6):2375–8.
67. L'esperance JO, Marguet CG, Walters RC, et al. Do nonspecific deep corticomedullary sutures performed during partial nephrectomy adequately control major vascular and collecting system injury? BJU Int. Feb 2010;105(3):411–5. Epub 22 Jun 2009.
68. Zimmermann R, Janetschek G Complications of laparoscopic partial nephrectomy. World J Urol. Dec 2008;26(6):531–7.
69. Richstone L, Seideman C, Baldinger L, et al. Conversion during laparoscopic surgery: frequency, indications and risk factors. J Urol. Sep 2008;180(3):855–9.
70. Campbell SC, Novick AC, Streem SB, Klein E, Licht M Complications of nephron sparing surgery for renal tumors. J Urol. May 1994;151(5): 1177–80.
71. Kaouk JH, Goel RK. Single-port laparoscopic and robotic partial nephrectomy. Eur Urol. May 2009;55(5):1163–9. Epub 7 Jan 2009.

Chapter 5

Adult Robotic-Assisted Partial Nephrectomy for Renal Cell Carcinoma

Ronald S. Boris and Peter A. Pinto

This chapter contains a video segment which can be found at the URL: http://www.springerimages.com/ost

Historical Overview

The introduction of robotic surgery has revolutionized the treatment of urologic malignancy. Initially established for radical prostatectomy, robotic techniques are now being applied in the management of renal cancer. The feasibility and safety of robotic-assisted partial nephrectomy (RAPN) has been demonstrated in several small, single-institution studies [1–10]. Recently this technique has been applied successfully in patients with hilar, endophytic, and multiple renal masses [8–10]. Features of the da Vinci Surgical System (Intuitive Surgical Corp., Sunnyvale, California, USA) include 3D vision, articulating instruments, and motion scaling to reduce tremor. These amenities may allow the surgeon the ability to replicate established "open" maneuvers and allow for complex tumor extirpation and renal reconstruction which is challenging in a pure laparoscopic manner. A list of potential advantages and disadvantages of robotic-assisted partial nephrectomy is described in Table 5.1.

In 2008 in the United States, there were more than 55,000 new cases of renal cell cancer and over 13,000 deaths [11]. As the overall incidence of RCC continues to rise, the greatest increase has occurred in small, localized tumors, which represent up to 66% of all renal masses [12]. Historically, the gold standard for patients with kidney cancer has been radical nephrectomy. Today, data have shown that in select patients, cancer outcomes for partial nephrectomy are equivalent to those of radical nephrectomy [13, 14]. Once considered treatment of choice only in patients with solitary kidneys or preexisting renal insufficiency, nephron-sparing surgery or partial nephrectomy is now emerging as the standard of care for patients with T1a tumors. Recent publications also support extending the role of partial nephrectomy to select patients with T1b tumors or multifocal disease [15, 16]. Important considerations for partial nephrectomy include the presence of benign lesions among T1a masses and the association of chronic kidney disease as an independent risk factor for cardiovascular disease, hospitalization, and all-cause mortality [17, 18]. These findings underscore the importance of nephron-sparing surgery in patients with small renal masses. Robotic-assisted partial nephrectomy upholds three critical principles in the surgical management of renal malignancy: oncologic efficacy, renal preservation, and early convalescence.

P.A. Pinto (✉)
Urologic Oncology Branch, National Cancer Institute, Bethesda, MD, USA
e-mail: pintop@mail.nih.gov

M.C. Ost (ed.), *Robotic and Laparoscopic Reconstructive Surgery in Children and Adults*, Current Clinical Urology, DOI 10.1007/978-1-60327-914-7_5, © Springer Science+Business Media, LLC 2011

Table 5.1 Potential advantages and disadvantages of robotic-assisted surgery compared with conventional laparoscopic surgery

Features specific to robotic-assisted surgery	Potential advantages/disadvantages
3D vision, motion scaling, and tremor elimination to allow more exact movements	Advantage
Six degrees of freedom of wristed instruments to improve tumor excision and aid in complex suturing and renal reconstruction	Advantage
Improved surgeon's comfort, especially important during long and complex cases	Advantage
May improve the learning curve of minimally invasive partial nephrectomy for novice laparoscopic surgeons	Advantage
Increased cost	Disadvantage
Absence of haptic feedback	Disadvantage
Need for a bedside assistant experienced in laparoscopy	Disadvantage

Indications and Contraindications

Patient selection is critical for the success of robotic-assisted partial nephrectomy, especially early in one's experience. Favorable tumors include exophytic, well-circumscribed lesions that are less than 4 cm. Recent literature has demonstrated the feasibility of robotic surgery for larger, deeper tumors that are hilar in their location as well as for multiple tumors in the hereditary renal population [9, 10]. However, these complex cases should be undertaken by an experienced team after completion of the initial learning curve has been met.

Because robotic surgery is a laparoscopic procedure, similar preoperative considerations should be taken into account prior to obtaining surgical consent. As with open partial nephrectomy, patients must be candidates to receive general anesthesia [19]. Severe pulmonary or cardiac disease may compromise the safety of the pneumoperitoneum, which can compromise ventilation and limit venous return [20, 21]. Prior abdominal surgery may limit access to necessary structures and impair critical surgical dissection as well as require laparoscopic lysis of adhesions, which can increase operative time and risk of visceral injury [22]. Obesity, although not a contraindication to laparoscopy or robotic-assisted surgery, has been shown to increase operative times, pulmonary and wound-related complications, and risk of rhabdomyolysis [23, 24]. However, the safety and efficacy of minimally invasive partial nephrectomy in the obese patient has been established [25]. Operating at lower insufflation pressures, using an alternative to carbon dioxide as an insufflant, or performing surgery through a retroperitoneal approach may be potential ways to minimize some of the hazards in higher risk patients [26].

Patient Preparation

All patients at our institution undergoing robotic-assisted partial nephrectomy obtain blood work including electrolyte chemistry, BUN and creatinine, complete blood count, basic coagulation profile, and a type and screen prior to surgery. Cross-matched blood may be reserved at the surgeon's discretion. All patients undergo adequate renal imaging including either an abdominal computed tomography (CT) or a magnetic resonance imaging (MRI). Imaging of the renal vasculature and three-dimensional reconstruction may be of assistance in certain cases. An electrocardiogram and chest radiograph may be obtained prior to surgery as indicated. Further medical clearance or additional blood work can be obtained on a case-by-case basis according to the patient's history and physical exam. We typically administer a bowel prep in all of our patients undergoing abdominal surgery but this may be left to the surgeon's preference. However, we strongly encourage bowel prep in obese patients and patients with prior abdominal surgery in whom lysis of adhesions may be anticipated. Intravenous antibiotic should be administered in the preoperative holding area to ensure delivery before the initial skin incision.

Ureteral Catheter Placement and Patient Positioning

Pneumatic compression stockings are placed on each calf prior to the induction of general anesthesia. A 5-Fr open-ended ureteral catheter is placed over a guidewire via a flexible cystoscope if extensive collecting system reconstruction is anticipated. The ureteral catheter is then connected to a syringe of methylene blue solution that can be accessed by the circulating nurse during the case. A 16-Fr Foley catheter is used in all cases.

The patient is then turned onto the table in a modified lateral decubitus position similar to positioning for laparoscopic transperitoneal flank procedures. We place a thin long gel pad on the operating room table prior to positioning and do not use beanbags or other stabilizing devices. The patient is shifted to the center of the table with his/her flank over the break. Two large jelly rolls are used for support of the neck, back, and hips as the body lays comfortably at about 30–45° tilt. The lower leg is placed in a bent knee position and the upper leg remains naturally straight. Pillows are placed between the legs longitudinally and all pressure points are sufficiently padded and supported.

A small axillary roll is properly placed. Anesthesia assists in obtaining a comfortable height and position for the patient's head and neck. A traditional arm rest is used to secure the down (contralateral) arm roughly perpendicular from the patient's body. The chest, hips, and legs are padded and taped safely and securely to the operating room table. The table is flexed to the minimum angle that adequately opens up the flank to maximize operating space. A vascular arm rest is secured to the table and positioned to allow the ipsilateral shoulder and arm to rest comfortably without tension at a minimal distance above the patient's chest. This will avoid any stretch injuries to the arm or the shoulder while allowing the robot arms to be safely docked and function without collision. The arm is secured using a Kerlix wrap and tape. Anterior and posterior views of standard patient positioning for transperitoneal robotic-assisted partial nephrectomy are demonstrated in Fig. 5.1 a, b. A photo of a patient positioned in preparation for right-sided surgery is seen in Fig. 5.2. It is important to note the position of the ipsilateral arm when the robot is docked, as it is in close proximity to the robotic instruments. The arm needs to be far enough cephalad to prevent limiting the range of motion of the subcostal robotic arm. When performing robotic-assisted partial nephrectomy using

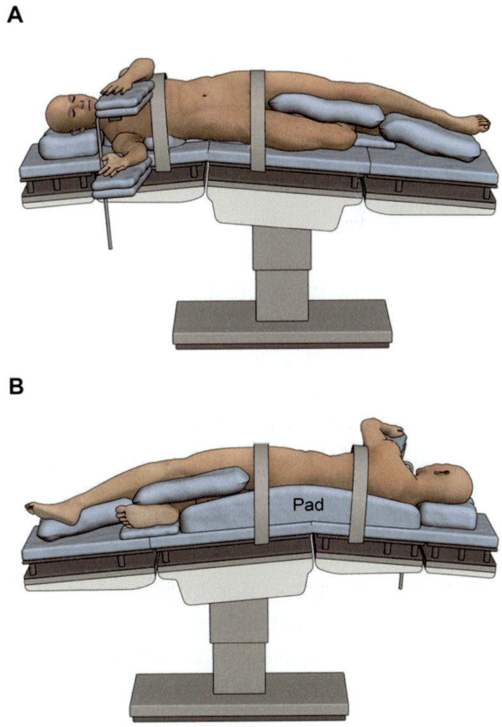

Fig. 5.1 Patient positioning for robotic-assisted partial nephrectomy: (**a**) anterior view; (**b**) posterior view

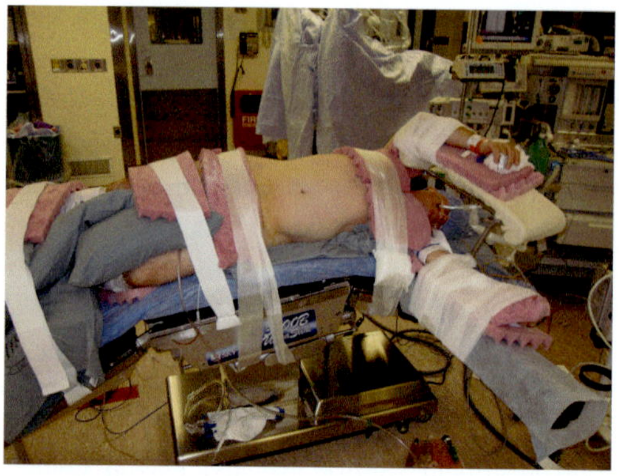

Fig. 5.2 Photo of patient properly positioned and padded in preparation for right-sided robotic-assisted partial nephrectomy

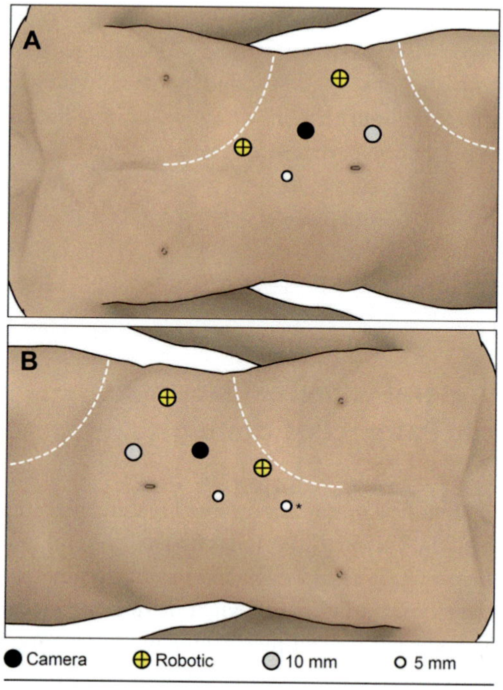

Fig. 5.3 Diagrams of port placement for robotic-assisted partial nephrectomy: (**a**) left side template; (**b**) right-side template. * additional 5-mm port for liver retraction

a retroperitoneal approach, the patient should be placed and supported in true flank position. Retroperitoneal access is obtained using standard retroperitoneoscopic technique and the robot is then docked over the head and the ipsilateral shoulder. With either approach, the safety of the patient's position is tested by rotating the table in either direction ensuring that he/she is well secured and protected.

Access, Port Placement, Robot Docking

Pneumoperitoneum is created using the Veress needle technique. The safety of this technique with optical trocar entry, even in patients with previous abdominal surgery, has been documented [27]. A Hassan technique may be used at the discretion of the surgeon. The first port placed is the 10/12-mm camera port placed under vision over a 0° 10-mm laparoscope. Once entry into the peritoneum is achieved, a 30° laparoscopic camera is exchanged prior to placement of the remainder of the ports. Diagnostic laparoscopy is performed to assess for distant disease. Port placement diagrams for both left- and right-sided approaches are displayed in Fig. 5.3a, b. A photograph of our port placement for a

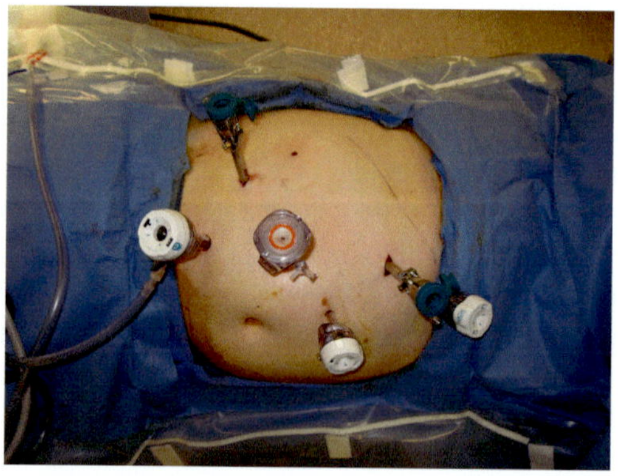

Fig. 5.4 Photo of port placement for right-sided robotic-assisted partial nephrectomy

standard right-sided robotic partial nephrectomy is demonstrated in Fig. 5.4. For larger, deeper patients or patients with primarily upper pole lesions, the ports should be shifted cephalad and medially. An additional 5-mm port is placed for right-sided cases to allow fixed retraction of the liver. Although this may not always be necessary, we advocate placing this port initially since placing ports under vision once the robot is docked can be challenging and cumbersome.

We use a three-arm approach and the standard system at our center for robotic-assisted partial nephrectomy. A four-arm approach with the da Vinci S® has been advocated by some surgeons for assistance with retraction, renal positioning, and clip application [28]. The robot is then docked over the ipsilateral shoulder aligned such that the robot center point or "sweet spot" is directed toward the camera port and the renal hilum. An example of proper robot docking is viewed in Fig. 5.5. Depending on the anatomy, either a 0° or a 30° downward lens can be used. We typically begin with a 30° downward lens in most instances. The pneumoperitoneum is typically set at 20 mmHg to start the case and lowered to 15 mmHg once all the ports are placed. The right robot arm is seated with a monopolar hot shears and the left arm is seated with a Maryland bipolar instrument for the initial dissection. The monopolar heat is typically set to 30 Hz and the bipolar set to 30 Hz. The bedside assistant stands or sits on the side opposite to the docked robot and the vision system is usually placed at the foot of the bed at a comfortable distance from the assistant. A bird's-eye view of the operating room setup demonstrating orientation and position of patient, surgeon, assistant, anesthesiologist, and robot is shown in Fig. 5.6. The role of the bedside assistant is to provide a variety of maneuvers throughout the case: retraction, suctioning, placement, and/or removal of lap pads, clips, bulldog or Satinsky clamps, sutures and needle, and hemostatic agents. An open tray is always present in the room in case of the need for conversion.

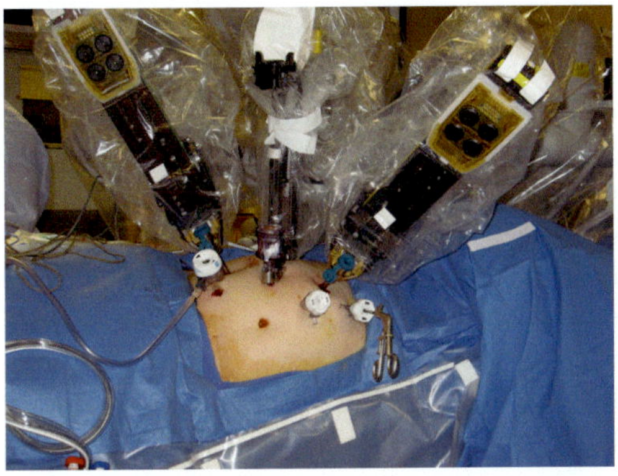

Fig. 5.5 Photo of robot docked in preparation for right-sided partial nephrectomy

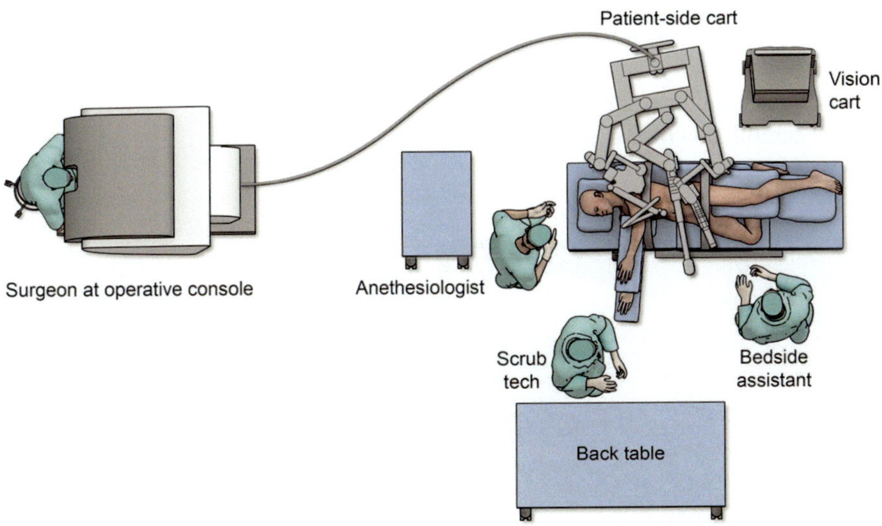

Fig. 5.6 Bird's-eye view of operating room setup for robotic-assisted partial nephrectomy

Bowel Mobilization and Hilar Dissection

Some have reported a hybrid technique of laparoscopic bowel and renal mobilization followed by robotic assistance for just the tumor extirpation and renorrhaphy. In our institution, we utilize the advantages of the da Vinci robotic system for the entire case. The overlying colon is identified and mobilized robotically by incising the white line of Toldt sharply and identifying the plane between the posterior mesocolon and the anterior Gerota's fascia (Fig. 5.7). Careful identification of this boundary is paramount to enter into the correct avascular, anatomic space. This maneuver may be aided with downward and medial retraction by the bedside assistant to help expose the correct layer. The triangular ligament in divided and the liver is freed laterally from its attachments to the side wall. A fixed liver retractor can be used once the liver is mobilized to improve exposure of the upper pole of the kidney, adrenal gland, and supra-hilar vena cava. For a right-sided procedure the duodenum is then identified and Kocherized to expose the inferior vena cava (Fig. 5.8). This can be safely performed without cautery by carefully lifting Gerota's fat with the left hand while sharply incising duodenal attachments with the scissors in the right hand. This maneuver should allow the duodenum to drop away medially as the IVC comes into view. The assistant can sometimes facilitate this with careful downward sweeps using a laparoscopic suction device once all attachments are meticulously incised by the console surgeon.

For a left-sided procedure it is imperative to perform complete splenic mobilization to maximize hilar exposure and operative working space. This is performed following left-sided colon mobilization by first identifying splenic sidewall attachments, which can be incised sharply. Be mindful of using cautery near the diaphragm because inadvertent pleural space entry can occur here. Dividing the splenorenal attachments is typically performed using sequential bipolar cautery with the left hand and sharp monopolar scissors using the right hand. The diaphragm should become visible as these attachments are divided. This dissection will allow proper mobilization of the spleen and pancreas away from the operative field and will facilitate subsequent steps of the operation. If visibility remains obscured even after performing these steps, one or two laparotomy pads can be passed into the abdomen through a 12-mm port and positioned to pack the spleen and pancreas away from the kidney.

The next step is hilar identification and posterior renal dissection. We typically begin this by identifying the ureter and gonadal vessels, which are easily seen at the lower pole of the kidney. The robotic surgeon enters a plane between these structures and the psoas muscle to enter and sweep this posterior plane (Fig. 5.9). The dissection proceeds cranially until the lower border of the renal vein is seen. For left-sided procedures

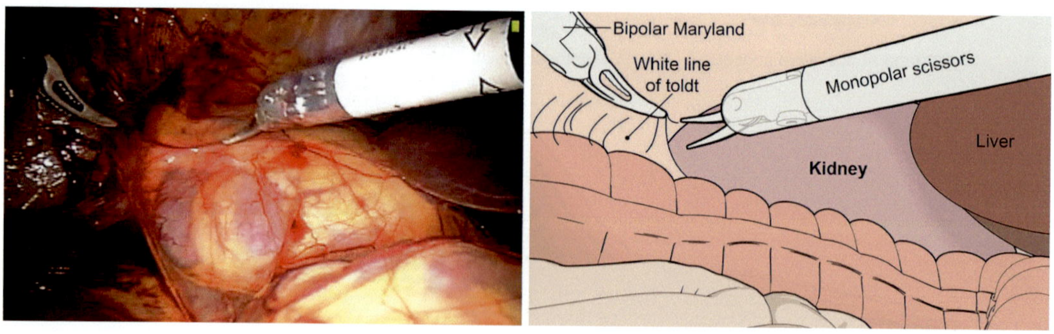

Fig. 5.7 Colon mobilization

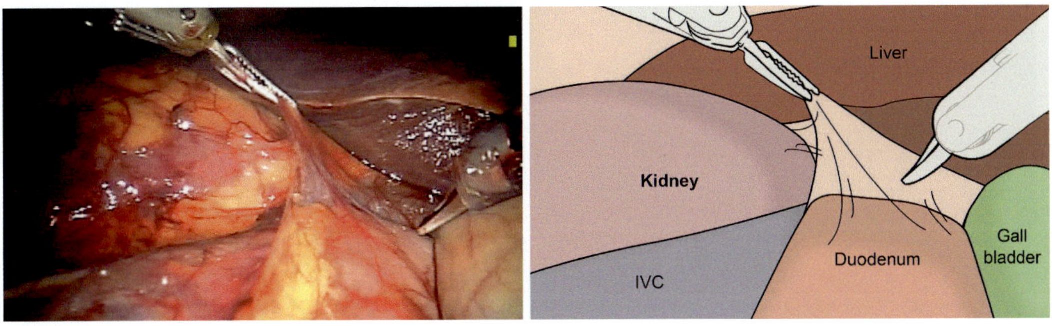

Fig. 5.8 Kocherization of duodenum

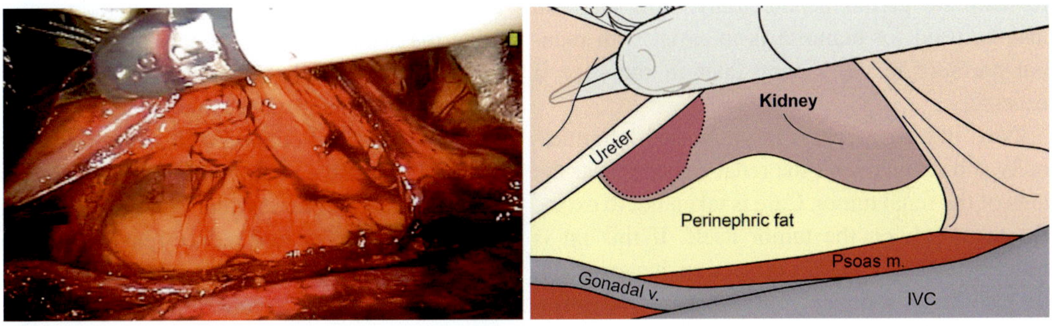

Fig. 5.9 Identification of ureter and renal hilum with dissection of posterior kidney

this can be facilitated by tracing the course of the gonadal vein to its entry point into renal vein. It may be necessary to ligate and divide the lumbar vein to expose the left renal hilum. Careful identification of the renal artery is then performed. Adequate space caudal and cranial to the renal hilum is created to allow placement of the bulldog clamps or laparoscopic Satinsky clamp.

Renal Mobilization, Tumor Identification, and Exposure

A number of factors will determine the amount of kidney mobilization required to perform robotic-assisted partial nephrectomy including tumor location, number, size, as well as the patient's prior surgical history and overall anatomy. The goal of renal dissection is to ensure adequate vision and maneuverability with the robot around key areas of anatomic interest including the renal hilum, the exposed renal tumor, and surrounding renal parenchyma, prior to the start of warm ischemia. In our experience, patients with posterior tumors, upper pole tumors, and multiple tumors require complete renal mobilization so that the kidney is entirely freed from its upper, lateral, and inferior poles as well as its adrenal attachments. This should allow the posterior renal surface to be exposed and situated, when needed, in direct view of the console surgeon. Patients who have had prior ipsilateral retroperitoneal surgery—i.e., partial nephrectomy, adrenalectomy, renal ablation, or percutaneous nephrolithotomy—have a higher propensity for renal scarring and we recommend meticulous dissection in these cases to ensure adequate mobilization and exposure to avoid later difficulties [29, 30]. Prior to hilar clamping, a laparotomy pad should be passed into the abdomen to stabilize the kidney in position

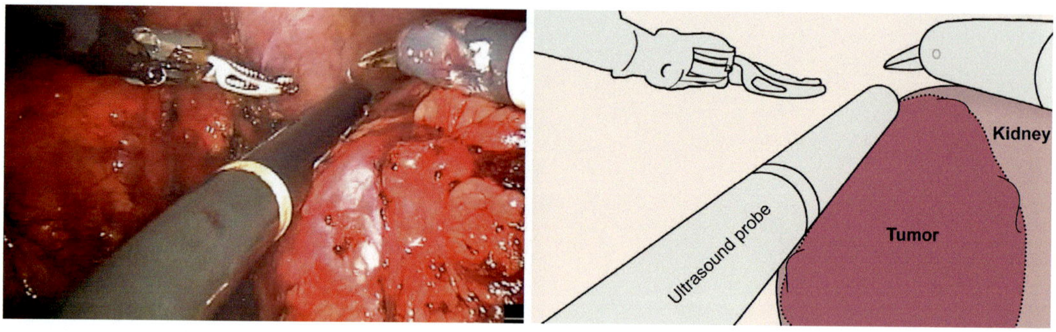

Fig. 5.10 Laparoscopic ultrasound of kidney and renal mass

to facilitate partial nephrectomy. This pad can also be used for hemostasis to assist with manual pressure to the kidney later in the case if necessary.

Next, the perinephric fat is incised longitudinally and divided over the renal capsule, near the area of the renal tumor. Care is taken not to excise the fat overlying the tumor itself. If this fat is removed during Gerota's dissection, it can be sent to pathology separately. A laparoscopic ultrasound probe is then introduced via the assistant port by the bedside assistant. Vascular anatomy, tumor size, extension, and depth are identified with ultrasound assistance (Fig. 5.10). The renal capsule can be scored with the monopolar hot scissors using ultrasound to identify the appropriate borders of the dissection. Doppler color flow is used to note the location of branch vessels in relationship to the tumor. Even with easily identifiable exophytic tumors, we recommend thorough intraoperative renal ultrasound, which can aid in dissection and ensure the absence of incipient lesions that may have been missed on preoperative scans [31].

Hilar Control and Tumor Extirpation

Prior to the initiation of warm ischemia, a "test run" should be performed including hilar exposure, bedside assistant clamp placement, and tumor access. A careful operating room check of instruments, sutures, hemostatic agents, and emergency equipment should be made. We typically use bulldog clamping over Satinsky clamping for a number of reasons including obviating the need for an additional port, eliminating the risk of catastrophic external dislodging of the Satinsky clamp, and allowing the ability to remove individual occlusion of the renal vein in cases of excessive renal congestion. Mannitol is administered before vascular clamping to create an osmotic diuresis and reduce renal injury. The clamps are then placed on the renal hilum, first on the renal artery followed by the renal vein (Fig. 5.11). The kidney should blanch quickly—if this is not appreciated, consideration should be given to inadequate clamping or additional hilar vessels. The starting time of warm ischemia should be recorded.

The tumor should be excised sharply respecting the principles of open surgery. The capsule is incised broadly and the tumor should be approached initially by maneuvering circumferentially before diving deeply into the renal parenchyma. This will help to avoid inadvertent entry into the tumor. The Maryland bipolar, ProGrasp, or fenestrated bipolar instrument can be used to help lift and elevate the tumor as the monopolar scissor is used with the right hand to sharply incise along the margin of dissection (Fig. 5.12). A cold curved scissors can be exchanged for the monopolar hot scissors because this tends to improve sharp cutting and can expedite tumor extirpation. The bedside assistant should use a suction and grasper in each hand to help expose the correct plane and provide adequate counter traction for the console surgeon. In cases of multifocal disease or hereditary renal disease, an enucleating technique can be utilized

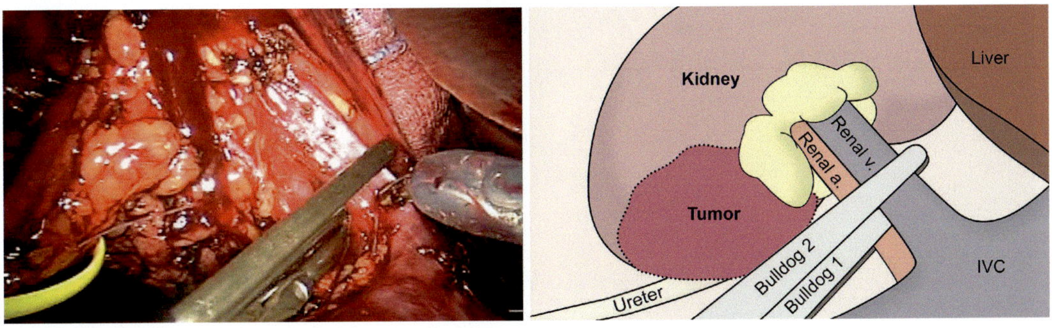

Fig. 5.11 Bulldog clamping of renal hilum

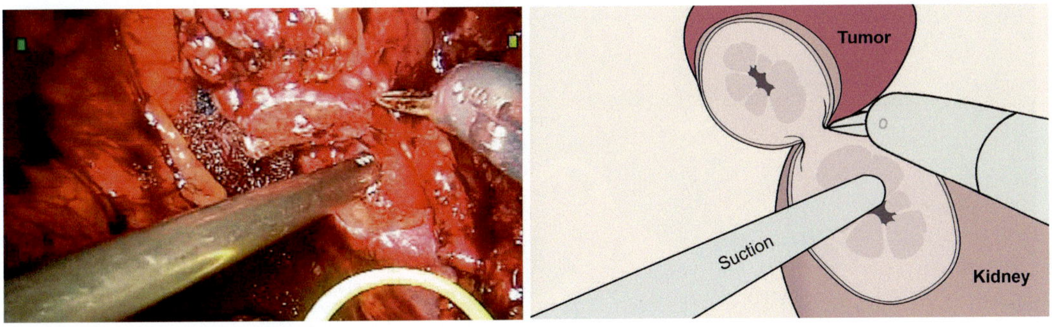

Fig. 5.12 Extirpation of renal mass

by incising the renal capsule and maintaining the plane between the tumor's pseudocapsule and the renal parenchyma [32, 33].

Once the tumor is completely excised, it should be inspected intracorporeally, especially at its base. We do not typically take frozen sections of the base unless we identify iatrogenic entry of the tumor or the tumor appears to be projecting through the capsule and violating the plane of dissection. In these rare circumstances, we will re-resect the base and continue with renal reconstruction in an effort to limit warm ischemia.

Renorrhaphy, Specimen Retrieval, and Closure

We exchange the scissor for a robotic needle driver and suture ligate open vessels with a 3-0 Vicryl on an RB-1 needle with a Lapra-Ty® (Ethicon, Cincinnati, OH) clip. This can usually be performed in figure of eight fashion. For deep tumors where entry into the collection system is anticipated, we next retrograde inject the pre-placed ureteral catheter with methylene blue to inspect for remaining defects. The open collecting system base is closed with a running 3-0 Vicryl suture on an RB-1 or an SH needle (Fig. 5.13). We next use a series of 2-0 Vicryl sutures on either a SH or a CT-1 needle cut to 7 in. with a Lapra-Ty® placed at the knot at the cut end. These are placed in interrupted fashion and the renal defect is closed by taking full needle bites of the renal capsule but avoiding unnecessary passes deep into the renal parenchyma (Fig. 5.14). Usually a series of two or three sutures are sufficient to incorporate the length of the repair and the defect is then filled with premade oxidized cellulose bolsters and injected with hemostatic sealant (Fig. 5.15). Next the bedside assistant places a second Lapra-Ty® clip on the needle end after the console surgeons apply his/her own tension against the renal parenchyma.

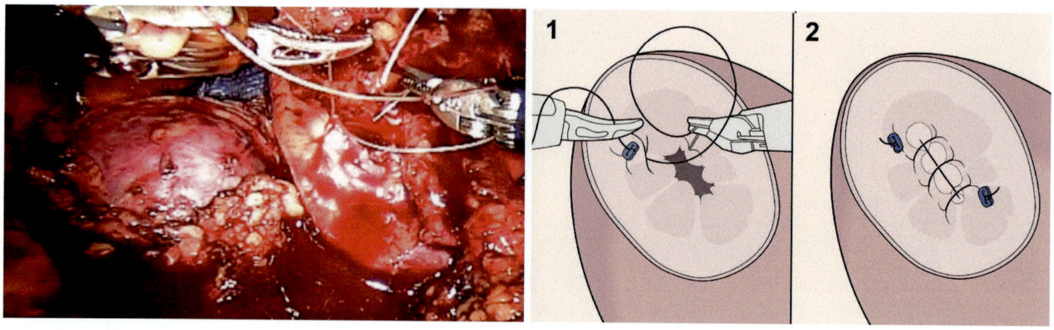

Fig. 5.13 Running closure of renal base

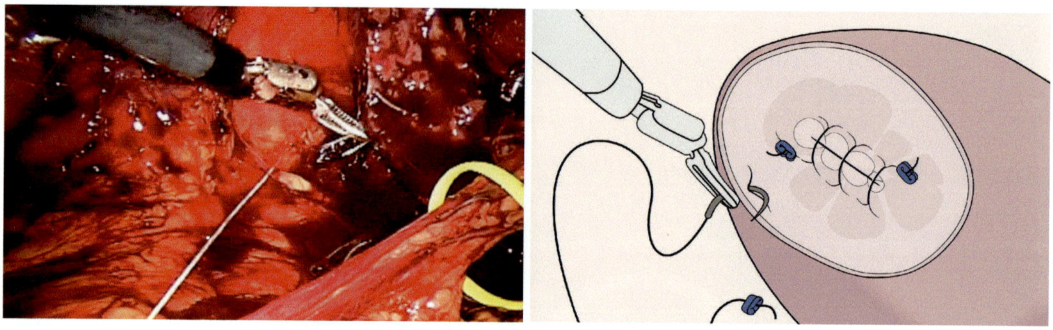

Fig. 5.14 Placement of capsular suture

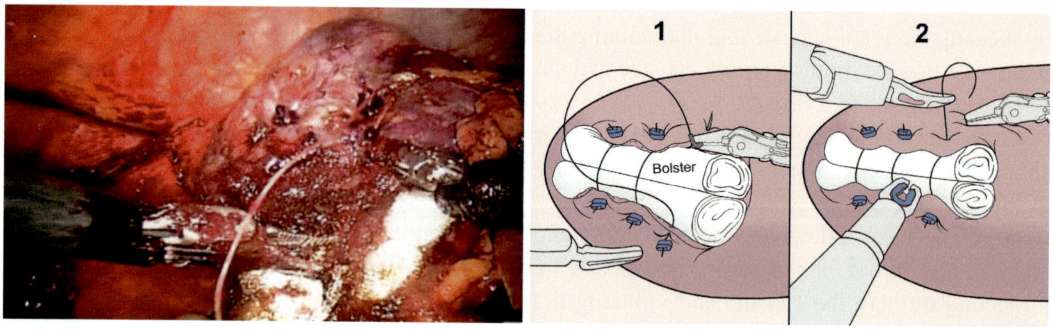

Fig. 5.15 Placement of final capsular suture over Surgicel® bolster and application of final Lapra-Ty® to complete renorrhaphy

This will tighten the capsular sutures and visually close the renal gap. The console surgeon must be careful to pull away from the kidney in the direction of the suture to ensure that he does not tear the renal capsule. This can be repeated sequentially to the remaining capsular sutures (Fig. 5.15). Alternatively, in a technique described by Benway et al. [34], a Hem-o-Lock® clip can be placed on the needle side of the capsular suture and used by the robotic surgeon to visibly apply tension to the repair by sliding it down against the parenchyma. Additionally, in an attempt to decrease warm ischemic time, some surgeons have performed bolstered renorrhaphy in an off-clamp fashion [35].

The hilar clamps are removed and time is noted. A lap pad is typically placed over the repair and pressure is held for several minutes if bleeding is noted. Once the kidney has restored its normal turgor, the defect is inspected. If minimal oozing exists, the kidney can be again observed with direct manual pressure and re-inspected. If bleeding is persistent, additional sutures can be placed, this time more deeply in the area of presumed location. Complete peritoneoscopy is performed to inspect for injury or bleeding. The lap pad is carefully removed under vision through the assistant port. The Gerota's fascia is closed with a running Vicryl suture and the kidney is returned to its most orthotopic position. The specimen is placed in a retrieval sac and removed through one of the assistant ports. All robotic instruments are removed and the robot is de-docked. We recommend repeat inspection after specimen removal to ensure adequate hemostasis. A closed suction drain is placed through the most inferior and lateral trocar site and is laid posterior to the kidney. All trocars are removed under direct vision and the incisions are closed. The ureteral catheter, if placed initially, is removed on the completion of the case.

Postoperative Course

Complete blood count and chemistries are obtained in the recovery room and once daily as required. Patients remain on bed rest until the following morning when they initiate ambulation. Liquid diet is advanced to regular diet as tolerated. Pain is managed with intravenous morphine or opiate alternative for the initial 12–24 h and converted to an oral substitute shortly thereafter. The Foley catheter is removed after ambulation commences and postvoid residuals are checked 4–6 h later to ensure adequate bladder emptying. We usually withhold the removal of the closed suction drain until the day of hospital discharge is anticipated and the drain creatinine level is in the normal serum range. When a urinary leak is suspected secondary to an elevated drain creatinine, we recommend pulling the drain back slightly and placing it to dependent drainage off self-suction. The patient's recorded outputs and drain creatinine level can be managed on an outpatient basis. It has been our experience that most leaks will resolve with expectant management within 7–14 days. In rare cases of persistent urinary leakage despite continued conservative measures weeks after surgery, we recommend cystoscopy and retrograde pyelogram to rule out a distal ureteral obstruction or excluded calyx followed by ureteral stenting and Foley catheter placement.

Results

Robotic-assisted partial nephrectomy was initially developed and promoted with the idea of broadening the utilization of nephron-sparing surgery while still providing the advantages of minimally invasive surgery [9]. This alternative to laparoscopic partial nephrectomy may aid in the learning curve and facilitate in the reconstructive aspects of what is a technically demanding operation. Established advantages of minimally invasive techniques for partial nephrectomy include decreased postoperative pain, decreased hospital stay, and shorter convalescence compared with standard open technique [36].

Head-to-head comparisons of laparoscopic and robotic techniques have been limited but have been described. Aron et al. [37] from Cleveland Clinic retrospectively compared 12 matched patients undergoing partial nephrectomy by either robotic-assisted or laparoscopic techniques. Overall, there were no differences in perioperative variables (ischemia time, blood loss, operative time, and length of stay) and renal functional outcomes, transfusion rates, and complication rates were similar. A larger study from Wang and Bhayani [38] studied 102 consecutive patients, comparing outcomes from 40 robotic-assisted partial nephrectomies (RAPNs) and 62 laparoscopic partial nephrectomies (LPNs). They noted similar outcomes in blood loss, tumor size, margin rate but noted that operative times, warm ischemia times, and length of stay were significantly shorter in the robotic group. Our NCI series comparing the first 36 RAPNs versus the most recent 33 LPNs, all for complex, challenging renal masses, also

Table 5.2 Comparison of robotic-assisted partial nephrectomy (RAPN) and laparoscopic partial nephrectomy (LPN) at the National Cancer Institute

	RAPN	LPN	*p* value
N	36	33	
Hereditary syndrome (%)	26 (72)	27 (82)	0.345
Multiplicity of tumors (%)	10 (32)	11 (33)	0.772
Mean tumor number (range)	1.5 (1–4)	1.5 (1–5)	0.945
Mean tumor size (cm)	2.8	2.5	0.278
Endophytic location (%)	33 (70)	22 (48)	0.049
Hilar location	9 (19)	3 (7)	0.062
Operative time, min (range)	335 (165–520)	365 (210–600)	0.264
Warm ischemia time, min (range)	26 (0–61)	27 (0–46)	0.759
Blood loss, ml (range)	492 (100–2,700)	502 (50–1,800)	0.938
Positive margins	1	0	
Complications (%)	13 (36)	10 (30)	0.558

showed comparable results (Table 5.2). Tumors in the robotic cohort tended to be more hilar and endophytic in their location. There were no major complications in the robotic group and one bowel injury in the laparoscopic group that necessitated open re-exploration. Cost and reliability on an experienced bedside assistant were described as disadvantages of the robotic technique.

Data from published experiences of robotic-assisted partial nephrectomy are listed in Table 5.3. A variety of information including tumor number, size, operative time, warm ischemia time, blood loss, and hospital stay are reported from over 10 institutions. A total of 309 tumors were removed from 303 patients undergoing robotic-assisted partial nephrectomy. The average tumor size was 2.86 cm. Cases

Table 5.3 Operative results of published series of robotic-assisted partial nephrectomy

Series	Patient number	Tumor number	Tumor size (cm)	Op time (min)	WIT (min)	Mean EBL (ml)	Mean hospital stay (days)
Gettman et al. [7]	13	13	3.5	215	22.0	170	4.3
Phillips et al. [6]	12	12	1.8	265	26.0	240	2.7
Kaul et al. [4]	10	10	2.3	155	21.0	92	1.5
Rogers et al. [10]	8	14	3.6	192	31.0	230	2.6
Aron et al. [37]	12	12	2.4	242	23.0	329	4.7
Deane et al. [3]	10	10	3.1	229	32.1	115	2.0
Michli et al. [1]	20	20	2.7	142	28.1	263	2.8
Ho et al. [2]	20	20	3.5	83	21.7	189	4.8
Rogers et al. [42] (multi-institutional)	148	148	2.8	197	27.8	183	1.9
Benway et al. [34]	50	50	2.7	145	17.8	140	2.5
Totals	303	309	2.84	186	25.0	185	2.98

WIT, warm ischemia time; EBL, estimated blood loss

took 186 min on average with 25 min of warm ischemia and 185 ml of blood loss. Patients were discharged on average on postoperative day 3.

Conversions and Complications

Complications are a known consequence of surgical intervention. Even in the most experienced hands, untoward events can occur at each step of the operation. The majority of complication data for partial nephrectomy have been described in the laparoscopic literature. The largest studied series of laparoscopic surgery for urological cancer was published on 1,867 patients undergoing surgery at the Cleveland Clinic [39]. They described an overall complication rate of 12.4%, 3.5% were intraoperative and 8.9% were postoperative. Less than 1% of the described cases were converted to open surgery. Laparoscopic partial nephrectomy was an independent risk factor for complication.

Reported complications in robotic partial nephrectomy appear similar to the laparoscopic series but case volume is less and the data remain immature. Positive margin, open conversion or conversion to traditional laparoscopy, and complication rates are described amongst various institutions in Table 5.4. The overall average complication rate reported from the current published experiences on robotic-assisted partial nephrectomy is 7.9% with a conversion rate of 2.6%. The average positive margin rate reported was 2.6%.

Robotic Surgery for Complex Tumors and Future Directions

As we advocate performing nephron-sparing surgery in increasingly more patients with more complex renal tumors, we are hopeful that robotic assistance may aid in transferring this philosophy

Table 5.4 Positive margins, conversions, and complication rates of published series

Series	Positive margins (%)	Conversion number (%)	Complication number (%)	Listed complications
Gettman et al. [7]	1 (7.7)	Number (0)	1 (7.7)	Ileus
Phillips et al. [6]	None	3 (25)	3 (25)	Bleeding, 2; urine leak, 1
Kaul et al. [4]	None	None (0)	2 (20)	Bleeding, 1; urine leak, 1
Rogers et al. [9]	None	None	None	
Aron et al. [37]	None	2 (17)	None	
Deane et al. [3]	None	None	1 (10)	Bleeding
Michli et al. [1]	None	None	3 (15)	Lost needle/exploration, 1; perirenal abscess, 1; pulmonary embolus, 1
Ho et al. [2]	None	None	None	
Rogers et al. [42] (multi-institutional)	6 (4)	2 (1.3)	9 (6)	Ileus, 3; pulmonary embolus, 2; urine leak, 2; bleeding, 1; rhabdomyolysis, 1
Benway et al. [34]	1 (2)	1 (2)	5 (10)	DVT, 1; myocardial infarction, 1; hypertensive crisis, 1; perirenal hematoma, 1; post-op anemia, 1
Totals	8 of 303 (2.6)	8 of 303 (2.6)	24 of 303 (7.9)	

Table 5.5 Current advances and future directions for robotic renal surgery

RAPN for endophytic and hilar tumors [9, 10]
RAPN for multiple tumors and patients with hereditary renal disease [8]
RAPN after prior open retroperitoneal surgery
Robotic-assisted radical nephrectomy for renal vein thrombus [43]
Robotic renal single-site surgery [40]
Robotic NOTES (natural orifice translumenal endoscopic surgery) [41]

into the minimally invasive arena. A published report from our group at the National Cancer Institute described the safety and feasibility of robotic-assisted partial nephrectomy in select patients with complex masses including hilar and endophytic tumors [9]. More recently at the NCI we have described our experience utilizing this technique successfully in 10 patients with hereditary renal disease and multifocal renal masses [8]. Due to concerns regarding the potential long-term effects of ischemia times, we have performed "off-clamp" robotic partial nephrectomy with encouraging results in a selected few patients with hereditary renal disease in whom reoperation in the future may be anticipated. Surgeons are now performing surgeries using robotic assistance via single-port access and have developed robotic NOTES (natural orifice translumenal endoscopic surgery) in reconstructive urology using an animal model [40, 41]. A list of current developments and the expanding role of robotic-assisted renal surgery are listed in Table 5.5.

Summary and Conclusion

Partial nephrectomy has shown equivalent outcomes and improved preservation of long-term renal function in comparison with radical nephrectomy. It is becoming more evident that partial nephrectomy should be offered as the treatment for patients with solid renal masses whenever technically feasible. The details of our technique of robotic-assisted partial nephrectomy and report of early outcomes using this technique have been outlined in this chapter.

Robotic surgery for renal cancer remains in its infancy. As urologists we should seek to expand the role of minimally invasive surgery not to replace existing surgical techniques but to offer equally effective procedures that will further reduce the impact of treatment on the patient. The growing acceptance and utilization of robotic-assisted partial nephrectomy underscores the ultimate goal in the management of localized kidney cancer: oncologic efficacy, renal preservation, and return of convalescence.

Critical Operative Steps

- Place 5-Fr open-ended ureteral catheter secured to Foley catheter for cases in which collecting system entry is anticipated. Catheter can be connected to methylene blue syringe and utilized to identify areas of pelvicalyceal violation after tumor is resected.
- Ensure padding and proper positioning of patient's neck, arms, and shoulders prior to docking of robot.
- Perform adequate renal dissection and tumor exposure prior to hilar clamping and tumor extirpation to maximize vision and maneuverability with robotic instruments.
- Utilize intraoperative ultrasound to identify boundaries of tumor and properly investigate any insipient lesion.
- Perform a "test run" including a mimicking of hilar clamping with bedside assistant and a back table instrument and material check with scrub tech prior to hilar clamping and tumor resection.
- Proceed swiftly but meticulously during tumor removal using mostly cold cutting and inspect

tumor and resection bed with 3D vision after resection is complete.

- Run base of resection site with Vicryl suture and then interrogate collection system by injection of methylene blue through ureteral catheter.
- Complete reconstruction by sliding capsular sutures over Surgicel® bolsters and cinching these down robotically under direct vision. Secure with Lapra-Ty® clips.
- Remove clamps and allow adequate time for kidney to reperfuse. Specimen can be placed in retrieval bag. Ports should be removed under direct vision.
- Jackson–Pratt drain is placed posteriorly to kidney and secured to skin.

Critical Instruments and Supplies

- da Vinci Surgical System® instruments: monopolar hot scissors, Maryland bipolar, ProGrasp, two robotic needle drivers.
- Veress needle, 10–12-mm trocars (2), 5-mm trocars (1 or 2), 8-mm robotic trocars (two or three depending on the role of the fourth arm and use of da Vinci S system®), 5-Fr open-ended ureteral catheter, and 60 cm^3 syringe with methylene blue.
- Bedside assistant instruments: laparoscopic suction irrigator, laparoscopic grasper, laparoscopic scissors, bulldog or Satinsky clamps, 10- and 5-mm Hem-o-Lock® clips and applicator, Lapra-Ty® clips and applicator.
- Laparoscopic pad or sponge that can be placed into the surgical field to assist with kidney exposure and positioning and assist with manual pressure of kidney if necessary.
- Laparoscopic ultrasound transducer and console (Aloka Diagnostic Ultrasound Systems®).
- *Sutures*:

  Resection base—5-in. 3-0 Vicryl SH needle with Lapra-Ty® on knotted end (1–2).

  Small collection system opening or open-end vessels—5-in. 4-0 Vicryl RB needle (2).

  Capsule closure—7-in. 2-0 Vicryl SH or CT needle with Hem-o-Lock® and Lapra-Ty® on knotted end (2–4).

  Gerota's closure—7-in. 2-0 Vicryl SH or CT needle (1).
- Surgicel® cigar-shaped bolsters (2–5) and Flo-seal applicator.
- EndoCatch specimen removal bag (10 mm), Carter-Thomason® closing instrument, 10-Fr round Jackson–Pratt drain.

References

1. Michli EE, Parra RO. Robotic-assisted laparoscopic partial nephrectomy: initial clinical experience. Urology. Feb 2009;73(2):302–5.
2. Ho H, Schwentner C, Neururer R, Steiner H, Bartsch G, Peschel R. Robotic-assisted laparoscopic partial nephrectomy: surgical technique and clinical outcomes at 1 year. BJU Int. Mar 2009;103(5):663–8.
3. Deane LA, Lee HJ, Box GN, et al. Robotic versus standard laparoscopic partial/wedge nephrectomy: a comparison of intraoperative and perioperative results from a single institution. J Endourol. May 2008;22(5):947–52.
4. Kaul S, Laungani R, Sarle R, et al. da Vinci-assisted robotic partial nephrectomy: technique and results at a mean of 15 months of follow-up. Eur Urol. Jan 2007;51(1):186–91; discussion 191–2.
5. Caruso RP, Phillips CK, Kau E, Taneja SS, Stifelman MD. Robot assisted laparoscopic partial nephrectomy: initial experience. J Urol. Jul 2006;176(1): 36–9.
6. Phillips CK, Taneja SS, Stifelman MD. Robot-assisted laparoscopic partial nephrectomy: the NYU technique. J Endourol. May 2005;19(4):441–5; discussion 445.
7. Gettman MT, Blute ML, Chow GK, Neururer R, Bartsch G, Peschel R. Robotic-assisted laparoscopic partial nephrectomy: technique and initial clinical experience with DaVinci robotic system. Urology. Nov 2004;64(5):914–8.
8. Boris R, Proano M, Linehan WM, Pinto PA, Bratslavsky G. Initial experience with robot assisted partial nephrectomy for multiple renal masses. J Urol. 13 Aug 2009.
9. Rogers CG, Singh A, Blatt AM, Linehan WM, Pinto PA. Robotic partial nephrectomy for complex renal tumors: surgical technique. Eur Urol. Mar 2008;53(3):514–21.
10. Rogers CG, Metwalli A, Blatt AM, et al. Robotic partial nephrectomy for renal hilar tumors: a multi-institutional analysis. J Urol. Dec 2008;180(6): 2353–6.

11. Jemal A, Siegel R, Ward E, et al. Cancer statistics, 2008. CA Cancer J Clin. Mar–Apr 2008;58(2):71–96.
12. Volpe A, Jewett MA. The natural history of small renal masses. Nat Clin Pract Urol. Aug 2005;2(8):384–90.
13. Fergany AF, Hafez KS, Novick AC. Long-term results of nephron sparing surgery for localized renal cell carcinoma: 10-year follow-up. J Urol. Feb 2000;163(2):442–5.
14. Belldegrun A, Tsui KH, deKernion JB, Smith RB. Efficacy of nephron-sparing surgery for renal cell carcinoma: analysis based on the new 1997 tumor-node-metastasis staging system. J Clin Oncol. Sep 1999;17(9):2868–75.
15. Dash A, Vickers AJ, Schachter LR, Bach AM, Snyder ME, Russo P. Comparison of outcomes in elective partial vs radical nephrectomy for clear cell renal cell carcinoma of 4–7 cm. BJU Int. May 2006;97(5):939–45.
16. Leibovich BC, Blute ML, Cheville JC, Lohse CM, Weaver AL, Zincke H. Nephron sparing surgery for appropriately selected renal cell carcinoma between 4 and 7 cm results in outcome similar to radical nephrectomy. J Urol. Mar 2004;171(3):1066–70.
17. Boorjian SA, Uzzo RG. The evolving management of small renal masses. Curr Oncol Rep. May 2009;11(3):211–7.
18. Go AS, Chertow GM, Fan D, McCulloch CE, Hsu CY. Chronic kidney disease and the risks of death, cardiovascular events, and hospitalization. N Engl J Med. 23 Sep 2004;351(13):1296–305.
19. Monk TG, Saini V, Weldon BC, Sigl JC. Anesthetic management and one-year mortality after noncardiac surgery. Anesth Analg. Jan 2005;100(1):4–10.
20. Hodgson C, McClelland RM, Newton JR. Some effects of the peritoneal insufflation of carbon dioxide at laparoscopy. Anaesthesia. Jul 1970;25(3):382–90.
21. Lew JK, Gin T, Oh TE. Anaesthetic problems during laparoscopic cholecystectomy. Anaesth Intensive Care. Feb 1992;20(1):91–2.
22. Chen RN, Moore RG, Cadeddu JA, et al. Laparoscopic renal surgery in patients at high risk for intra-abdominal or retroperitoneal scarring. J Endourol. Apr 1998;12(2):143–7.
23. Fazeli-Matin S, Gill IS, Hsu TH, Sung GT, Novick AC. Laparoscopic renal and adrenal surgery in obese patients: comparison to open surgery. J Urol. Sep 1999;162(3 Pt 1):665–9.
24. Troppmann C, Perez RV. Rhabdomyolysis associated with laparoscopic live donor nephrectomy and concomitant surgery: a note of caution. Am J Transplant. Nov 2003;3(11):1457–8.
25. Colombo JR Jr., Haber GP, Aron M, Xu M, Gill IS. Laparoscopic partial nephrectomy in obese patients. Urology. Jan 2007;69(1):44–8.
26. Wolf JS Jr.. Pathophysiologic effects of prolonged laparoscopic operation. Semin Surg Oncol. Mar–Apr 1996;12(2):86–95.
27. Thomas MA, Rha KH, Ong AM, et al. Optical access trocar injuries in urological laparoscopic surgery. J Urol. Jul 2003;170(1):61–3.
28. Rogers CG, Laungani R, Bhandari A, et al. Maximizing console surgeon independence during robot-assisted renal surgery by using the Fourth Arm and TilePro. J Endourol. Jan 2009;23(1):115–21.
29. Johnson A, Sudarshan S, Liu J, Linehan WM, Pinto PA, Bratslavsky G. Feasibility and outcomes of repeat partial nephrectomy. J Urol. Jul 2008;180(1):89–93; discussion 93.
30. Turna B, Aron M, Frota R, Desai MM, Kaouk J, Gill IS. Feasibility of laparoscopic partial nephrectomy after previous ipsilateral renal procedures. Urology. Sep 2008;72(3):584–8.
31. Pautler SE, Choyke PL, Pavlovich CP, Daryanani K, Walther MM. Intraoperative ultrasound aids in dissection during laparoscopic partial adrenalectomy. J Urol. Oct 2002;168(4 Pt 1):1352–5.
32. Carini M, Minervini A, Lapini A, Masieri L, Serni S. Simple enucleation for the treatment of renal cell carcinoma between 4 and 7 cm in greatest dimension: progression and long-term survival. J Urol. Jun 2006;175(6):2022–6; discussion 2026.
33. Herring JC, Enquist EG, Chernoff A, Linehan WM, Choyke PL, Walther MM. Parenchymal sparing surgery in patients with hereditary renal cell carcinoma: 10-year experience. J Urol. Mar 2001;165(3):777–81.
34. Benway BM, Wang AJ, Cabello JM, Bhayani SB. Robotic partial nephrectomy with sliding-clip renorrhaphy: technique and outcomes. Eur Urol. Mar 2009;55(3):592–9.
35. Nguyen MM, Gill IS. Halving ischemia time during laparoscopic partial nephrectomy. J Urol. Feb 2008;179(2):627–32; discussion 632.
36. Gill IS, Kavoussi LR, Lane BR, et al. Comparison of 1,800 laparoscopic and open partial nephrectomies for single renal tumors. J Urol. Jul 2007;178(1):41–6.
37. Aron M, Koenig P, Kaouk JH, Nguyen MM, Desai MM, Gill IS. Robotic and laparoscopic partial nephrectomy: a matched-pair comparison from a high-volume centre. BJU Int. Jul 2008;102(1):86–92.
38. Wang AJ, Bhayani SB. Robotic partial nephrectomy versus laparoscopic partial nephrectomy for renal cell carcinoma: single-surgeon analysis of >100 consecutive procedures. Urology. Feb 2009;73(2):306–10.
39. Colombo JR Jr., Haber GP, Jelovsek JE, et al. Complications of laparoscopic surgery for urological cancer: a single institution analysis. J Urol. Sep 2007;178(3 Pt 1):786–91.

40. Stein RJ, White WM, Goel RK, Irwin BH, Haber GP, Kaouk JH. Robotic laparoendoscopic single-site surgery using GelPort as the access platform. Eur Urol. Jan 2010;57(1):132–6.
41. Haber GP, Crouzet S, Kamoi K, et al. Robotic NOTES (natural orifice translumenal endoscopic surgery) in reconstructive urology: initial laboratory experience. Urology. Jun 2008;71(6):996–1000.
42. Rogers C, Menon M, Weise E, et al. Robotic partial nephrectomy: a multi-institutional analysis. J Robot Surg. 2008;2:141–3.
43. Rogers CG, Linehan WM, Pinto PA. Robotic nephrectomy for kidney cancer in a horseshoe kidney with renal vein tumor thrombus: novel technique for thrombectomy. J Endourol. Aug 2008;22(8):1561–3; discussion 1563.

Chapter 6

Pediatric Laparoscopic and Robotic Upper Pole Nephrectomy for Nonfunctioning Moieties

Glenn M. Cannon and Richard S. Lee

This chapter contains a video segment which can be found at the URL: http://www.springerimages.com/ost

Introduction

In 1993, Jordan and Winslow described laparoscopic upper pole partial nephrectomy in a 14-year-old girl with bilateral duplicated collecting systems [1]. Since that time, there has been a substantial amount of literature devoted to laparoscopic renal surgery in children. Prior to and including 2009, there have been 28 case series of retroperitoneal laparoscopic nephrectomy [2–29], 26 case series of transperitoneal laparoscopic nephrectomy [2, 11, 28, 30–52], and 3 case series of robotic-assisted laparoscopic nephrectomy [53–55]. Regardless of the approach taken, the literature reveals that laparoscopic renal ablative surgery in children is safe and effective [56].

Indications

The most common indication for laparoscopic partial nephrectomy in children is a nonfunctioning renal moiety secondary to obstruction or vesicoureteral reflux [44]. Obstruction may result from ureteral ectopia, ureterocele, or obstruction at the ureteropelvic or ureterovesical junction. Vesicoureteral reflux (VUR) may be associated with renal dysplasia or severe scarring in the affected moiety of a duplicated system. Although the most common indication for laparoscopic partial nephrectomy in adults is a suspected renal malignancy, this is a rare indication in the pediatric population.

Preoperative Evaluation

Children with a nonfunctioning renal moiety may have a variety of presentations. Prenatal or postnatal hydronephrosis, flank pain, hypertension, hematuria, urinary tract infections, vaginal discharge, change in bowel habits, palpable abdominal mass, and urinary incontinence in girls from an ectopic ureter have all been described as possible presentations for a nonfunctional renal moiety [1, 34, 44]. Renal ultrasound is often the initial diagnostic test that helps define anatomy as well as visualize the degree of parenchymal thickness/echogenicity and ureteral dilatation (Fig. 6.1). A voiding cystourethrogram is necessary to identify VUR in the ipsilateral moieties or contralateral kidney (Fig. 6.2). Identification of VUR in the other renal moieties may alter overall therapy or require therapy beyond heminephrectomy. Determination of function of the affected moiety is critical to help determine salvage reconstruction versus heminephrectomy. Dimercaptosuccinic acid nuclear

R.S. Lee (✉)
Department of Urology, Harvard Medical School, Children's Hospital Boston, Boston, MA 02115, USA
e-mail: richard.lee@childrens.harvard.edu

M.C. Ost (ed.), *Robotic and Laparoscopic Reconstructive Surgery in Children and Adults*, Current Clinical Urology, DOI 10.1007/978-1-60327-914-7_6, © Springer Science+Business Media, LLC 2011

A. B.

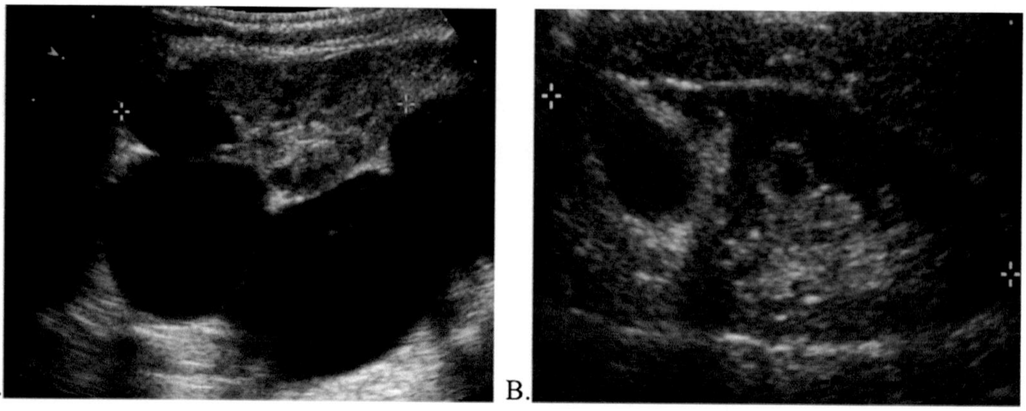

Fig. 6.1 (**a**) Renal ultrasound revealing dilated right upper pole with thin parenchyma and significantly dilated upper pole ureter. (**b**) Dilated left upper pole with hyperechoic parenchyma

A. B.

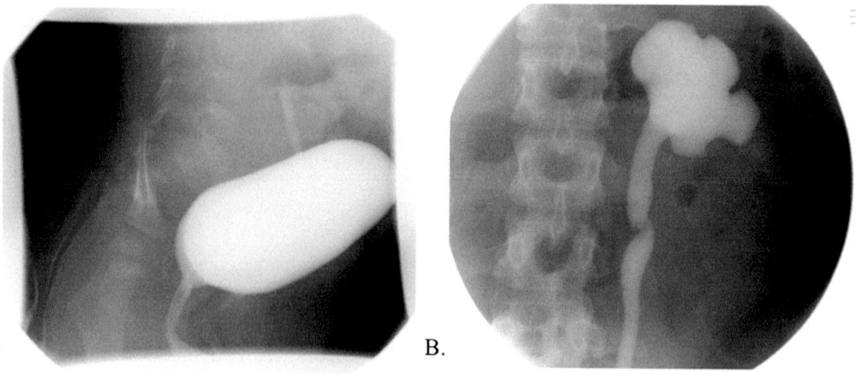

Fig. 6.2 (**a**) VCUG from patient in Fig. 6.1a. Ipsilateral VUR is not present but contralateral Grade I VUR is present. (**b**) VCUG from patient in Fig. 6.1b. VUR is present in the dilated left upper pole

A. B.

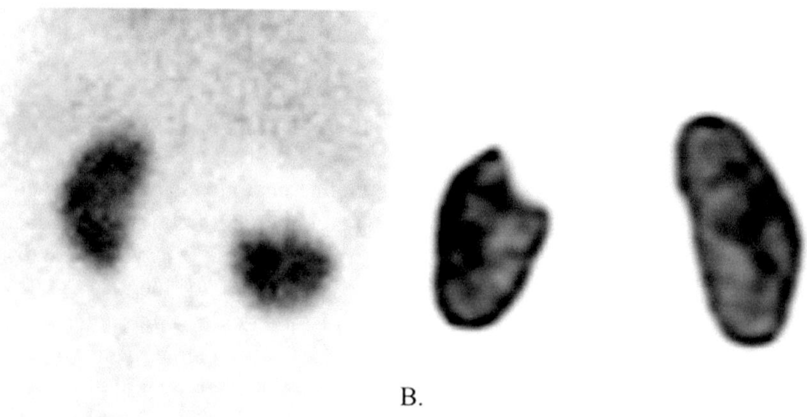

Fig. 6.3 (**a**) DMSA scan from patient in Fig. 6.1a revealing lack of function in the right upper moiety. (**b**) DMSA scan from patient in Fig. 6.1b revealing lack of function in the left upper pole moiety

renography (DMSA) is the gold standard to determine function in the affected moiety (Fig. 6.3). Further imaging in children is usually not necessary; however, if the diagnosis is still unclear, MR urography or intravenous pyelography may be informative.

Surgical Approach

The first published reports of laparoscopic partial nephrectomy in children were performed through a transperitoneal approach [2, 11, 28, 30–52]. Since then, the retroperitoneal approach has been demonstrated [2–29]. Advocates of the transperitoneal approach frequently quote the larger working space and more familiar surgical anatomy as advantages [2, 11, 28, 30–52]. Advocates of the retroperitoneal approach note the short distance to the kidney, the theoretical reduction in postoperative intraabdominal adhesions, and improved containment of complications such as a urine leak as favorable factors [2–29]. With the advent of robotic-assisted laparoscopy, a robotic-assisted approach has also gained in popularity [53–55]. Regardless of the approach chosen, mean operative times, hospital stay, and overall complication are similar and appear to be trending toward the open experience [56]. Table 6.1 lists advantages and disadvantages of each approach.

Surgical Technique—Robotic-Assisted Transperitoneal Approach

At our institution it is our preference to perform laparoscopic upper pole nephrectomy utilizing a robotic-assisted transperitoneal approach. Appropriate room setup is critical to help facilitate operative flow. Prior to the patient's arrival in the operating room, the robot is positioned on the

Table 6.1 Advantages and disadvantages of each approach to laparoscopic partial nephrectomy in children

Surgical approach	Advantages	Disadvantages
Transperitoneal	• Large working space • Familiar surgical anatomy • Potentially less manipulation of lower moiety [27] • Second incision not needed for ureterectomy • Option to perform concomitant ureteral reimplantation if necessary • Postoperative intraabdominal adhesions are usually not clinically significant [57, 58]	• Theoretical risk of postoperative intraabdominal adhesions [59, 60] • Possible difficulty in patients with previous intraperitoneal surgery • Urine leakage and bleeding is not confined
Retroperitoneal	• Short distance to kidney • Avoids colonic dissection • Less interference from surrounding organs (liver, spleen) • Theoretical reduction in postoperative adhesions • Straightforward conversion to open approach if necessary • Urine leakage and bleeding is confined to the retroperitoneal space	• Limited working space • Unfamiliar surgical anatomy • Greater degree of manipulation of normal lower moiety [27] • Risk of balloon rupture and need for fragment retrieval if balloon dilator is utilized to develop space

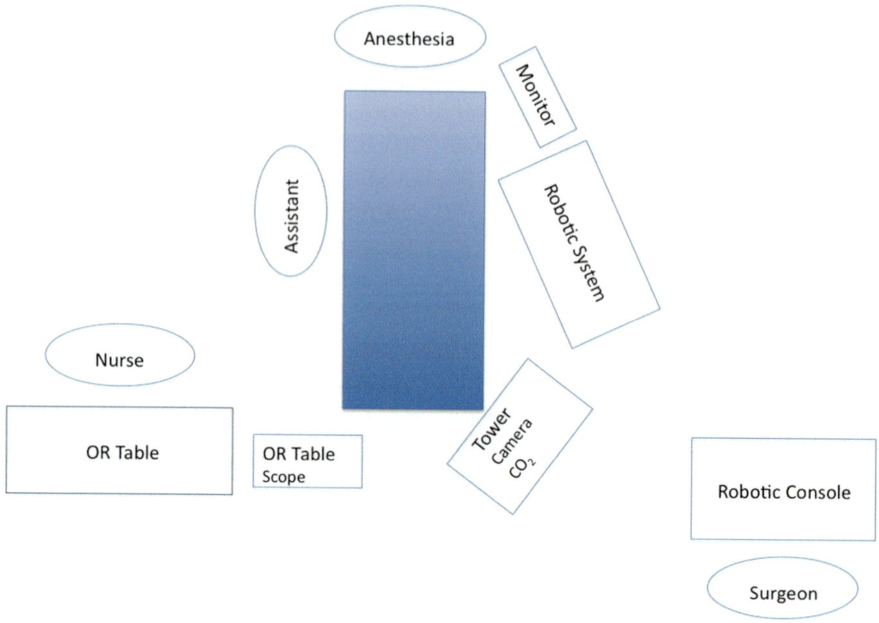

Fig. 6.4 Operating room setup for a left robotic-assisted upper pole nephrectomy

ipsilateral shoulder of the pathological side. The laparoscopic tower is placed at the foot of the bed on the side of the pathology. The surgical cart is positioned beyond the foot of the bed (Fig. 6.4). This room setup helps avoid excessive traveling of the surgical cart during positioning.

After the induction of general anesthesia, the patient receives preoperative antibiotic prophylaxis, orogastric tube, and urethral catheter. The patient is then positioned in a modified flank position with the affected side elevated 30° off the table with a gel roll. The bottom leg is bent at the knee and any area of pressure is padded with foam. Axillary padding is utilized. The patient is secured to the table at multiple points utilizing 3-in. silk tape as well as a safety strap over the legs. At this point, test rolling of the table is performed to the extreme right and left limits of the table to insure that the patient is secure and that the anesthesia team is satisfied with the security of the head, neck, and endotracheal tube.

The surgical table is initially rolled toward the affected side to make the abdomen as flat as possible. Access to the peritoneum is gained at the umbilicus with a Veress needle or a modified Hasson technique. After abdominal insufflation, either an 8- or a 12-mm camera port is placed at the umbilicus. The size of the camera port depends on the size of the child and it is our preference to place this using a plastic trocar through a DaVinci camera port. After the camera port is in the abdomen, the DaVinci laparoscope (positioned 30° down) is immediately inserted into the abdomen to inspect for evidence of visceral or vascular injury. Next two additional 8-mm robotic ports are placed under direct vision. One port is placed directly in the midline about 10 cm superior to the umbilicus. The second port is placed inferolateral 45° and 10 cm away from the umbilical port (Fig. 6.5).

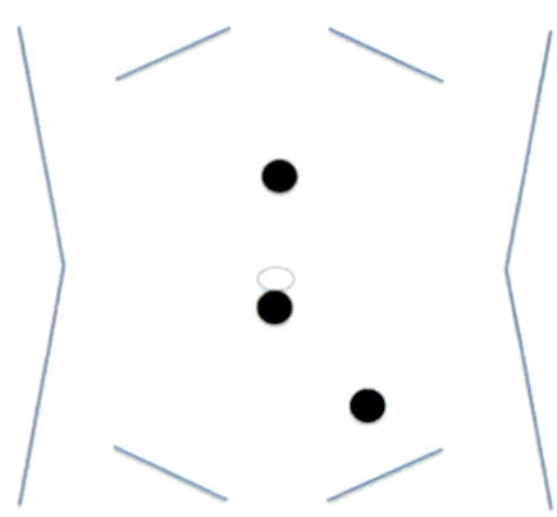

Fig. 6.5 Location of port placement for left transperitoneal upper pole nephrectomy

At this point, it is our practice to point the laparoscope at the kidney and hold this view in place while positioning the DaVinci surgical cart. The center post of the surgical cart lines up directly in line with the laparoscope. It is important to remember that the center post of the cart will travel beyond the laparoscope in a superior direction prior to turning the cart toward the patient. Once satisfied with the surgical cart position, the table is rolled to its extreme opposite side of the pathology to facilitate movement of the small bowel and colon away from the kidney. The surgical cart is brought toward the patient and the robotic arms are docked to the camera and working ports. A DeBakey forceps is placed in the left hand and the monopolar cautery scissors in the right hand.

If standard laparoscopy is to be performed, the patient position and port locations should be the same as the robotic-assisted technique. However, 5- or 3-mm working ports are typically utilized. The remaining steps will occur in an identical fashion to a robotic-assisted procedure.

The dissection is begun by mobilizing the colon along the white line of Toldt and reflecting it in a medial direction (Fig. 6.6). The perirenal fascia is opened and the ureters are then identified medial to the psoas muscle. After identification of the upper pole ureter, it is separated from the lower pole ureter and dissected in an inferior direction, while taking care to preserve as much adventitia and blood supply to the normal lower pole ureter (Fig. 6.7). The upper pole ureter is dissected as far as possible in a distal direction and divided. If there is reflux into the upper pole ureter, the ureteral stump is sutured closed.

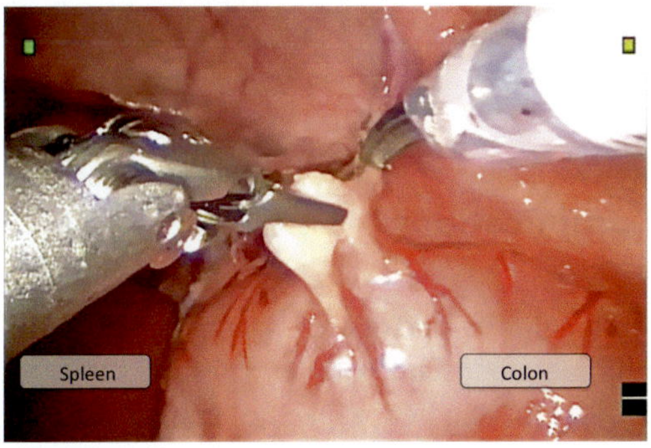

Fig. 6.6 Mobilization of the colon

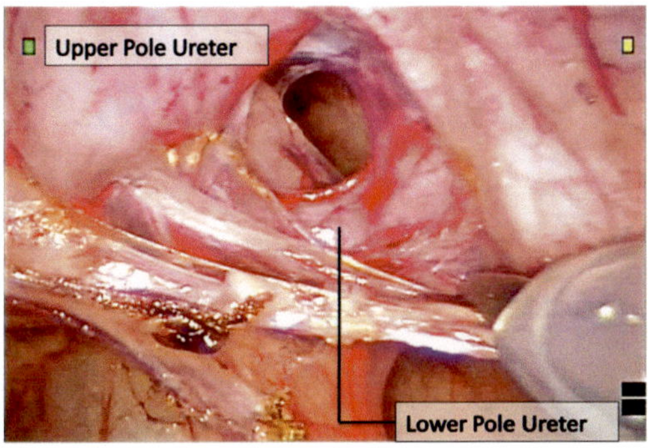

Fig. 6.7 Separation of the upper and lower pole ureters

The upper pole ureter is then dissected in a superior direction up to the lower pole hilum. Once the lower pole hilum is identified, dissection of the upper pole ureter superior to the lower pole hilum is performed to allow passage of the upper pole ureter posterior to the lower pole vessels (Fig. 6.8). Cephalad traction can then be placed on the upper pole ureter to facilitate access to the nonfunctioning upper moiety. Care must be exercised in this maneuver so as not to avulse small vessels to the upper pole. Dissection is carried in a superior direction until the upper pole hilar vessels are identified and divided.

After ligation and division of the vessels to the upper pole (Fig. 6.9), a clear demarcation

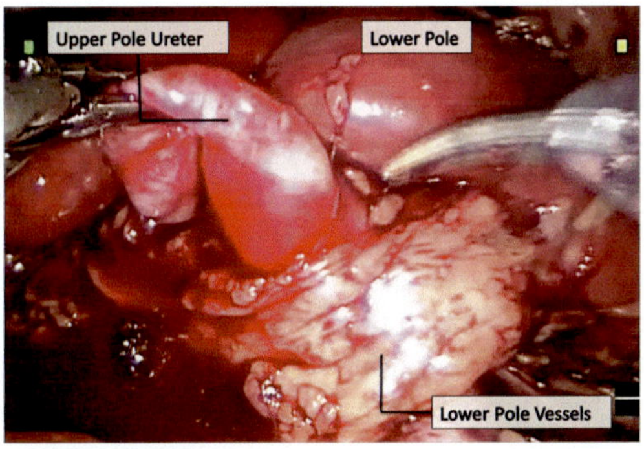

Fig. 6.8 Transposition of the upper pole ureter beneath the lower pole vessels

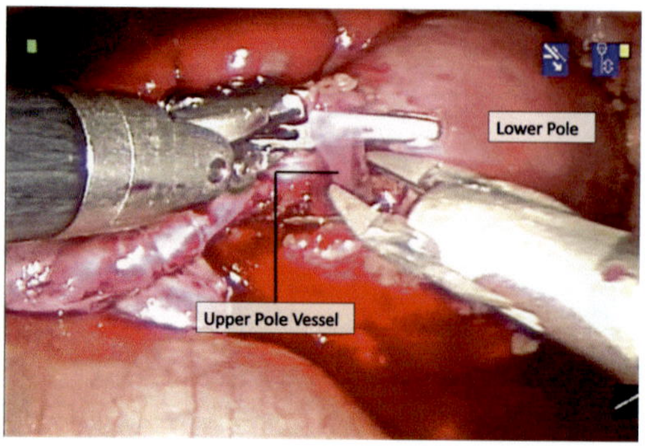

Fig. 6.9 Ligation of the upper pole vasculature

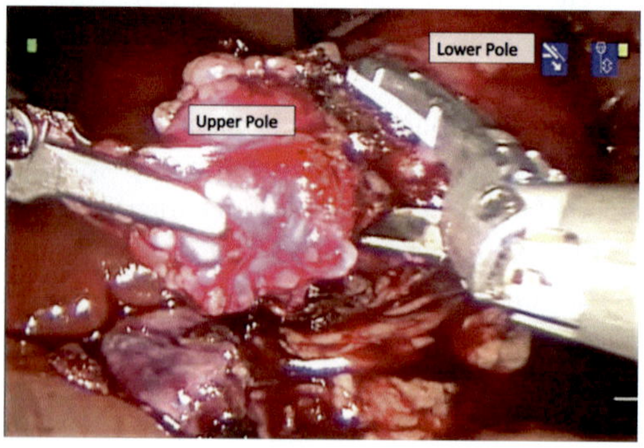

Fig. 6.10 Excision of upper pole with harmonic scalpel

between the hydronephrotic upper pole and the normal lower pole should be visualized. The nonfunctioning upper pole is then excised utilizing electrocautery or a harmonic scalpel (Fig. 6.10). We choose to err on the side of leaving nonfunctioning upper pole parenchyma versus removing functioning lower pole parenchyma. Any collecting system injury to the lower pole should be closed immediately with absorbable suture such as 4-0 or 5-0 Vicryl (Ethicon, Somerville, NJ). The renal capsule is then closed over a piece of fat or gel foam bolster with a running absorbable suture such as 3-0 or 4-0 Vicryl (Ethicon, Somerville, NJ). A hemostatic agent such as Tisseel fibrin sealant (Baxter Healthcare Corporation, Mansfield, MA) is then placed over the closed renal capsule. If the surgeon desires, a drain can be placed at this point.

Surgical Technique—Retroperitoneal Prone and Lateral

Either a prone or a flank approach can be utilized to obtain retroperitoneal access to the kidney. For the prone approach, initial access to the retroperitoneum is gained by an open technique. Dissection of the retroperitoneal space is performed utilizing balloon dilatation with 15–20 mmHg of pressure. Three trocars are inserted at the costovertebral angle near the paraspinous muscle and the 12th rib, just above the iliac crest at the posterior clavicular line and just medial to the paraspinous muscle above the iliac crest. Identification of the psoas muscle as a landmark is crucial to avoid peritoneal tears.

The abnormal upper pole, ureter, and supplying vasculature are identified. Minimal mobilization of the normal pole and vasculature should be performed to prevent vasospasm. The vasculature and the ureter to the upper pole are divided and the ureter can be used as a handle for manipulation of the upper pole parenchyma. The upper pole is then excised attempting to avoid collecting system injury. The parenchymal edges of the remaining lower are then sutured over bolsters. It is our practice to place a drain within the retroperitoneum.

The flank approach is similar except that the first trocar is inserted 3 cm below the top of the 12th rib. The peritoneum is dissected away from the anterior abdominal wall. The next two trocars are placed in the costovertebral angle and in the anterior axillary line 1 cm superior to the iliac crest (Fig. 6.11). The remainder of the procedure is identical to the retroperitoneal prone approach.

Complications

Although the incidence is low [61], complications can occur with any laparoscopic procedure in children. Specific complications of laparoscopic upper pole nephrectomy include bleeding, collecting system injury, injury to the

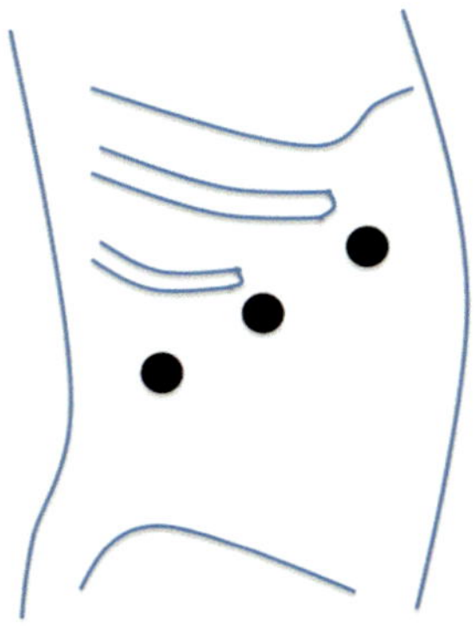

Fig. 6.11 Port locations for a right flank retroperitoneal heminephrectomy

normal pole ureter or vasculature, loss of the remaining moiety, peritoneal perforation during retroperitoneoscopy, and equipment failure [62]. Argon beam coagulation has been associated with diaphragmatic injury and pneumothorax [63]. Urologists must also be aware that there are significant hemodynamic and respiratory changes that occur during pediatric laparoscopic surgeries such as elevated end tidal CO_2, respiratory rate, peak airway pressure, and heart rate [64].

Critical Operative Steps

1. Mobilization of the colon in a medial direction
2. Identification and separation of the upper and lower pole ureters with care to preserve as much tissue as possible on the lower pole ureter
3. Dissection and transposition of the upper pole ureter around the lower pole vasculature
4. Ligation and division of the vasculature to the upper pole
5. Resection of the upper pole with care to avoid injury to the lower pole parenchyma or the collecting system

Critical Instruments and Supplies

- Gel rolls and pillows for positioning
- 30° laparoscope
- 8 mm robotic DeBakey forceps, microforceps, monopolar scissors
- 5 mm laparoscopic harmonic scalpel
- 10 mm laparoscopic specimen bag
- Hemostatic agent

References

1. Jordan GH, Winslow BH. Laparoendoscopic upper pole partial nephrectomy with ureterectomy. J Urol. Sep 1993;150(3):940–3.
2. Hamilton BD, Gatti JM, Cartwright PC, Snow BW. Comparison of laparoscopic versus open nephrectomy in the pediatric population. J Urol. Mar 2000;163(3):937–9.
3. Diamond DA, Price HM, McDougall EM, Bloom DA. Retroperitoneal laparoscopic nephrectomy in children. J Urol. Jun 1995;153(6):1966–8.
4. Luque Mialdea R, Martin-Crespo Izquierdo R, Navascues del Rio JA, Barrientos Fernandez G, Arrojo Vila F. Retroperitoneal laparoscopic nephrectomy in children. Actas Urol Esp. Jun 1997;21(6):637–9.
5. Chee-Awai RA, Chandhoke PS, Koyle MA. Laparoscopic nephrectomy in children. Semin Laparosc Surg. Mar 1998;5(1):47–54.
6. Kobashi KC, Chamberlin DA, Rajpoot D, Shanberg AM. Retroperitoneal laparoscopic nephrectomy in children. J Urol. Sep 1998;160(3 Pt 2):1142–4.
7. El-Ghoneimi A, Valla JS, Steyaert H, Aigrain Y. Laparoscopic renal surgery via a retroperitoneal approach in children. J Urol. Sep 1998;160(3 Pt 2):1138–41.
8. Borer JG, Cisek LJ, Atala A, Diamond DA, Retik AB, Peters CA. Pediatric retroperitoneoscopic nephrectomy using 2 mm instrumentation. J Urol. Nov 1999;162(5):1725–9; discussion 1730.
9. El-Ghoneimi A, Sauty L, Maintenant J, Macher MA, Lottmann H, Aigrain Y. Laparoscopic retroperitoneal nephrectomy in high risk children. J Urol. Sep 2000;164(3 Pt 2):1076–9.
10. Miyazato M, Hatano T, Miyazato T, Kagawa H, Yonou H, Ogawa Y. Retroperitoneoscopic heminephrectomy of the right upper collecting system emptying into an ectopic ureterocele in a 5-year-old girl: a case report. Hinyokika Kiyo. Jun 2000;46(6):413–6.
11. Figenshau RS, Yu MK. Laparoscopic nephrectomy and nephroureterectomy in the pediatric patient. Urol Clin North Am. Feb 2001;28(1):53–60.
12. Shanberg AM, Sanderson K, Rajpoot D, Duel B. Laparoscopic retroperitoneal renal and adrenal

surgery in children. BJU Int. Apr 2001;87(6): 521–4.
13. Borzi PA. A comparison of the lateral and posterior retroperitoneoscopic approach for complete and partial nephroureterectomy in children. BJU Int. Apr 2001;87(6):517–20.
14. Wu WJ, Chiang PH, Huang CH. Retroperitoneal laparoscopic nephrectomy in the treatment of incontinence from ectopic ureter with renal hypoplasia in the child—a case report. Kaohsiung J Med Sci. Dec 2001;17(12):626–9.
15. Urbanowicz W, Wieczorek M, Sulislawski J. Retroperitoneoscopic nephrectomy in the prone position in children (point of technique). Eur Urol. Nov 2002;42(5):516–9.
16. Lapointe SP, Houle AM, Barrieras D. Retroperitoneoscopic left nephrectomy in a horseshoe kidney with the use of the harmonic scalpel. Can J Urol. Oct 2002;9(5):1651–2.
17. Luque Mialdea R, Martin-Crespo Izquierdo R. Laparoscopy in pediatric urology. Arch Esp Urol. Jul–Aug 2002;55(6):737–47.
18. Farhat W, Khoury A, Bagli D, McLorie G, El-Ghoneimi A. Mentored retroperitoneal laparoscopic renal surgery in children: a safe approach to learning. BJU Int. Oct 2003;92(6):617–20; discussion 620.
19. Capolicchio JP, Jednak R, Anidjar M, Pippi-Salle JL. A modified access technique for retroperitoneoscopic renal surgery in children. J Urol. Jul 2003;170(1):204–6.
20. Valla JS, Breaud J, Carfagna L, Tursini S, Steyaert H. Treatment of ureterocele on duplex ureter: upper pole nephrectomy by retroperitoneoscopy in children based on a series of 24 cases. Eur Urol. Apr 2003;43(4):426–9.
21. El-Ghoneimi A, Farhat W, Bolduc S, Bagli D, McLorie G, Khoury A. Retroperitoneal laparoscopic vs open partial nephroureterectomy in children. BJU Int. Apr 2003;91(6):532–5.
22. Tarrado X, Rovira J, Garcia L, Morales L. Retroperitoneoscopy: minimally invasive renal surgery. Cir Pediatr. Oct 2003;16(4):189–92.
23. Kawauchi A, Fujito A, Naito Y, et al. Retroperitoneoscopic heminephroureterectomy for children with duplex anomaly: initial experience. Int J Urol. Jan 2004;11(1):7–10.
24. Ku JH, Yeo WG, Choi H, Kim HH. Comparison of retroperitoneal laparoscopic and open nephrectomy for benign renal diseases in children. Urology. Mar 2004;63(3):566–70; discussion 570.
25. Lee RS, Retik AB, Borer JG, Diamond DA, Peters CA. Pediatric retroperitoneal laparoscopic partial nephrectomy: comparison with an age matched cohort of open surgery. J Urol. Aug 2005;174(2):708–11; discussion 712.
26. Song SH, Lee SB, Yoo DS, Kim KS. Fluoroscopy-assisted retroperitoneal laparoscopic renal surgery in children. J Endourol. Apr 2006;20(4): 256–9.
27. Wallis MC, Khoury AE, Lorenzo AJ, Pippi-Salle JL, Bagli DJ, Farhat WA. Outcome analysis of retroperitoneal laparoscopic heminephrectomy in children. J Urol. Jun 2006;175(6):2277–80; discussion 2280–2.
28. Castellan M, Gosalbez R, Carmack AJ, Prieto JC, Perez-Brayfield M, Labbie A. Transperitoneal and retroperitoneal laparoscopic heminephrectomy—what approach for which patient? J Urol. Dec 2006;176(6 Pt 1):2636–9; discussion 2639.
29. Leclair MD, Vidal I, Suply E, Podevin G, Heloury Y. Retroperitoneal laparoscopic heminephrectomy in duplex kidney in infants and children: a 15-year experience. Eur Urol. Aug 2009;56(2): 385–9.
30. York GB, Robertson FM, Cofer BR, Bomalaski MD, Lynch SC. Laparoscopic nephrectomy in children. Surg Endosc. May 2000;14(5):469–72.
31. Koyle MA, Woo HH, Kavoussi LR. Laparoscopic nephrectomy in the first year of life. J Pediatr Surg. May 1993;28(5):693–5.
32. Ehrlich RM, Gershman A, Fuchs G. Laparoscopic renal surgery in children. J Urol. Mar 1994;151(3):735–9.
33. Seibold J, Janetschek G, Bartsch G. Laparoscopic surgery in pediatric urology. Eur Urol. 1996;30(3):394–9.
34. Janetschek G, Seibold J, Radmayr C, Bartsch G. Laparoscopic heminephroureterectomy in pediatric patients. J Urol. Nov 1997;158(5):1928–30.
35. Fahlenkamp D, Winfield HN, Schonberger B, Mueller W, Loening SA. Role of laparoscopic surgery in pediatric urology. Eur Urol. 1997;32(1):75–84.
36. Davies BW, Najmaldin AS. Transperitoneal laparoscopic nephrectomy in children. J Endourol. Oct 1998;12(5):437–40.
37. Abe T, Banya Y, Fujisawa H, Sugimura J, Fujioka T. A case of laparoscopic nephrectomy for ectopic vaginal ureter in a child. Hinyokika Kiyo. Mar 1998;44(3):175–7.
38. Ushiyama T, Kageyama S, Mugiya S, Suzuki K, Fujita K. Laparoscopic nephrectomy in children: two case reports. Int J Urol. Mar 1998;5(2): 181–4.
39. Prabhakaran K, Lingaraj K. Laparoscopic nephroureterectomy in children. J Pediatr Surg. Apr 1999;34(4):556–8.
40. Yao D, Poppas DP. A clinical series of laparoscopic nephrectomy, nephroureterectomy and heminephroureterectomy in the pediatric population. J Urol. May 2000;163(5):1531–5.
41. Horowitz M, Shah SM, Ferzli G, Syad PI, Glassberg KI. Laparoscopic partial upper pole nephrectomy in infants and children. BJU Int. Apr 2001;87(6): 514–6.
42. Andersen RD, Van Savage JG. Laparoscopic nephrectomy of the lower kidney for crossed fused ectopia. J Urol. Jun 2000;163(6):1902–3.

43. Kurokawa Y, Kanayama HO, Anwar A, et al. Laparoscopic nephroureterectomy for dysplastic kidney in children: an initial experience. Int J Urol. Nov 2002;9(11):613–7.
44. Kim HH, Kang J, Kwak C, Byun SS, Oh SJ, Choi H. Laparoscopy for definite localization and simultaneous treatment of ectopic ureter draining a dysplastic kidney in children. J Endourol. Aug 2002;16(6):363–6.
45. Robinson BC, Snow BW, Cartwright PC, De Vries CR, Hamilton BD, Anderson JB. Comparison of laparoscopic versus open partial nephrectomy in a pediatric series. J Urol. Feb 2003;169(2):638–40.
46. Wang DS, Bird VG, Cooper CS, Austin JC, Winfield HN. Laparoscopic upper pole heminephrectomy for ectopic ureter: initial experience. Can J Urol. Feb 2004;11(1):2141–5.
47. Mulholland TL, Kropp BP, Wong C. Laparoscopic renal surgery in infants 10 kg or less. J Endourol. Apr 2005;19(3):397–400.
48. Sydorak RM, Shaul DB. Laparoscopic partial nephrectomy in infants and toddlers. J Pediatr Surg. Dec 2005;40(12):1945–7.
49. Piaggio L, Franc-Guimond J, Figueroa TE, Barthold JS, Gonzalez R. Comparison of laparoscopic and open partial nephrectomy for duplication anomalies in children. J Urol. Jun 2006;175(6):2269–73.
50. Jesch NK, Metzelder ML, Kuebler JF, Ure BM. Laparoscopic transperitoneal nephrectomy is feasible in the first year of life and is not affected by kidney size. J Urol. Sep 2006;176(3):1177–9.
51. Fuchs J, Luithle T, Warmann SW, Haber P, Blumenstock G, Szavay P. Laparoscopic surgery on upper urinary tract in children younger than 1 year: technical aspects and functional outcome. J Urol. Oct 2009;182(4):1561–8.
52. Figenshau RS, Clayman RV, Kerbl K, McDougall EM, Colberg JW. Laparoscopic nephroureterectomy in the child: initial case report. J Urol. Mar 1994;151(3):740–1.
53. Olsen LH, Jorgensen TM. Robotically assisted retroperitoneoscopic heminephrectomy in children: initial clinical results. J Pediatr Urol. Apr 2005;1(2):101–4.
54. Lee RS, Sethi AS, Passerotti CC, et al. Robot assisted laparoscopic partial nephrectomy: a viable and safe option in children. J Urol. Feb 2009;181(2):823–8; discussion 828–9.
55. Pedraza R, Palmer L, Moss V, Franco I. Bilateral robotic assisted laparoscopic heminephroureterectomy. J Urol. Jun 2004;171(6 Pt 1):2394–5.
56. Kim C, McKay K, Docimo SG. Laparoscopic nephrectomy in children: systematic review of transperitoneal and retroperitoneal approaches. Urology. Feb 2009;73(2):280–4.
57. Hedican SP, Schulam PG, Docimo SG. Laparoscopic assisted reconstructive surgery. J Urol. Jan 1999;161(1):267–70.
58. Pattaras JG, Moore RG, Landman J, et al. Incidence of postoperative adhesion formation after transperitoneal genitourinary laparoscopic surgery. Urology. Jan 2002;59(1):37–41.
59. Moore RG, Kavoussi LR, Bloom DA, et al. Postoperative adhesion formation after urological laparoscopy in the pediatric population. J Urol. Mar 1995;153(3 Pt 1):792–5.
60. Moore RG, Partin AW, Adams JB, Kavoussi LR. Adhesion formation after transperitoneal nephrectomy: laparoscopic v open approach. J Endourol. Jun 1995;9(3):277–80.
61. Peters CA. Complications in pediatric urological laparoscopy: results of a survey. J Urol. Mar 1996;155(3):1070–3.
62. Esposito C, Lima M, Mattioli G, et al. Complications of pediatric urological laparoscopy: mistakes and risks. J Urol. Apr 2003;169(4):1490–2; discussion 1492.
63. Shanberg AM, Zagnoev M, Clougherty TP. Tension pneumothorax caused by the argon beam coagulator during laparoscopic partial nephrectomy. J Urol. Nov 2002;168(5):2162.
64. Halachmi S, El-Ghoneimi A, Bissonnette B, et al. Hemodynamic and respiratory effect of pediatric urological laparoscopic surgery: a retrospective study. J Urol. Oct 2003;170(4 Pt 2):1651–4; discussion 1654.

Part III
Laparoscopic and Robotic Reconstructive Renal Pelvis Surgery

Chapter 7

Adult Laparoscopic and Robotic-Assisted Pyeloplasty for Ureteropelvic Junction Obstruction

Sarah P. Conley and Benjamin R. Lee

This chapter contains a video segment which can be found at the URL: http://www.springerimages.com/ost

Introduction

Historically the gold standard for the management of ureteropelvic junction obstruction (UPJO) has been open pyeloplasty. However, since laparoscopic-assisted pyeloplasty was first described by Schuessler et al. in 1993, the minimally invasive approach has gained wide popularity and acceptance among both academic and community urologists [1, 2]. The goal of correcting a UPJO is not to reverse damage which the kidney has already sustained but to prevent further deterioration of function and to relieve symptoms. Laparoscopic or robotic approaches to correction of UPJO have been well documented in the literature, including reduction in hospital stay, decreased postoperative analgesic requirements, and reduced incision size and amount of esthetically undesirable scarring [3]. The da Vinci® robotic surgical system (Intuitive Surgical, Sunnyvale, CA) offers additional advantages over laparoscopy including optimal needle angle placement and better visualization in difficult anatomic locations. Additional benefits of depth perception and easier intracorporeal suturing allow initiation and completion of the anastomosis in an efficient, coordinated fashion. While the robotic-assisted procedures lack haptic feedback, visual cues from dissection of the tissues overcome this issue. Other factors to consider are longer operative times that decrease with experience, a steep learning curve, and higher costs compared to open and pure laparoscopic approaches [4].

S.P. Conley (✉)
Department of Urology, Tulane University School of Medicine, New Orleans, LA, USA
e-mail: sconley2009@gmail.com

Indications

The indications for robotic-assisted laparoscopic pyeloplasty are identical for both the open and pure laparoscopic approach, namely symptomatic UPJO, progressive impairment of renal function with a prolonged $t_{1/2}$ time on renal scan greater than 20 min, and/or differential function less than 40%. In addition, concomitant upper tract stones are a factor in approach.

Contraindications

Any patient who is a candidate for open ureteropelvic junction (UPJ) repair or laparoscopic UPJ repair is a candidate for the robotic approach.

M.C. Ost (ed.), *Robotic and Laparoscopic Reconstructive Surgery in Children and Adults*, Current Clinical Urology, DOI 10.1007/978-1-60327-914-7_7, © Springer Science+Business Media, LLC 2011

Absolute contraindications to minimally invasive surgery include irreversible coagulopathy, abdominal wall infection, bowel obstruction, massive hemoperitoneum, and malignant ascites [5]. Relative contraindications include severe COPD, pregnancy, morbid obesity, extensive prior abdominal surgery, pelvic fibrosis, iliac or aortic aneurysms, and hernias (diaphragmatic or umbilical).

Preoperative Preparation and Positioning

Preoperative evaluation includes a diuretic MAG3 nuclear renal scan to evaluate differential function and $t_{1/2}$. A prolonged $t_{1/2}$ time of greater than 20 min together with differential function less than 40% indicates a clinically significant UPJO. Abdominal imaging with a computed tomography (CT) urogram is helpful to evaluate renal anatomy, including crossing vessels, but it is not mandatory prior to surgery as a careful dissection of the anterior renal pelvis will identify any crossing vessels in this location. A renal ultrasound is acceptable in children in order to avoid unnecessary radiation exposure. Preoperative tests such as complete blood count, basic metabolic panel, coagulation studies, chest X-ray, and EKG should be obtained in appropriate patients. Anticoagulants should be held for 7–10 days prior to surgery. Informed consent must always be obtained and includes a discussion of the risks of bleeding, infection, injury to adjacent organs, stricture, and possible conversion to open or pure laparoscopic procedure. Thromboembolic stockings and pneumatic compression devices should be placed on both lower extremities prior to the induction of anesthesia. A single dose of intravenous antibiotics, such as a first-generation cephalosporin, should be administered 30 min prior to incision. A negative urine culture should be obtained prior to the procedure.

Preoperative cystoscopy and retrograde pyelogram followed by placement of double J ureteral stent is then performed (Fig. 7.1). Some surgeons choose to place a 6-Fr open-ended ureteral catheter (or 4–5 Fr in children) in the proximal ureter to promote ureteral dilation and identification of the ureter. If a straight open-ended ureteral catheter is used, it should be prepped into the surgical field in order to allow retrograde placement of a double pigtail ureteral stent during the procedure. A 16-Fr Foley catheter is placed in the bladder prior to positioning for the robotic portion of the case.

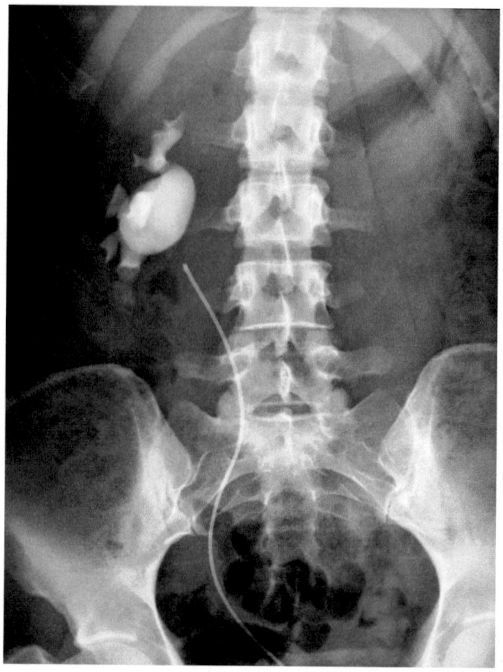

Fig. 7.1 Retrograde pyelogram demonstrating a classic right ureteropelvic junction obstruction with a 6-Fr open-ended ureteral catheter in the proximal ureter

The patient is then repositioned in a 45° modified flank position with the ipsilateral kidney elevated. In this modified lateral position, an axillary roll is not necessary. All pressure points should be padded and the patient should be secured to the table with 3-in. silk tape in three fixation points. The upper arm is placed on a pillow or a foam padding and care is taken to avoid compressing the ulnar nerve. In addition, the table is rotated prior to draping to confirm no slippage or movement of the patient.

Surgical Technique

We favor a transperitoneal approach with a preference for the Anderson–Hynes dismembered pyeloplasty. In the setting of a high insertion of the ureter into the renal pelvis, a Heineke–Mikulicz repair can be performed. Pneumoperitoneum is achieved in standard fashion using a Veress needle until an intraabdominal pressure of 15 mmHg is achieved. Opening pressures should be less than 10 mmHg in order to confirm proper intraperitoneal location. A 12-mm camera port is placed. The remainder of the ports are placed under direct visualization and include two 8-mm right and left robotic ports in a standard V configuration approximately 8 cm from the camera port. A 12-mm assistant port is placed subxiphoid to aid with retraction, suction, and passing suture in and out of the surgical field.

The initial dissection and mobilization of the kidney can be performed in a pure laparoscopic fashion with standard laparoscopic instruments or after docking the robot. Our preference is complete robotic mobilization. We recommend using Maryland bipolar forceps in the left robotic instrument port and monopolar scissors in the right. We prefer complete robotic mobilization of the white line of Toldt and colorenal ligaments in order to reflect the bowel medially. The lower pole of the kidney is elevated and the ureter is identified. Gentle dissection of the ureter is carried out superiorly toward the renal hilum with care to preserve the ureteral blood supply. It is important to mobilize the entire renal pelvis both anteriorly and posteriorly to the level of the renal sinus. A stay suture can be placed on the renal pelvis above the level of obstruction using a 3-0 Vicryl suture on a Keith needle, passing the needle directly through the abdominal wall, through the renal pelvis, then back through the abdominal wall. This hitch stitch helps to stabilize the renal pelvis and maintain orientation. The cause of obstruction should be identified as either a crossing vessel or an intrinsic stenosis. Preservation of the crossing vessel is crucial in maintaining renal function (Fig. 7.2).

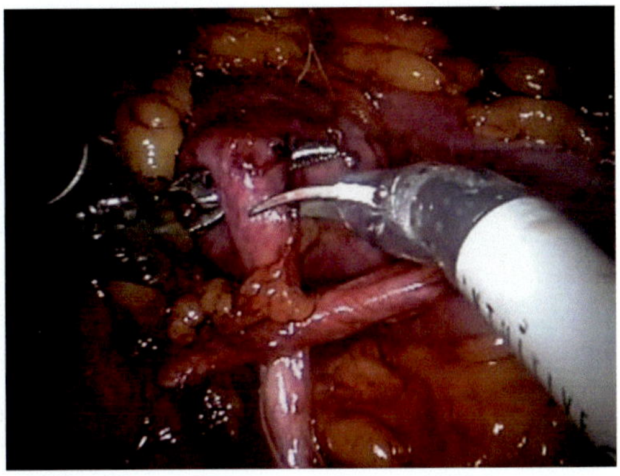

Fig. 7.2 A crossing vessel visualized anterior to the renal pelvis at the level of the ureteropelvic junction obstruction is preserved

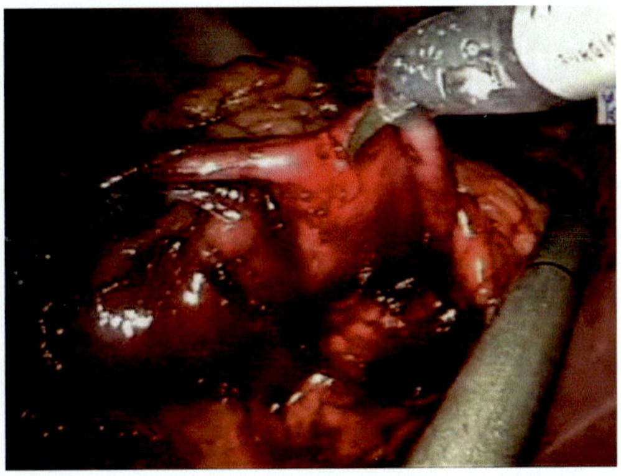

Fig. 7.3 Transection of ureteropelvic junction with monopolar scissors

The ureter is transected sharply with scissors at the level of the renal pelvis, leaving the indwelling ureteral stent intact (Fig. 7.3). Prior to complete transaction, the ureter is spatulated laterally in order to maintain proper orientation (Fig. 7.4). Sufficient spatulation should be performed in order to excise any stenotic ureter. If there is significant hydronephrosis, the renal pelvis can be reduced and tapered after the anastomosis is completed. Once the ureter is completely transected, a 4-0 Vicryl suture on a tapered SH needle is used to reapproximate the apex of the ureteral spatulation to the most dependent portion of the renal pelvis (Fig. 7.5). Although there is no haptic feedback on the da Vinci robot, visual cues can be used to gauge

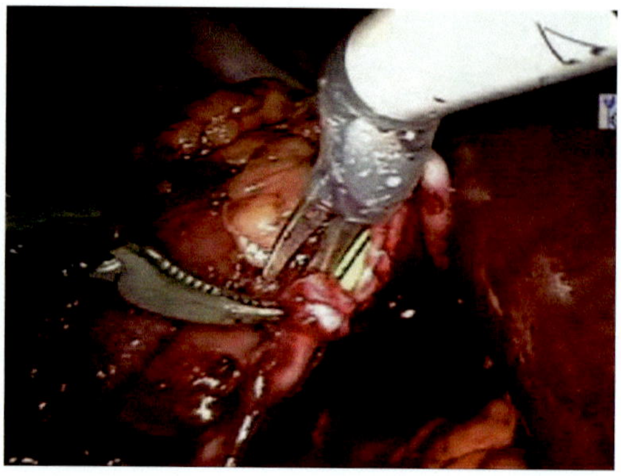

Fig. 7.4 Spatulation of proximal ureter on the lateral aspect after transecting the ureteropelvic junction

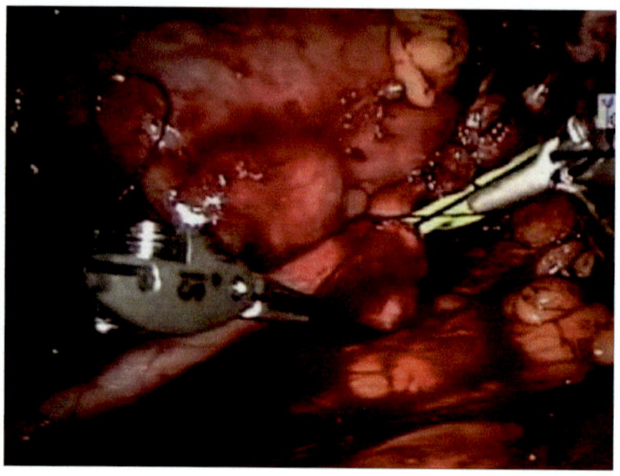

Fig. 7.5 A running 4-0 Vicryl suture on a tapered SH needle is used to complete the anastomosis

tension on the suture and subsequent knot. If a crossing vessel is identified, the anastomosis should be located distal and anterior to the vessel. An interrupted lateral posterior knot is placed, and then subsequent completion of the lateral posterior aspect of the anastomosis is performed. The anterior suture line is then completed to achieve a mucosa-to-mucosa, watertight, tension-free anastomosis. The apical stay suture can be used to rotate the suture line in order to facilitate running the posterior suture line. Prior to completing the anastomosis, the proximal end of the double pigtail ureteral catheter is gently placed within the renal pelvis. If an open-ended ureteral catheter is initially placed, the bedside assistant exchanges the open-ended ureteral catheter for a 3.8–6-Fr double pigtail ureteral stent over a wire. Alternatively, a double pigtail ureteral stent can be placed in antegrade fashion with the bladder previously filled with indigo carmine to visualize when the distal aspect of the stent is positioned in the bladder. If the renal pelvis has not yet been closed, the same suture can be used to close the renal pelvis. After ensuring hemostasis, a closed surgical drain, such as a Jackson–Pratt drain, is placed nearby the anastomosis through one of the 8-mm ports. The fascia of the 12-mm ports and skin are then closed in a standard fashion.

Postoperative Care

The patients remain in the hospital overnight. Diet is advanced as tolerated. We routinely administer Ketorolac 15 mg IV every 6 h for up to the first 48 h postoperatively with supplemental oral and IV narcotics as needed. The Foley catheter is removed the morning of postoperative day #1. If the drain has minimal output, it can be removed on postoperative day #1 and the patient discharged home. In the setting of high-drain output, a drain creatinine can be checked to confirm source. If the value is consistent with serum creatinine, the drain is removed and the patient is dismissed.

The ureteral stent is removed in the office with a flexible cystoscope 4–6 weeks postoperatively. Children will require a general anesthetic for stent removal. A renal ultrasound and/or a diuretic MAG3 nuclear renal scan can be obtained 3 months, 6 months, and/or 12 months after surgery.

Technical Considerations

The da Vinci robotic surgical system offers many technical advantages during dismembered pyeloplasty. We prefer to perform a complete robotic dissection of the kidney including mobilization of the white line of Toldt and colorenal ligaments and identification of the ureter as opposed to performing the initial dissection with pure laparoscopic techniques. The lack of tactile feedback can result in suture breakage during the anastomosis if careful attention is not paid during needle handling [6]. In the event of technical failure of the robotic surgical system, the case can be completed with conventional laparoscopy rather than converting to an open procedure. It is therefore important to be facile with intracorporeal suturing by either free hand or Endo Stitch technique.

Crossing Vessels

Crossing vessels are encountered in 30–69% of pyeloplasties [7–12, 17] (Table 7.1). A preoperative CT can help identify crossing vessels and help with surgical planning, but is not necessary as crossing vessels can be identified during the dissection and mobilization of the ureter and anterior renal pelvis. Care should be taken to create the anastomosis anteriorly and inferiorly to the crossing vessel.

Secondary Pyeloplasties

Robotic-assisted laparoscopic pyeloplasty is a safe and effective procedure for patients who have undergone previously failed open pyeloplasty or endourologic procedures. In a multi-institutional review of robotic-assisted laparoscopic dismembered pyeloplasty, Mufarrij et al. included 23 patients in their series of 140 patients undergoing secondary pyeloplasties. They found no difference in any parameters when comparing patients undergoing primary or secondary repair with respect to operative time, estimated blood loss (EBL), complication rate, length of stay (LOS), radiographic resolution of obstruction postoperatively, and need for secondary procedures postoperatively [10]. Similarly, Hemal et al. [13] reported on nine patients who successfully underwent robotic-assisted laparoscopic pyeloplasty after failed open repair. There were no intraoperative complications and all patients had postoperative nuclear renal scans verifying unobstructed drainage. However, in a series of 92 patients undergoing robotic-assisted pyeloplasty, Schwentner et al. [11] reported a slightly lower success rate in the 12 patients who underwent secondary pyeloplasty compared to primary pyeloplasty (83.3 vs. 97.5%).

Table 7.1 Outcomes of robotic-assisted laparoscopic pyeloplasty

Study	n	Crossing vessels (%)	Mean OR time (min)	Mean anastomosis time (min)	Mean EBL (mL)	Mean LOS (days)	Mean success rate (%)	Mean follow-up (months)	Open conversion (%)	Complications (%)
Gettman et al. [6]	9	–	139	62	< 50	4.7	100	4.1	0	11.1
Patel et al. [7]	50	30	122	20	40	1.1	100	11.7	0	2.0
Palese [16]	35	–	216	63	74	2.9	94	7.9	0	11.4
Chammas et al. [8]	100	43	125	–	< 100	3.5	90	29	1.0	0
Yanke et al. [17]	29	69	196	–	39	2.2	100	11	6.9	6.9
Mufarrij et al. [10]	140	55	217	–	59	2.1	95.7	29	–	10.0
Schwentner et al. [11]	92	45	108	25	–	4.6	96.7	39.1	0	3.3
Mendez-Torres et al. [12]	32	44	300	–	52	1.1	88.9	8.6	0	3.1

An interesting study by Sergi et al. [14] analyzed the collagen type I and III content of UPJ tissue in patients who underwent Anderson–Hynes dismembered pyeloplasty following antegrade endopyelotomy and compared it to tissue in patients following primary pyeloplasty and patients without UPJO. Total collagen content was higher in both the primary and secondary pyeloplasty groups compared to controls. Staining for collage type III was statistically significantly higher in the secondary pyeloplasty group. They concluded that an inflammatory response following endopyelotomy resulted in deposition of more fibrous collagen III, thus limiting the success of the procedure.

In prospective animal study, Andreoni et al. [15] performed immunohistological staining on porcine ureters following Acucise endopyelotomy at time intervals ranging from 0 h to 8 weeks. The initial ureteral incision was sealed by blood clot and periureteral fat. The urothelium rapidly regenerated within 2 weeks; however, the muscle layer failed to bridge the circumference of the ureter at 8 weeks after surgery. The presence of urinoma delayed healing of both mucosal and muscle layers. They found that an abundance of myofibroblasts rather than smooth muscle cells in the healing ureteral defect suggested the wound may heal by contraction.

Concomitant Pyelolithotomy

Concomitant pyelolithotomy can be performed at the time of robotic pyeloplasty using laparoscopic grasping forceps or a 16-Fr flexible cystoscope placed through the 12-mm assistant port with nitinol endoscopic basket in order to render the patients stone free [10, 16, 17]. In the multi-institutional series of 140 patients by Mufarrij et al. [10], 13 patients underwent simultaneous stone extraction without any difference in operative time, EBL, LOS, or need for secondary procedures. Care must be taken to suction the irrigant following flexible nephroscopy.

Horseshoe Kidney

Robotic-assisted laparoscopic pyeloplasty in horseshoe kidney is feasible [11]. Positioning of the trocars more inferior is necessary for optimal dissection. Bowel retraction may be aided by Trendelenburg position and assistant retraction with a fan retractor. It is critical to identify and preserve any aberrant renal vessels.

Body Habitus

Patient body habitus can also influence ease of operation. In small patients or young children, the two robotic working arms may need to be placed closer to the camera port, necessitating frequent realignment. For obese patients the standard V configuration of port placement may need to shift laterally in order to effectively work in the retroperitoneum. A second assistant port may also be placed for obese patients.

Bilateral UPJO

Patients with bilateral UPJO can undergo staged robotic-assisted laparoscopic pyeloplasties. In a case report by Kumar et al. [18], one patient successfully underwent simultaneous bilateral robotic-assisted dismembered pyeloplasties. Total operative time was 305 min and there were five adverse events, including subcutaneous emphysema, two incorrect suture placements, and two suture breakages during know tying.

Outcomes

Success rates of laparoscopic and robotic-assisted pyeloplasties are similar to open surgery [19–22]. In a retrospective series, Bauer et al. [19] compared 42 laparoscopic pyeloplasties to 35 open pyeloplasties and found equivalent outcomes in terms of pain relief, relief of obstruction, and return to activity levels. In another series comparing open to endourologic approaches to UPJO, Brooks et al. [20] also reported that success rates (100%) and complication rates (0%) were similar among the patients undergoing open and laparoscopic dismembered pyeloplasties. Postoperative analgesic use, LOS, and recovery time were significantly shorter for the laparoscopic group. In the pediatric population, Lee et al. [3] also demonstrated decreased hospital stay and decreased postoperative analgesic in the robotic-assisted group use compared to open group. Mean operative times were similar among the two groups (open 181 min, robotic 281 min, $p = 0.031$).

As with most surgical procedures, operative times and efficiency improve with case repetition. In their series of 50 patients who underwent robotic-assisted laparoscopic dismembered pyeloplasty, Patel and colleagues [7] demonstrated that mean operative time decreased from 194 min during the first 10 cases to 91 min during the last 10 cases. Robot docking time similarly decreased from 21 to 4 min.

Cost is an important factor when considering a new procedure. Recent studies have demonstrated that robotic-assisted laparoscopic pyeloplasties are not as cost effective as laparoscopic pyeloplasty [4, 23]. Although total in room time was shorter for robotic pyeloplasty (176 vs. 210 min) in Bahayani and colleagues' series, total cost was higher than that of laparoscopic pyeloplasty when including mean setup and take-down times, disposable instrument cost and depreciation, and maintenance of the da Vinci system [4]. Link et al. reported that robotic-assisted laparoscopic pyeloplasty is 2.7 times more costly than conventional laparoscopy [23]. Even after eliminating the depreciation of capital equipment, the robotic procedure was still 1.7 times more costly than a pure laparoscopic procedure.

Complications

The reported intraoperative and postoperative complication rates for robotic-assisted laparoscopic pyeloplasty are very low (0–11.4%) [3, 6–12, 16] (Table 7.1). Reported complications include pyelonephritis, flank pain, hematuria, stent migration, gluteal compartment syndrome, febrile urinary tract infection, minor intraoperative splenic laceration, and urine leak.

Conclusions

The da Vinci robotic system can be successfully used to perform laparoscopic Anderson–Hynes pyeloplasty with minimal morbidity and similar outcomes as the gold standard open approach.

Critical Operative Steps

- Preoperative cystoscopy and placement of double pigtail ureteral stent
- Positioning for robotic pyeloplasty
- Insufflation, access, trocar placement, and docking the robot
- Initial identification and dissection of the ureter and the renal pelvis
- Dismemberment of the ureteropelvic junction
- Reconstruction
- Drain placement
- Closure

Critical Instruments and Supplies

- da Vinci® robotic surgical system
- Maryland bipolar forceps
- Monopolar cautery scissors
- Needle holders
- Keith needle
- Suction/irrigation system
- 4-0 Vicryl running suture on an SH needle
- Indwelling double pigtail ureteral stent
- Closed drainage system (Jackson–Pratt)

References

1. Schuessler WW, Grune MT, Tecuanhuey LV, Preminger GM. Laparoscopic dismembered pyeloplasty. J Urol. 1993;150:1795–9.
2. Tan BJ, Rastinehad AR, Marcovich R, Smith AD, Lee BR. Trends in ureteropelvic junction obstruction management among urologists in the United States. Urology. 2005;65:260–4.
3. Lee RS, Retik AB, Borer JG, Peters CA. Pediatric robot assisted laparoscopic dismembered pyeloplasty: comparison with a cohort of open surgery. J Urol. 2006;175:683–7.
4. Bhayani SB, Link RE, Varkarakis JM, Kavoussi LR. Complete daVinci versus laparoscopic pyeloplasty: cost analysis. J Endourol. 2005;19: 327–32.
5. McDougall EM, Finley D, Clayman RV, et al. Basic urologic laparoscopy: a standardized guideline for training programs. AUA 2005.
6. Gettman MT, Neururer R, Bartsch G, Peschel R. Anderson–Hynes dismembered pyeloplasty performed using the da Vinci robotic system. Urology. 2002;60:509–13.
7. Patel V. Robotic-assisted laparoscopic dismembered pyeloplasty. Urology. 2005;66:45–9.
8. Chammas MF Jr, Hubert J, Patel VR. Robotically assisted laparoscopic pyeloplasty: a transatlantic comparison of techniques and outcomes. BJU Int. 2007;99:1113–7.
9. Yanke BV, Lallas CD, Pagnani C, McGinnis DE, Bagley DH. The minimally invasive treatment of ureteropelvic junction obstruction: a review of our experience during the last decade. J Urol. 2008;180:1397–402.
10. Mufarrij PW, Woods M, Shah OD, et al. Robotic dismembered pyeloplasty: a 6-year, multi-institutional experience. J Urol. 2008;180:1391–6.
11. Schwentner C, Pelzer A, Neururer R, et al. Robotic Anderson–Hynes pyeloplasty: 5-year experience of one centre. BJU Int. 2007;100:880–5.
12. Mendez-Torres F, Woods M, Thomas R. Technical modifications for robot-assisted laparoscopic pyeloplasty. J Endourol. 2005;19:393–6.
13. Hemal AK, Mishra S, Mukharjee S, Suryavanshi M. Robot assisted laparoscopic pyeloplasty in patients of ureteropelvic junction obstruction with previously failed open surgical repair. Int J Urol. 2008;15: 744–6.
14. Sergi F, Flammia GP, Alcini A, et al. Collagen changes in the ureteropelvic junction after failed antegrade endopyelotomy. J Endourol. 2007;21: 103–7.
15. Andreoni CR, Lin HK, Olweny E, Landman J, Lee D, Bostwick D, Clayman RV. Comprehensive evaluation of ureteral healing after electrosurgical endopyelotomy in a porcine model: original report and review of the literature. J Urol. 2004;171:859–69.
16. Palese MA, Stifelman MD, Munver R, et al. Robot-assisted laparoscopic dismembered pyeloplasty: a combined experience. J Endourol. 2005;19:382–6.
17. Yanke BV, Lallas CD, Pagnani C, Bagley DH. Robot-assisted laparoscopic pyeloplasty: technical considerations and outcomes. J Endourol. 2008;22: 1291–6.
18. Kumar R, Yadav R, Kolla SB. Simultaneous bilateral robot-assisted dismembered pyeloplasties for bilateral ureteropelvic junction obstruction: technique and literature review. J Endourol. 2007;21:750–3.
19. Bauer JJ, Bishoff JT, Moore RG, Chen RN, Iverson AJ, Kavoussi LR. Laparoscopic versus open pyeloplasty: assessment of objective and subjective outcome. J Urol. 1999;162:692–5.
20. Brooks JD, Kavoussi LR, Preminger GM, Schuessler WW, Moore RG. Comparison of open and endourologic approaches to the obstructed ureteropelvic junction. Urology. 1995;46:791–5.
21. Ost MC, Kaye JD, Guttman MJ, Lee BR, Smith AD. Laparoscopic pyeloplasty versus antegrade endopyelotomy: comparison in 100 patients and a new algorithm in the minimally invasive treatment of ureteropelvic junction obstruction. Urology. 2005;66:47–51.
22. Soulie M, Thoulouzan M, Seguin P, et al. Retroperitoneal laparoscopic versus open pyeloplasty with a minimal incision: comparison of two surgical approaches. Urology. 2001;57:443–7.
23. Link RE, Bhayani S, Kavoussi LR. A prospective comparison of robotic and laparoscopic pyeloplasty. Ann Surg. 2006;243:486–91.

Chapter 8

Pediatric Laparoscopic (Infant, Pre-pubertal, and Teenager) Pyeloplasty for Ureteropelvic Junction Obstruction

Danielle D. Sweeney and Steven G. Docimo

This chapter contains a video segment which can be found at the URL: http://www.springerimages.com/ost

Introduction

Laparoscopy has been utilized in pediatric urology for over 30 years, dating back to Cortesi, who first described using the modality for the evaluation of non-palpable testes [1]. Nevertheless, acceptance of pediatric urologic laparoscopy has generally lagged behind when compared to its adult counterpart, in large part due to the nature of the practice of pediatric urology [2]. Fortunately, there has been a shift in the paradigm. Pediatric laparoscopy has recently benefited from improvement in equipment and technology, as well as an increase in experienced laparoscopic surgeons entering the field. The techniques that were developed in adults have been refined for the pediatric population, allowing for the expansion of the technique from diagnostic procedures to complex reconstructive surgeries.

Laparoscopic pyeloplasty for treatment of ureteropelvic junction obstruction (UPJO) in children has followed a similar evolution as other forms of pediatric laparoscopic surgery. For many decades, open dismembered pyeloplasty had been the gold standard in the treatment of UPJO, in both the adult and pediatric populations, with success rates greater than 90% [3, 4]. However, there was a desire to find less invasive treatment options. In 1993, Schuessler published the first adult laparoscopic pyeloplasty series in which all patients had successful surgical outcomes [5]. This was followed by Peters in 1995, who reported the first pediatric case [6]. Since these initial publications, a variety of techniques and approaches have been described and utilized. Surgical outcomes and success rates for laparoscopic pyeloplasty have been found to be equivalent to the open procedure [4], and additional advantages include less incisional discomfort, a quicker convalescence, and excellent surgical cosmesis.

Etiology and Presentation of Ureteropelvic Junction Obstruction

Ureteropelvic junction obstruction is the functional impairment of urinary transport from the renal pelvis to the proximal ureter. The incidence of UPJO is approximately 1:500 with a male:female ratio of 2:1 [7]. It is more common on the left side than the right side and is reported to be bilateral in 10–40% [7]. It is the most common cause of hydronephrosis in newborns and young children [8]. If left untreated,

D.D. Sweeney (✉)
Pediatric Urology, Dell Children's Hospital, Austin, TX, USA
e-mail: danielledsweeney@gmail.com

M.C. Ost (ed.), *Robotic and Laparoscopic Reconstructive Surgery in Children and Adults*,
Current Clinical Urology, DOI 10.1007/978-1-60327-914-7_8, © Springer Science+Business Media, LLC 2011

this condition may cause progressive dilation of the renal collecting system, with subsequent deterioration of renal function and loss of the renal unit. UPJO is not uniform in its age of presentation; patients can present with a congenital UPJO diagnosed prenatally or a UPJO that is not apparent until late adolescence or early adulthood. Less commonly it can be linked to secondary causes such as infection, vesicoureteral reflux, recurrent stone passage, or iatrogenic strictures from previous surgery [9].

The etiology of UPJO is varied depending on the age of presentation. In infants and children, UPJO is usually primary or congenital in nature, related to intrinsic developmental abnormalities of the ureteropelvic junction. Intrinsic causes include an aperistaltic segment of the proximal ureter, congenital ureteral strictures due to excessive collagen deposition at a narrowed site, and ureteral fibroepithelial polyps (Fig. 8.1) [10]. In older children, adolescents, and young adults, UPJO can be caused by extrinsic compression from anatomic variants. Primary extrinsic causes include ureteral kinking and, more frequently, vessels to the lower pole of the kidney that pass anterior to the ureteropelvic junction and intermittently cause obstruction (Fig. 8.2) [11].

The presentation of UPJO can be as varied as the etiologies of the disease. In the infant population, hydronephrosis is usually diagnosed prenatally with maternal ultrasonography, and of this group, approximately 44% are found to have UPJO on postnatal evaluation [12]. In older children the presentation is typically characterized by a symptomatic episode of abdominal or flank pain and nausea and vomiting, called a Dietl's crisis. Cyclic vomiting alone can also be a sign of intermittent UPJO; however, this symptom complex is often misdiagnosed as gastrointestinal in origin. Less common presentations include urinary tract infection, hematuria, nephrolithiasis, and rarely hypertension. With the increased use of radiographic imaging, incidental diagnosis of asymptomatic UPJO is also becoming more prevalent.

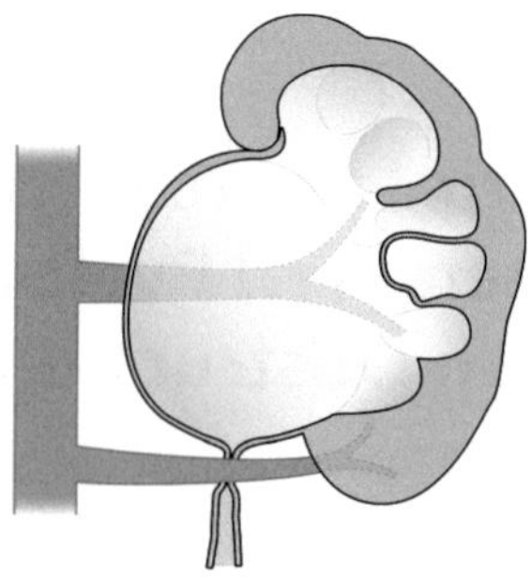

Fig. 8.2 Extrinsic compression from anatomic variants such as vessels to the lower pole of the kidney

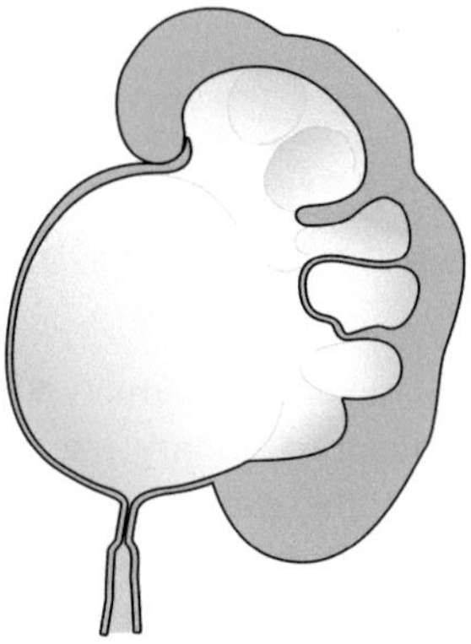

Fig. 8.1 Intrinsic causes of UPJO: aperistaltic segment of proximal ureter, congenital ureteral strictures due to excessive collagen deposition, and ureteral fibroepithelial polyps

Diagnostic Assessment

Ultrasonography

For infants who have been diagnosed prenatally with hydronephrosis, a renal ultrasound should be obtained neonatally to reassess the dilatation of the renal collecting system. Renal ultrasonography does not diagnose obstruction or predict resolution; however, it can correlate with a clinically relevant obstructive process. When the anterior posterior diameter of the renal pelvis is >15 mm, it is suggestive of the presence of obstruction, as is a trend of worsening hydronephrosis over

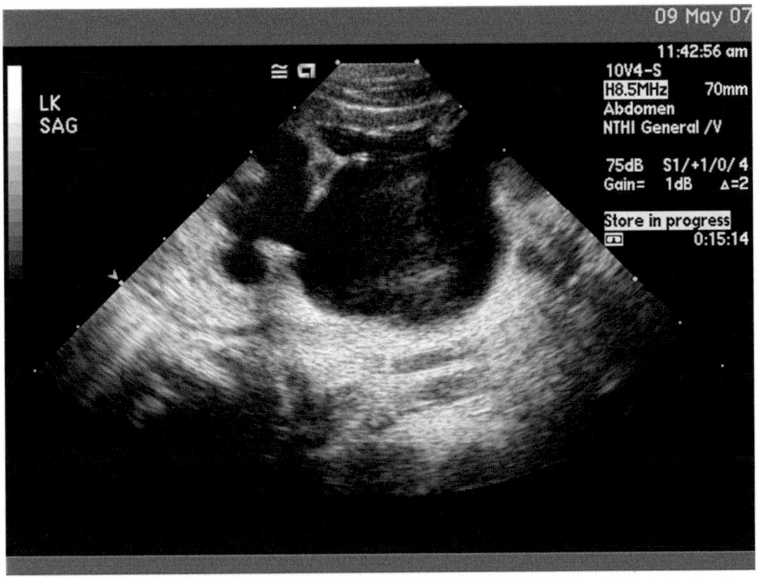

Fig. 8.3 Typical appearance of a UPJO on ultrasonography

time (Fig. 8.3). Renal size should be measured in the affected kidney and contralateral kidney over a period of time. As obstruction worsens, there tends to be an overall decrease in function and growth of the affected kidney with a compensatory hypertrophy of the contralateral healthy kidney. Ultrasonography is also a useful tool in older children who present acutely. This modality is a relatively simple, non-invasive test that can monitor dilation over time. It can be easily done in the office setting.

Computerized Tomography

Computerized tomography (CT) has not been the first-line imaging modality for the diagnosis of hydronephrosis or UPJO in children, particularly infants. This is primarily due to the radiation exposure risk of CT and the relative ease and accuracy of renal ultrasonography. However, many older children with UPJO who present with non-specific complaints of abdominal pain or nausea and vomiting are evaluated with a CT scan to differentiate other possible causes of their symptoms such as appendicitis or bowel obstruction. The typical CT scan appearance of UPJO is significant hydronephrosis without the presence of a dilated ureter (Fig. 8.4). CT can also be beneficial in defining retroperitoneal anatomy, particularly aberrant lower pole crossing vessels to the kidney. When performed with IV contrast, an overall functional assessment of the kidney can also be made; however, the benefits of this modality often do not outweigh the radiation risk or cost of the study. CT as a primary imaging study should be evaluated on an individual basis after the risks and benefits have been considered.

Intravenous Pyelogram

Intravenous pyelography (IVP) has fallen out of favor in the workup of hydronephrosis and suspected UPJO due to its high radiation exposure and the ease and accuracy of other imaging modalities such as ultrasonography. IVP can still be useful in those cases with unclear anatomy and a confusing clinical picture. The ideal timing for this study would be during an acute episode of obstruction.

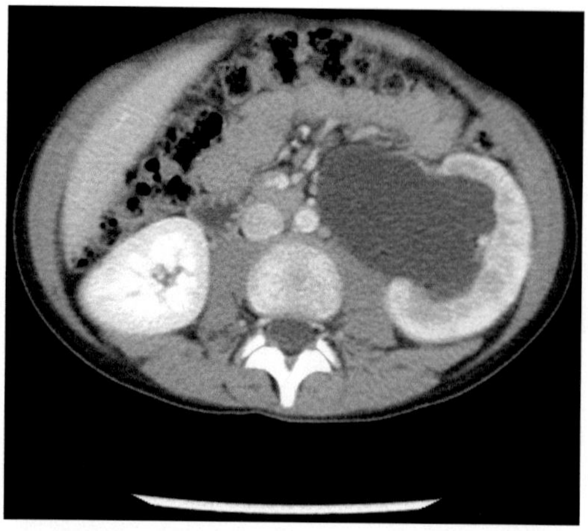

Fig. 8.4 The typical CT scan appearance of UPJO: significant hydronephrosis without the presence of a dilated ureter

Voiding Cystourethrogram

A voiding cystourethrogram (VCUG) should be performed in all children with prenatally diagnosed hydronephrosis to evaluate for the presence of vesicoureteral reflux (VUR) even if UPJO is suspected as the cause of collecting system dilatation. VUR is present in 40% of children with UPJO, although it is usually low grade [9]. In older children, this testing modality is not necessary.

Diuretic Radionuclide Renography

Radionuclide renography is an objective study that is able to suggest the diagnosis of obstruction by analyzing quantitative data regarding differential renal function. When performed in conjunction with the administration of a diuretic, this test is able to assess the velocity of washout of the radioisotope from each kidney, hence a direct measurement of renal collecting system emptying. This test is mainly performed with mercaptoacetyltriglycine (MAG3), which is excreted mostly by the proximal renal tubules and provides an indirect means of measuring estimated renal plasma flow. The measurement of the excretory curve of the renogram will correlate with the efficiency of emptying of the renal pelvis. In an obstructed system, the radioisotope is not as effectively cleared from the kidney. Furosemide is usually given to promote diuresis and emptying. When the kidney does not respond to the diuretic, it is assumed that there is a loss of renal function and/or significant renal obstruction [13]. The relative standard would be to perform this test in a well-hydrated child with a catheter draining the bladder, as a full bladder can lead to vesicoureteral reflux in the susceptible ureter or poor emptying in an otherwise unobstructed system. It is our preference that the diuretic be administered 20–30 min after the renogram ($F + 20–30$) or when the renal pelvis is filled with contrast, whichever is later. Following administration of the diuretic, the time to washout suggests the degree of obstruction.

The analysis of the drainage curve should take into consideration the technique and the time to diuretic administration. A general standard in analyzing the curve is to report the time it takes for the radioisotope activity to decrease by 50% ($T_{1/2}$). If the $T_{1/2}$ is less than 10 min, the study is determined to be normal. When the $T_{1/2}$ is between 10 and 20 min, the study is equivocal, and if the $T_{1/2}$ is greater than 20 min the kidney reportedly is obstructed (Fig. 8.5). Caution must be observed when taking these results at absolute face value, as the technique, the drainage curves, and the clinical condition of the child must be taken into consideration in the analysis. It should be noted that diuretic renography should not generally be performed in infants less than a month of age, as false-positive results may be obtained with an immature kidney.

Pressure Flow Study

A pressure flow study is an invasive test that measures the intrapelvic pressure during infusion of a fluid into the renal pelvis and the subsequent decrease in intrapelvic pressure over time. This

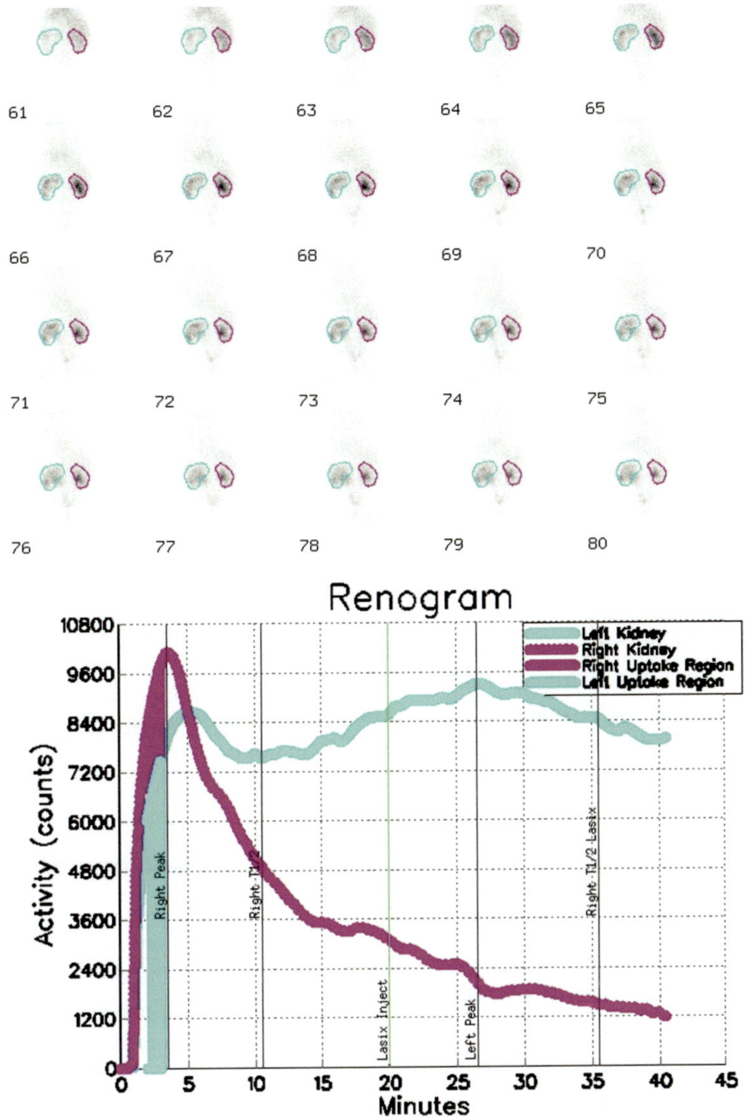

Fig. 8.5 Mag 3 Lasix scan drainage curve in the setting of UPJO

is termed as the pressure decay. The pressure decay represents the efficiency of urine transport as well as the relative compliance and volume of the collecting system [14]. A rapid pressure decay indicates a non-obstructed system, while a slow pressure decay demonstrates obstruction. Pressure flow studies are not routinely performed in the pediatric population and are usually used in equivocal clinical situations after a prior repair.

Patient Management: Asymptomatic vs. Symptomatic

Asymptomatic patients are typically diagnosed prenatally or in infancy. Older management schemes included surgical intervention within the first few months of life. Because many of these kidneys will improve spontaneously, most infants are currently managed expectantly with close monitoring and follow-up. The goal is to prevent children from having unnecessary surgery while balancing the need to intervene on the population that will deteriorate without intervention.

There are general guidelines that determine which infant is appropriate for observation. Typically patients with greater than 40% split function of the affected kidney, stable hydronephrosis over time, stable renal function and no urinary tract infections can be monitored closely without intervention. Our protocol is to perform renal ultrasounds every 3–4 months for the first year of life, followed by every 6 months for the next 2 years, then annually. If there is a change in the renal ultrasound, diuretic radionuclide renography should be obtained. If there is greater than a 10% decline in overall function of the affected kidney, surgical intervention should be considered.

Children who do not present prenatally, have progressing hydronephrosis on serial exams, have less than 40% function of the affected kidney, or who present clinically with colic, hematuria, stones, or infection should undergo operative intervention for the management of UPJO.

Surgical Management

Open dismembered pyeloplasty has been the gold standard treatment of UPJO for decades; however, recent outcomes of laparoscopic pyeloplasty in children are consistent with those of open pyeloplasty [15–17], and this has become our preferred technique in the management of UPJO in the pediatric population. Laparoscopic pyeloplasty in children has followed a similar evolution as other forms of laparoscopic renal surgery, in that the techniques and equipment that were developed in adults have been refined for the pediatric population. The benefits of the laparoscopic technique include improved cosmesis, reduced postoperative morbidity, shorter convalescence, and increased magnification and visualization.

Transperitoneal, retroperitoneal, and robotic approaches for laparoscopic pyeloplasty have all been described in the literature, with advocates for each procedure [15, 18, 19]. In the end, the approach used should be based on the experience and comfort of the operating surgeon. In this section we will describe each procedure in detail as well as surgical outcomes.

Pre-operative Assessment

Upon initial evaluation, a thorough history and physical exam must be obtained. Antenatal history for hydronephrosis should be elicited. The presence of a palpable kidney, as well as a personal or family history of other urologic issues, should be noted. In our practice, age is not an exclusion factor for a laparoscopic pyeloplasty. Our youngest patient to date has been less than 3 months of age.

Instruments in Pediatric Laparoscopy

There are two basic types of instruments used in pediatric urology: those used to gain access to the patient and those used to perform the actual operation. Access can be gained in a variety of ways. Common approaches include the Veress needle technique, which allows for CO_2 insufflation of the working space followed by blind insertion of a trocar, and a variety of open techniques, which include the Hassan cannula system [20, 21]. The options for working elements for pediatric laparoscopic pyeloplasty include scissors, needle drivers, graspers, forceps, retractors, and cautery devices, such as the harmonic scalpel (Ethicon, Cincinnati). These instruments are mainly 5 mm in size, with some instruments 3 mm in diameter. These instruments are now made with shorter shaft lengths, specifically for pediatric indications. Suture-assist devices, often used in adult pyeloplasty, are not suitable for reconstruction in children, given their instrument and suture size. Laparoscopic devices are constantly evolving, and the choices available to the practitioner are expanding; however, a balance between cost effectiveness and practicality should be considered in deciding their utility.

Transperitoneal Laparoscopic Pyeloplasty

Transperitoneal laparoscopic pyeloplasty in the pediatric population was the first approach described in the literature [6]. Although there is a theoretical risk of intra-abdominal injury while performing a transabdominal technique, in fact this is rare [22]. Advocates of this approach have suggested that the retroperitoneal technique provides less working space often making the procedure difficult in smaller children and infants [22]. There is also some question as to whether crossing vessels are more easily missed [22]. Transperitoneal laparoscopic pyeloplasty is the preferred technique at our institution, and in this section we will describe in detail the operative procedure and also discuss surgical outcomes.

Technique

Open communication with the anesthesia team is essential. Inhaled NO_2 should not be used in order to avoid bowel distention, and an oral gastric tube should be inserted to maximize visualization in the intra-abdominal cavity. After induction of general anesthesia, the patient is placed in the dorsal lithotomy position and rigid cystoscopy is performed. A retrograde pyelogram of the affected side is performed to get an assessment of the anatomy. A guidewire is placed into the renal pelvis under fluoroscopic guidance, and a double-J ureteral stent is inserted into the kidney. An appropriate sized Foley catheter is inserted for the duration of the case. The patient is then repositioned into a 45° flank position. We do not believe that an axillary roll is necessary in the pediatric patient if the child is properly positioned and supported with either pressure or stretch placed on the axilla. The patient is secured to the bed with wide tape at the level of the chest and low thigh. Care is taken to place the tape without tension over the chest and legs and not to restrict ventilation. Securing the child to the table permits Trendelenburg or laterally rolled positions. When prepping and draping, plan for an open procedure and drape accordingly.

Access into the peritoneum is achieved in an open fashion at the umbilicus. Blind access for pneumoperitoneum with a Veress needle or a trocar is less commonly used in the pediatric population as an overly compliant abdomen may increase the risk of injury to intra-abdominal structures. It is our preference to use the Bailez Technique for open access [23], modified to employ the use of a radially dilating trocar. For this technique, a 2-0 Vicryl suture is placed in the umbilicus to provide continual anterior tension. A 3-mm hidden infraumbilical incision is made in the skin and a scissor is then used at an approximate 15–20° angle cephalad to cut through the umbilical fascia into the underlying adherent peritoneum. Alternatively, the rectus fascia and underlying peritoneum may be entered sharply at 90° under direct vision.

For the umbilical camera port, we utilize a 5-mm radially dilating trocar to accommodate a 5-mm camera with either a 30 or a 0° lens. The patient's abdomen is insufflated at 1–2 l/min to a pressure of 10–12 cmH_2O. A general survey of the abdomen is undertaken, inspecting the underlying bowel for injury that might have occurred during port placement.

For left-sided procedures, the ureteropelvic junction (UPJ) is accessed via a transmesenteric approach in most cases, and for the right-sided procedures, access is gained by mobilizing the colon to the level of the hepatic flexure (Fig. 8.6). The renal pelvis is usually readily identifiable, even after placement of a double-J ureteral stent. If the renal pelvis is not evident, the ureter can be identified and traced proximally to the UPJ and the renal pelvis. After the UPJ has been dissected clear of the surrounding tissues, complete transection and excision of the abnormal segment can be performed (Fig. 8.7). Dissection can be

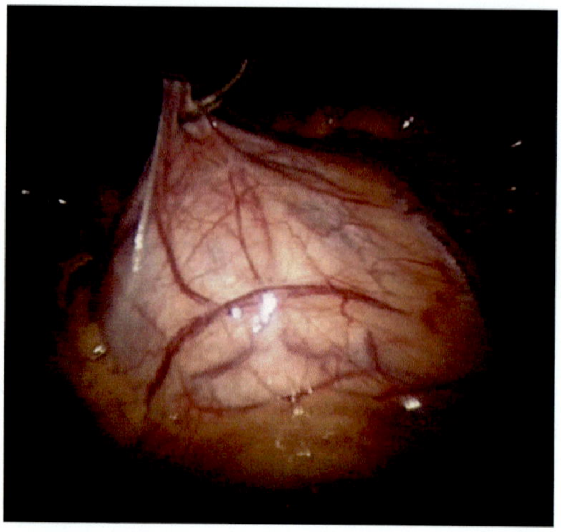

Fig. 8.6 Obtaining access to left UPJO through the mesentary

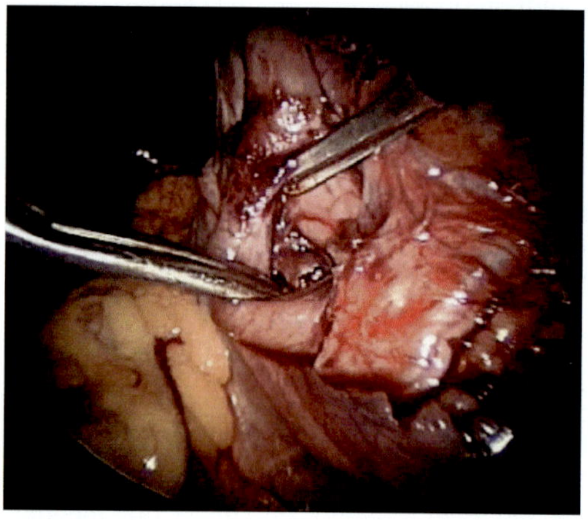

Fig. 8.7 Exposure of the UPJO

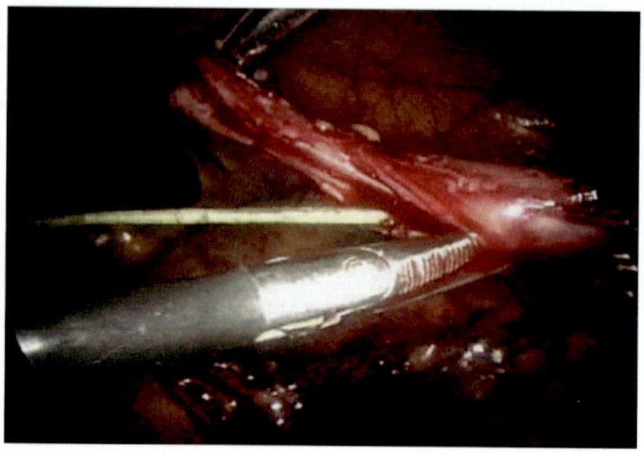

Fig. 8.8 Spatulation of the ureter after dismemberment

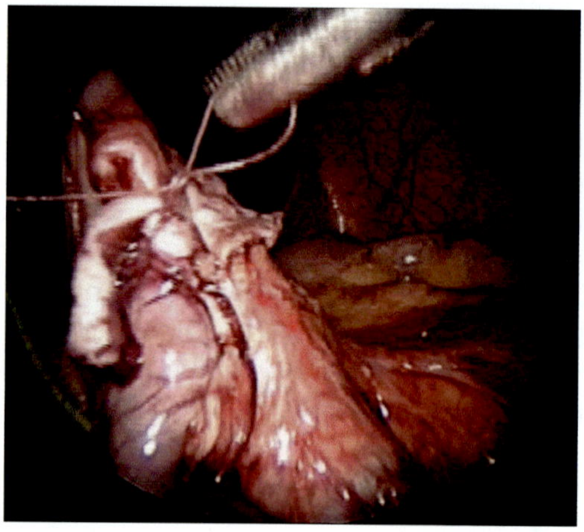

Fig. 8.9 Intracorporeal suturing of the anastomosis

aided by early placement of an anterior pelvic stay suture through the anterior abdominal wall. If there is no crossing vessel, the pelvis can be divided just above the UPJ to leave a "handle" of distal pelvis on the ureter. If there are crossing vessels, the pelvis is exposed above the vessels, and the space behind the vessels is developed. The ureter may be divided just above the UPJ, and then the UPJ is lifted anterior to the vessels for anastomosis. The ureter is spatulated laterally (Fig. 8.8), and intracorporeal suturing using 5-0 or 6-0 absorbable suture is performed to anastomose the two segments (Fig. 8.9). An indwelling double pigtail ureteral stent is placed into its final position prior to completion of the anastomosis. In rare occasions the stent is placed antegrade over a guidewire if the ureteral stent was unable to be placed retrograde at the beginning of the case. After completion of the anastomosis, the hitch stitch is removed and the renal pelvis is placed back into orthotopic position. Prior to closing the ports, excess urine and fluid, which normally settles in the gravity-dependent portions of the intraperitoneal cavity, are suctioned to minimize bowl irritation and post-op ileus.

The abdomen is surveyed a final time and the pneumoperitoneum pressure is lowered. Any occult bleeding should be identified and addressed at this point. While maintaining pneumoperitoneum, the two accessory ports are removed sequentially and inspected for bleeding. The fascial layers of these trocar sites are closed with 2-0 Vicryl suture. The laparoscopic view is maintained on the port sites during closure to ensure that it is airtight and free of any intra-abdominal contents (i.e., bowel or omentum). Through the umbilical port the pneumoperitoneum is evacuated. Larger tidal volumes given by the anesthesiologist and mild abdominal pressure help with the expulsion of CO_2. The umbilical trocar and camera are removed while inspecting for bleeding. Fascial sutures are placed in the umbilical port, the skin is closed, and dressings are applied.

A Foley catheter is left overnight in all of these cases. Generally, the patient stays overnight in the hospital and is discharged home on a regular diet. The stent is removed 4–6 weeks postoperatively. An office ultrasound is performed 1 and 6 months after stent removal if the patient remains symptom free. We do not routinely perform a Lasix renal scan and reserve this test for children who remain symptomatic or children who do not have improvement of their hydronephrosis on ultrasound.

Outcomes

The first transperitoneal laparoscopic dismembered pyeloplasty series of 18 children was reported in 1999 by Tan [24]. Mean laparoscopic time was 89 min and no patient required conversion to an open procedure, although two patients continued to have persistent obstruction and required repeat laparoscopic pyeloplasty [24]. Other series have demonstrated that transperitoneal pyeloplasty has comparable efficacy and success rates to the open procedure [15–17, 24, 25]. In a series of 46 children, Metzelder [26] reported that transperitoneal laparoscopic pyeloplasty was safe and effective in children from infancy until 18 years of age. In a series of eight infants aged 3–5 months, Kutikov [27] demonstrated that a transperitoneal approach was safe and effective in children less than 6 months of age.

In our series, 112 patients underwent transperitoneal laparoscopic pyeloplasty for the treatment of symptomatic or radiographic UPJO, from 2001 to 2009. Mean patient age was 9.4 years (0.2–20.5 years), and 15 patients were under 18 months of age. Follow-up was available on all 112 patients with a mean duration of 15.3 months (0.6–84.5 months). There was one open conversion in the series, for an open conversion rate of 0.8%. Total laparoscopic operative time was 254 min (102–525 min). One intraoperative complication was reported (0.8%), which resolved without any long-term sequelae. There were 12 (10.8%) postoperative complications; most were relatively minor with complete resolution without long-term sequelae. Postoperative ultrasound has been performed in 102 patients, with 99 (97%) patients demonstrating improvement of the UPJO. Three patients (4%) continued to have symptomatic and/or radiographic evidence of obstruction which necessitated the need for adjunctive procedures, which included laser endopyelotomy in two patients and a re-do open pyeloplasty in one patient. Of those cases that were completed laparoscopically, the overall success rate was 97.2% (Sweeney et al., Laparoscopic pyeloplasty in the pediatric population: evolution of technique, Not Published, 2009).

Retroperitoneal Approach

Retroperitoneal laparoscopic pyeloplasty is a well-described technique with advocates suggesting an easier dissection of the UPJ [22]. However, the working space is small and this can become problematic in younger children, particularly when performing the ureteropelvic anastomosis [24, 28]. Because of these limitations, some surgeons have made modifications to the technique including a laparoscopic-assisted procedure that performs extracorporeal suturing of the anastomosis at the level of the skin [29, 30]. In this section we will discuss the various techniques and the outcomes associated with them.

Technique

The retroperitoneal laparoscopic dismembered pyeloplasty, as reported by Yeung, will be described [31]. The modifications advocated by other authors will be discussed later in the chapter [18]. The patient is placed in a semi-prone position with the flank at a 45° angle. A 1-cm incision is made over the mid-axillary line about 4 cm above the iliac crest, and the retroperitoneal space is entered and developed using a glove balloon. A 5-mm laparoscope is used, and two additional working ports (3 or 5 mm) are inserted above and below the camera port. A fourth port on occasion is necessary and is typically inserted below the 12th rib, lateral to the paraspinus muscle.

The kidney is identified and Gerota's fascia is entered and the lower pole of the kidney is exposed. At this point the renal pelvis and proximal ureter are identified and are dissected free. A 4-0 Prolene hitch stitch is passed percutaneous through the abdominal wall and is used to elevate the renal pelvis to aid in dissection. The UPJ is then dismembered, and the ureter is spatulated prior to starting the anastomosis. The anastomosis is completed with 6-0 Vicryl suture in a running fashion. If a double-J ureteral stent is not placed at the beginning of the case, it is inserted antegrade prior to completion of the anterior layer of the anastomosis. The hitch stitch is removed and the reconstructed UPJ is placed in its orthotopic position. The retroperitoneum is deinsufflated and the ports are closed in the previously described manner.

El Ghoneimi [18] described his retroperitoneal laparoscopic approach in a series that was published 2003. His modifications include placing the first port 1 cm from the lower border of the tip of the 12th rib and dissecting down to Gerota's fascia through a muscle-splitting incision. Gerota's fascia is opened under direct vision and the first trocar is placed inside this layer. Dissection of Gerota's fascia is made by insufflating with CO_2. A 0° laparoscope is inserted into this port. A second 3-mm port is inserted posteriorly near the costovertebral angle, and the third 3-mm port is inserted 1 cm superior to the top of the iliac crest in the anterior axillary line. Dissection of the UPJ is carried out as described above; however, they recommend dismembering the UPJ in the most dependent location so as to leave a handle of renal pelvis and ureter connected to minimize tension of the repair when the anastomosis is being sewn. This handle of tissue is resected at the conclusion of the anastomosis.

Outcomes

In Yeung's initial series of retroperitoneal laparoscopic dismembered pyeloplasty, there was one open conversion out of 13 patients [31]. Mean laparoscopic time was 143 min, and there were no intraoperative or postoperative complications [31]. Of the 12 completed cases, all demonstrated an improvement in the radiographic imaging of the UPJO [31]. In the largest series to date, El Ghoneimi [18] reported a series of 22 cases with four open conversions. Mean operative time was 228 min, and average hospital stay was 2.5 days [18]. In the only retrospective comparison published to date between retroperitoneal laparoscopic pyeloplasty and open pyeloplasty, Bonnard reported a significant decrease in both hospital stay (2.4 vs. 5 days) and postoperative acetaminophen requirement for patients undergoing retroperitoneal laparoscopic pyeloplasty. However, when compared to the open group, the laparoscopic group had a significantly longer mean operative time (219 vs. 96 min) [22].

Due to the limitations of the retroperitoneal technique, Farhat describes a retroperitoneal-assisted laparoscopic pyeloplasty technique that has the advantage of the laparoscopic UPJ dissection but performs the dismembered anastomosis in an extracorporeal fashion [30]. This approach is based on the principles of the dorsal lumbotomy incision. In this technique a urethral catheter is placed and connected to an infusion of methylene blue-tinted saline. The patient is placed in the flank position, and a 1 cm incision is made inferior to the tip of the 12th rib. To minimize gas leakage from the retroperitoneum, 2-0 absorbable sutures are placed in a purse-string fashion in the abdominal fascial layers. A 10-mm Hassan trocar with a blunt tip is inserted into this incision around the perinephric space, and the retroperitoneal space is insufflated with CO_2. Posterior mobilization of the kidney is performed bluntly using the laparoscope, and two additional 5-mm ports are placed: one anterior to the paraspinal muscles and the other superior to the anterior superior iliac spine. Once these ports are placed, further dissection of the kidney and UPJ is performed. A 5-0 Prolene stay suture is placed through the 10-mm trocar into the atretic segment of the UPJ and the needle end is brought through the same trocar. At this point a portion of the renal pelvis and UPJ is brought through the 10-mm port incision after removal of the Hassan trocar. Multiple stay sutures are recommended to lessen the tension placed during manipulation. Prior to bringing the UPJ to the level of the skin, the ureter is transected below the level of the obstruction, and the renal pelvis and the ureter are brought to the level of the skin separately. Completion of the anastomosis with 6-0 PDS is accomplished extracorporeally, and prior to completion of the anastomosis, a double-J ureteral stent is placed antegrade. Efflux of methylene blue from the stent indicates correct position of the distal portion into the bladder. A Penrose drain is placed through one of the 5-mm port sites, the UPJ is returned into the retroperitoneum, and the flank and port sites are closed.

Outcomes

In Farhat's initial series,this procedure was performed successfully in 10 patients, with an average operative time of 160 min [30]. There were two open conversions and postoperative urine leak in one patient. All patients demonstrated improvement in their obstruction post-procedure as measured by diuretic renography [30]. In the largest series to date, using this technique with some minor modifications, Abraham reported 39 procedures, with a mean operative time of 147 min. All cases were completed in the retroperitoneal-assisted laparoscopic fashion with no open conversions [29]. There was improved function of the kidney in 37 patients, no improvement in 1 patient, and deterioration of renal function in 1 patient, for an overall success rate of 94.8% [29].

Robotic-Assisted Laparoscopic Pyeloplasty

Technological advances in the field of laparoscopic surgery have allowed for the application of robotic technology, which was first described by Partin [32] in the adult urologic population. There are few studies that have examined its use in pediatric population. Robotic-assisted laparoscopy allows three-dimensional visualization and seven degrees of freedom, making suturing and fine motor movements more intuitive; however, there is loss of tactile feedback. Moreover, the use of the robot often requires additional and larger ports as compared to standard laparoscopy. However, the technology continues to evolve, and 8- and 5-mm port sizes are now available. Compared to traditional laparoscopy, the overall cost of equipment and training is much higher for the robotic device, and the equipment is not universally available.

Laparoscopic pyeloplasty seems a natural candidate for a robotic assistance, given the delicate intracorporeal suturing required for the procedure. This procedure can be performed through either a transperitoneal or a retroperitoneal approach. The robot is most helpful to those early in the learning curve, and its major value will be in increasing access to minimally invasive procedures in centers lacking experience in complex laparoscopic technique. The following techniques are as described by Casale [33].

Robotic-Assisted Transperitoneal Approach

After cystoscopy and insertion of the double-J ureteral stent, the patient is placed in a modified flank position. The first robotic trocar is placed at the umbilicus, and a 0° robotic telescope is inserted. A robotic arm trocar is inserted subcostal and lateral to the ipsilateral rectus muscle, and the second robotic arm trocar is inserted 1 cm above the top of the iliac crest lateral to the ipsilateral rectus muscle. The UPJ dissection is performed in the identical manner as described in Section "Transperitoneal Laparoscopic Pyeloplasty." The anastomosis is similar to the transperitoneal laparoscopic technique in that it is performed in a running fashion with 6-0 absorbable suture.

Robotic-Assisted Retroperitoneal Approach

The patient is placed in either a modified semi-prone position for a left-sided operation or a 45° right lateral decubitus position for right-sided procedures. Retroperitoneal access is achieved by making a 1.5 cm muscle-splitting incision off the lower border of the tip of the 12th rib. The port is inserted and fixed with a purse-string suture around the abdominal fascial layers. The retroperitoneal space is created by insufflation of CO_2. The 8-mm robotic trocar is inserted posterior near the costovertebral angle, and the other 8-mm robotic trocar is inserted 10 mm above the top of the iliac crest at the anterior axillary line. The kidney is approached posteriorly and lower pole of the kidney is exposed by entering Gerota's fascia parallel to the psoas muscle. The UPJ is dissected free and stay sutures are placed to help keep orientation and to aid in manipulation. The renal pelvis is dismembered partially, at the most dependent part, and the ureter is partly divided and spatulated. The anastomosis is then performed in the identical manner as described in the previous section.

Outcomes

In a comparison between adult laparoscopic pyeloplasty performed with the da Vinci (Intuitive Surgical, Sunnyvale, CA) robotic system to procedures performed with standard laparoscopic techniques, Gettman [34] reported decreased operative times with robotic assistance. However, these results have not been duplicated. In a prospective comparison in adults, Link [35] reported that mean operative and total room times for robotic-assisted laparoscopic pyeloplasty were significantly longer than those of standard laparoscopic pyeloplasty by 19.5 and 39.0 min, respectively. Further, the robotic laparoscopic pyeloplasty was 2.7 times more costly than the laparoscopic pyeloplasty due to longer operative time, increased consumables costs, and depreciation of the da Vinci system [35]. Link concluded that for the experienced laparoscopist, application of the da Vinci robot resulted in no significant clinical advantage and added substantial cost to transperitoneal laparoscopic dismembered pyeloplasty [35]. Initial series in the pediatric urology literature have demonstrated that the robotic technique is technically feasible and safe; however, operative times did not approach those of the standard open procedure, and there was no clear advantage in the reduction of postoperative morbidity compared to the standard laparoscopic pyeloplasty [19, 36–38]. However, Olsen described his experience of robot-assisted retroperitoneoscopic pyeloplasty, over a 5-year period, and reported shorter operative times and complication rates comparable to the transperitoneal robotic-assisted pyeloplasty, standard laparoscopic pyeloplasty, and open pyeloplasty in the pediatric population [39].

Early results with robotic-assisted laparoscopy are encouraging and warrant further evaluation.

Hopefully, the technology will advance to a point where it becomes advantageous even to those with significant reconstructive experience.

Conclusion

The spectrum of laparoscopic urological surgery in children continues to expand, although it still lags behind its adult counterparts. Procedures such as laparoscopic pyeloplasty and laparoscopic reconstructive surgery have only recently been introduced and are primarily available at centers with advanced laparoscopic experience. Laparoscopic pyeloplasty for UPJO in the pediatric population is technically challenging; however, with experience, excellent success rates with few complications and reasonable operative times can be expected. Results are consistent with those for open pyeloplasty, with potentially less postoperative incisional discomfort, a quicker convalescence, and an excellent cosmetic outcome. In experienced hands, laparoscopic pyeloplasty should be considered an accepted technique for repair of ureteropelvic junction obstruction. As the field continues to evolve with improvement in technology and surgeons entering the profession with basic laparoscopic backgrounds, pediatric urologic laparoscopy will also continue to progress. It is our hope that minimally invasive approaches to urologic conditions will become more available to children in the near future.

Critical Operative Steps for Transperitoneal Laparoscopic Pyeloplasty

1. Cystoscopy and retrograde pyelogram of the affected side to assess the anatomy.
2. Double-J ureteral stent is inserted into the kidney.
3. The patient is then repositioned in a 45° flank position and the patient is secured to the bed with wide tape at the level of the chest and low thigh.
4. Access into the peritoneum is achieved in an open fashion at the umbilicus. For the umbilical camera port, we utilize a 5-mm radially dilating trocar to accommodate a 5-mm camera with either a 30° or a 0° lens.
5. The patient's abdomen is insufflated at 1–2 l/min to a pressure of 10–12 cmH_2O. A general survey of the abdomen is undertaken.
6. For left-sided procedures, the ureteropelvic junction (UPJ) is accessed via a transmesenteric approach, and for the right-sided procedures, access is gained by mobilizing the colon to the level of the hepatic flexure.
7. The UPJ is dissected clear of the surrounding tissues, and complete transection and excision of the abnormal segment can be performed. If there is no crossing vessel, the pelvis can be divided just above the UPJ to leave a "handle" of distal pelvis on the ureter. If there are crossing vessels, the pelvis is exposed above the vessels, and the space behind the vessels is developed. The ureter may be divided just above the UPJ, and then the UPJ is lifted anterior to the vessels for anastomosis.
8. The ureter is spatulated laterally and intracorporeal suturing using 5-0 or 6-0 absorbable suture is performed to anastomose the two segments.
9. An indwelling double pigtail ureteral stent is placed into its final position prior to completion of the anastomosis.
10. Renal pelvis is placed back into orthotopic position.
11. The abdomen is surveyed a final time and the pneumoperitoneum pressure is lowered. While maintaining pneumoperitoneum, the two accessory ports are removed sequentially and inspected for bleeding. The fascial layers

of these trocar sites are closed with 2-0 Vicryl suture.

12. Through the umbilical port the pneumoperitoneum is evacuated. The umbilical trocar and camera are removed while inspecting for bleeding. Fascial sutures are placed in the umbilical port, the skin is closed, and dressings are applied.

Critical Operative Steps for Retroperitoneal Laparoscopic Pyeloplasty

1. Cystoscopy performed as previously described for the transperitoneal approach.
2. The patient is placed in a semi-prone position with the flank at a 45° angle.
3. A 1-cm incision is made over the mid-axillary line about 4 cm above the iliac crest, and the retroperitoneal space is entered and developed using a glove balloon.
4. A 5-mm laparoscope is used, and two additional working ports (3 or 5 mm) are inserted above and below the camera port.
5. The kidney is identified and Gerota's fascia is entered and the lower pole of the kidney is exposed. At this point, the renal pelvis and proximal ureter are identified and are dissected free.
6. A 4-0 Prolene hitch stitch is passed percutaneously through the abdominal wall and is used to elevate the renal pelvis to aid in dissection.
7. The UPJ is then dismembered, and the ureter is spatulated prior to starting the anastomosis. The anastomosis is completed with 6-0 Vicryl suture in a running fashion.
8. If a double-J ureteral stent is not placed at the beginning of the case, it is inserted antegrade prior to completion of the anterior layer of the anastomosis.
9. The hitch stitch is removed and the reconstructed UPJ is placed in its orthotopic position.
10. The retroperitoneum is deinsufflated and the ports are closed in the previously described manner.

Critical Operative Steps for Retroperitoneal-Assisted Laparoscopic Pyeloplasty

1. A urethral catheter is placed and connected to an infusion of methylene blue-tinted saline.
2. The patient is placed in the flank position, and a 1-cm incision is made inferior to the tip of the 12th rib.
3. A 10-mm Hassan trocar with a blunt tip is inserted into this incision around the perinephric space, and the retroperitoneal space is insufflated with CO_2.
4. Posterior mobilization of the kidney is performed bluntly using the laparoscope, and two additional 5-mm ports are placed: one anterior to the paraspinal muscles and the other superior to the anterior superior iliac spine.
5. Dissection of the kidney and UPJ is performed. A 5-0 Prolene stay suture is placed through the 10-mm trocar into the atretic segment of the UPJ and the needle end is brought through the same trocar. A portion of the renal pelvis and UPJ is brought through the 10-mm port incision after removal of the Hassan trocar.
6. Multiple stay sutures are placed to lessen the tension placed during manipulation. Prior to bringing the UPJ to the level of the skin, the ureter is transected below the level of the obstruction, and the renal pelvis and ureter are brought to the level of the skin separately.
7. Completion of the anastomosis with 6-0 PDS is accomplished extracorporeally, and prior to completion of the anastomosis a double-J ureteral stent is placed antegrade.
8. Efflux of methylene blue from the stent indicates correct position of the distal portion into the bladder.
9. A Penrose drain is placed through one of the 5-mm port sites, the UPJ is returned into the

retroperitoneum, and the flank and port sites are closed.

Critical Operative Steps for Robotic-Assisted Transperitoneal Pyeloplasty

1. Cystoscopy and patient positioning performed in the same manner as the transperitoneal laparoscopic pyeloplasty.
2. The first robotic trocar is placed at the umbilicus, and a 0° robotic telescope is inserted.
3. A robotic arm trocar is inserted subcostal and lateral to the ipsilateral rectus muscle, and the second robotic arm trocar is inserted 1 cm above the top of the iliac crest lateral to the ipsilateral rectus muscle.
4. The UPJ dissection and anastomosis are performed in the identical manner as described for transperitoneal laparoscopic pyeloplasty.

Critical Operative Steps for Robotic-Assisted Retroperitoneal Pyeloplasty

1. The patient is placed in either a modified semi-prone position for a left-sided operation or a 45° right lateral decubitus position for right-sided procedures.
2. Retroperitoneal access is achieved by making a 1.5-cm muscle-splitting incision off the lower border of the tip of the 12th rib. The port is inserted and fixed with a purse-string suture around the abdominal fascial layers.
3. The retroperitoneal space is created by insufflation of CO_2.
4. The 8-mm robotic trocar is inserted posterior near the costovertebral angle, and the other 8-mm robotic trocar is inserted 10 mm above the top of the iliac crest at the anterior axillary line.
5. The kidney is approached posteriorly and the lower pole of the kidney is exposed by entering Gerota's fascia parallel to the psoas muscle.
6. The UPJ is dissected free and stay sutures are placed to help keep orientation and to aid in manipulation.
7. The renal pelvis is dismembered partially, at the most dependent part, and the ureter is partly divided and spatulated.
8. The anastomosis is then performed in the identical manner as described in the previous section.

Critical Instruments

1. Laparoscopic ports
2. Laparoscopic scissors with Bovie attachment
3. Laparoscopic needle drivers (3 or 5 mm)
4. Laparoscopic graspers and forceps (3 or 5 mm)
5. Laparoscopic cautery devices 5 mm (harmonic scalpel; Ethicon, Cincinnati).
6. da Vinci robot system (Intuitive Surgical, Sunnyvale, CA)
7. 5-0 or 6-0 absorbable suture for anastomosis

References

1. Cortesi N, Ferrari P, Zambarda E, et al. Diagnosis of bilateral abdominal cryptorchidism by laparoscopy. Endoscopy. 1976;8:33.
2. Peters CA. Laparoscopy in pediatric urology. Curr Opin Urol. 2004;14:67.
3. El Ghoneimi A. Laparoscopic management of hydronephrosis in children. World J Urol. 2004;22:415.
4. Jarrett TW, Chan DY, Charambura TC, et al. Laparoscopic pyeloplasty: the first 100 cases. J Urol. 2002;167:1253.
5. Schuessler WW, Grune MT, Tecuanhuey LV, et al. Laparoscopic dismembered pyeloplasty. J Urol. 1993;150:1795.
6. Peters CA, Schlussel RN, Retik AB. Pediatric laparoscopic dismembered pyeloplasty. J Urol. 1995;153:1962.
7. Sidhu G, Beyene J, Rosenblum ND. Outcome of isolated antenatal hydronephrosis: a systematic review and meta-analysis. Pediatr Nephrol. 2006;21:218.

8. Brown T, Mandell J, Lebowitz RL. Neonatal hydronephrosis in the era of ultrasonography. Am J Roentgenol. 1987;148:959.
9. Lebowitz RL, Blickman JG. The coexistence of ureteropelvic junction obstruction and reflux. Am J Roentgenol. 1983;140:231.
10. Hanna MK, Jeffs RD, Sturgess JM, et al. Ureteral structure and ultrastructure: part II. Congenital ureteropelvic junction obstruction and primary obstructive megaureter. J Urol. 1976;116:725.
11. Lowe FC, Marshall SF. Ureteropelvic junction obstruction in adults. Urology. 1984;23:331.
12. Reddy N, Mandell J. Prenatal diagnosis: therapeutic implications. Urol Clin North Am. 1998;25:171.
13. Gonzalez R, Schimke CM. Ureteropelvic junction obstruction in infants and children. Pediatr Clin North Am. 2001;1506.
14. Fung LCT, Khoury AE, McLorie GA, et al. Pressure decay half-life: a method for characterizing upper urinary tract urine transport. J Urol. 1996; 155:1045.
15. Piaggio LA, Franc-Guimond J, Noh PH, et al. Transperitoneal laparoscopic pyeloplasty for primary repair of ureteropelvic junction obstruction in infants and children: comparison with open surgery. J Urol. 2007;178:1579.
16. Lam PN, Wong C, Mulholland TL, et al. Pediatric laparoscopic pyeloplasty: 4 year experience. J Endourol. 2007;21:1467.
17. Lopez M, Guye E, Becmeur F, et al. Laparoscopic pyeloplasty for repair of pelviureteric junction obstruction in children. J Laparoendosc Adv Surg Tech. 2009;19:s91.
18. El Ghoneimi A, Farhat W, Bolduc S, et al. Laparoscopic dismembered pyeloplasty by a retroperitoneal approach in children. BJU. 2003;92.
19. Yee DS, Shanberg AM, Duel BP, et al. Initial comparison of robotic-assisted laparoscopic versus open pyeloplasty in children. Urology. 2006;67:599.
20. Cuellar DC, Kavoussi PK, Baker LA, et al. Open laparoscopic access using a radially dilating trocar: experience and indications in 50 consecutive cases. J Endourol. 2000;14:755.
21. Schulam PG, Hedican SP, Docimo SG. Radially dilating trocar system for open laparoscopic access. Urology. 1999;54:727.
22. Bonnard A, Fouquet V, Carricaburu E, et al. Retroperitoneal laparoscopic versus open pyeloplasty in children. J Urol. 2005;173:1710.
23. Docimo SG. Re: Experience with the Bailez technique for laparoscopic access in children. J Urol. 2004;171:806.
24. Tan HL. Laparoscopic Anderson–Hynes dismembered pyeloplasty in children. J Urol. 1999;162:1045.
25. Kojima Y, Sasaki S, Mizuno K, et al. Laparoscopic dismembered pyeloplasty for ureteropelvic junction obstruction in children. Int J Urol. 2009;16:472.
26. Metzelder ML, Schier F, Petersen C, et al. Laparoscopic transabdominal pyeloplasty in children is feasible irrespective of age. J Urol. 2006;175:688.
27. Kutikov A, Resnick M, Casale P. Laparoscopic pyeloplasty in the infant younger than 6 months – Is it technically possible. J Urol. 2006;175:1477.
28. Janestschek G, Peschel R, Altarac S, et al. Laparoscopic and retroperitoneoscopic repair of ureteropelvic junction obstruction. Urology. 1996;47:311.
29. Abraham MK, Rasheed AN, Bindu S, et al. Experience with laparoscopy-assisted retroperitoneal pyeloplasty in children. Pediatr Surg Int. 2009;25:601–605.
30. Farhat W, Afshar K, Papanikolaou F, et al. Retroperitoneal-assisted laparoscopic pyeloplasty in children: initial experience. J Endourol. 2004;18:879.
31. Yeung CK, Tam YH, Sihoe JDY, et al. Retroperitoneoscopic dismembered pyeloplasty for pelvi-ureteric junction in infants and children. BJU. 2001;87:509.
32. Partin AW, Adams JB, Moore RG, et al. Complete robot-assisted laparoscopic urologic surgery: a preliminary report. J Am Coll Surg. 1995;181:552.
33. Casale P. Robotic pyeloplasty in the pediatric population. Curr Urol Rep. 2009;10:55.
34. Gettman MT, Peschel R, Neururer R, et al. A comparison of laparoscopic pyeloplasty performed with the daVinci robotic system versus standard laparoscopic techniques: initial clinical results. Eur Urol. 2002;42:453.
35. Link RE, Bhayani SB, Kavoussi LR. A prospective comparison of robotic and laparoscopic pyeloplasty. Ann Surg. 2006;243:486.
36. Atug F, Woods M, Burgess SV, et al. Robotic assisted laparoscopic pyeloplasty in children. J Urol. 2005;174:1440.
37. Olsen LH, Jorgensen TM. Computer assisted pyeloplasty in children: the retroperitoneal approach. J Urol. 2004;171:2629.
38. Lee RS, Retik AB, Borer JG, et al. Pediatric robot assisted laparoscopic dismembered pyeloplasty: comparison with a cohort of open surgery. J Urol. 2006;175:683.
39. Olsen LH, Rawashdeh YF, Jorgensen TM. Pediatric robot assisted retroperitoneoscopic pyeloplasty: a 5 year experience. J Urol. 2007;178:2137.

Chapter 9

Pediatric Robotic (Infant, Pre-pubertal, and Teenager) Pyeloplasty for Ureteropelvic Junction Obstruction

Yoshiyuki Kojima and Pasquale Casale

Ureteropelvic junction obstruction (UPJO) is characterized by a functionally significant impairment of urinary transport caused by an intrinsic or an extrinsic obstruction in the area where the ureter joins the renal pelvis. This results in the gradual dilatation of the renal collecting system (hydronephrosis) and may lead to deterioration of renal function and pain. Therefore, the main goals of treatment are the preservation of renal function and the relief of symptoms.

Open pyeloplasty remains the standard surgical repair; however, conventional laparoscopic pyeloplasty has gained acceptance as a feasible and reliable treatment associated with minimal morbidity in the pediatric population, because it has several advantages over standard open pyeloplasty. The main advantages of conventional laparoscopic pyeloplasty include more rapid recovery, improved cosmetic outcome, less postoperative pain, and, consequently, lower analgesic requirements and shorter hospital stays. Even a 3–5 cm posterior lumbodorsal incision for open pyeloplasty necessitates several weeks before a return to normal activity and a flank incision requires even more time [1], because the muscle incision and damage seem to be more than anticipated and significant tissue retraction is needed to expose the operative field. On the other hand, conventional laparoscopic pyeloplasty needs only a 5–12 mm skin incision and less muscle damage corresponds to the skin incision and can be performed safely with good exposure. Other main advantage is that conventional laparoscopic pyeloplasty makes increased magnification improving visualization and control excellent. In addition, all medical staff, including the surgeons, assistants, anesthesiologist, nurses, residents, and medical students, share the same real-time operative view through the monitor. This enables us not only to avoid complications and technical insecurity but also to better educate inexperienced surgeons, residents, and medical students. However, the main disadvantage of conventional laparoscopic pyeloplasty is that operative times are significantly higher than open pyeloplasty [2, 3]. In particular, laparoscopic suturing for children is challenging and time consuming and requires a learning curve because of technical difficulty [2].

Robotic surgery may offer a significant benefit to those undertaking a pyeloplasty, especially when performing intracorporeal suturing for an anastomosis. The da Vinci Surgical System (Intuitive Surgical, Sunnyvale, CA, USA) provides movements of the robotic arm in real time with increased degree of freedom and a magnified three-dimensional (D) view. Impediments encountered with conventional laparoscopy in performing a pediatric pyeloplasty may be overcome by utilizing the da Vinci Surgical System.

P. Casale (✉)
Division of Urology, The Children's Hospital of Philadelphia, Philadelphia, PA, USA
e-mail: casale@email.chop.edu

M.C. Ost (ed.), *Robotic and Laparoscopic Reconstructive Surgery in Children and Adults*, Current Clinical Urology, DOI 10.1007/978-1-60327-914-7_9, © Springer Science+Business Media, LLC 2011

Consequently there may be a decrease in the learning curve encountered when performing a conventional laparoscopic pyeloplasty [4, 5]. However, no direct comparison study between pediatric conventional laparoscopic and robotic pyeloplasty has been performed to support this.

The purpose of this chapter is to discuss the role of robotics in performing a pyeloplasty in pediatric population. Technical aspects of the procedure are described.

Diagnosis

Hydronephrosis is the most common abnormal finding in the urinary tract on prenatal screening with ultrasounds. Although antenatal hydronephrosis can be the result of non-obstructive processes such as vesicoureteral reflux (VUR) and non-refluxing non-obstructed megaureters, 50% of these cases are UPJO. Therefore, neonates suspected to have this condition are usually evaluated for obstruction using renal ultrasounds and diuretic renograms. A diuretic renogram using ^{99m}Tc-diethylenetriaminepentaacetic acid (DTPA) or ^{99}Tc^{m}-mercaptoacetyltriglycine (MAG3) will usually help to determine the presence or the absence of an obstruction, providing an indication for surgical intervention in a hydronephrotic kidney(s).

We have recently performed MR urography (MRU) for children with UPJO, which can combine both anatomic and quantitative functional information of each kidney in a single test without radiation exposure [6, 7]. Anatomical assessment by MRU includes renal size, degree of hydronephrosis based on Society for Fetal Urology, renal pelvic dilation with ureteral narrowing, renal pelvis anterior–posterior diameter, and the diagnosis of crossing vessels. Preoperative assessment of a crossing vessel at the UPJO may be of importance for preoperative planning. On the other hand, functional assessment by MRU includes differential renal function, single kidney glomerular filtration rate (GFR) index, and renal transit time [6]. MRU is capable of providing a comprehensive evaluation of pediatric hydronephrosis and obstructive uropathy that could ultimately help select those patients most likely to benefit from surgical intervention.

Debate continues as to whether or not a voiding cystourethrogram might be utilized to rule out VUR and lower urinary anomalies as a cause of the hydronephrosis or as a concomitant finding [8]. Excretory urogram and retrograde pyelogram might be sometimes useful for children to demonstrate the anatomic details and other anomalies of the urinary tract system, but they are not routinely necessary before robotic pyeloplasty.

Symptoms of UPJO are typically seen in prepubertal or teenager but can be seen in infants and include any combination of back and flank pain, hematuria, failure to thrive, flank mass, constipation, and pyelonephritis [8].

Indications

The indications of robotic pyeloplasty, which are similar to those for open and conventional laparoscopic pyeloplasty, included an increasing degree of hydronephrosis, a low split renal function (<40%), an obstructive pattern on diuretic renogram, and/or progressive deterioration of renal function during follow-up associated with or without symptoms. The patients may have undergone percutaneous nephrostomy or double-J ureteral stent placement before surgery because of acute renal failure, abdominal pain, or enormous hydronephrosis.

Conventional laparoscopic pyeloplasty is safe and effective in small infants and can be performed with outcomes comparable to those of open pyeloplasty [9–11]. Although a larger sample size is needed, we previously presented our early small experience with robotic pyeloplasty in infants, demonstrating a successful outcome in nine infants (ages 3–8 months) who underwent robotic pyeloplasties [12].

A smaller working space can induce collision of the various parts of the robot and could be a limiting factor while performing complex manipulative procedure such as suturing an anastomosis between the renal pelvis and the ureter in a restricted space [13]. It is our opinion that robotic pyeloplasty is certainly technically possible yet challenging in small infants. At this time, open or conventional laparoscopic pyeloplasty may be a more acceptable option for small infants with UPJO. However, additional advancement in robotic technology will address this limitation when performing a robotic pyeloplasty in a smaller infant.

Instruments and Supplies

Typically, an open access technique is used for the 12-mm camera port. We usually place camera port in the superior aspect of the umbilicus. The abdomen is insufflated with CO_2 at a pressure of 10–15 mmHg with a flow rate of 10 l/min to observe the inside of the abdominal cavity clearly using a 12-mm, 0° telescope. A 5-mm endoscope is available but is monocular and cannot provide the 3D image of the larger scope. Two additional working 5-mm trocars are usually inserted. The robot has instruments that are available in both 8 and 5 mm sizes. A fourth arm is available for grasping and retraction. We utilize Maryland bipolar forceps as a grasper and either monopolar hook device or curved scissors during dissection. Robotic needle driver can make suturing easier. The techniques and technology have evolved allowing identical results and utilizing 5-0, 6-0, and 7-0 sutures as in open surgeries. We typically utilize 6-0 monofilament absorbable suture, but one can use any 5-0 or 6-0 suture depending on the size of the patient. We do not recommend anything larger than 6-0 for small children and infants.

Surgical Technique

General Procedures

The patient is placed in a modified flank position with a 60° elevation of the flank. The patient is placed as close to the edge of the bed as possible and secured with towels and silk tape. The urethral catheter is introduced into the operative field for intraoperative access to allow instillation of saline, with an indicator for verification of antegrade double-J pigtail stent placement in the bladder, as described below.

In pre-pubertal or teenager, ports are placed in the umbilicus for the camera port, midline above the umbilicus, and mid clavicular line below the umbilicus for the working ports. In infants, however, the upper working port should be placed sub-xiphoid in the midline and the lower working port as lateral as possible to the rectus muscle and close to the inguinal region (Fig. 9.1). After the port placement, it is helpful to use conventional laparoscopic instrumentation to manipulate the bowel and make additional plans for the surgical access. At this point in the operation, any necessary additional patient rotation or repositioning must be performed as it is nearly impossible to be done after robotic docking. The robotic device is docked from the ipsilateral side, and the robotic arms are engaged. The surgical procedures follow the same rules as the conventional laparoscopic approach. The choice of the transperitoneal or the retroperitoneal approach depends on the surgeon's experience. The UPJ is exposed transmesenterically on the left (Fig. 9.2) or by mobilizing the colon on the right. If one chooses colonic mobilization on the left, it must be taken medially over the aorta. A precise dissection of the UPJ is required to evaluate the cause of UPJO. Crossing vessels are often encountered. They may appear posteriorly or anteriorly from a lower pole artery; additional small arterial branches or small lumber or gonadal veins crossing the ureter may be encountered [14]. Any crossing vessel should be completely isolated. The ureter should also be fully freed from surrounding structures and periureteral bands. After exposure of UPJO, a hitch stitch is passed through the abdominal wall and is placed to elevate and stabilize the pelvis if so desired. We use a hitch stitch if a pyelolithotomy is necessary. The choice of the dismembered (Fig. 9.3) or non-dismembered pyeloplasty (Fig. 9.4) depends on the surgeon's

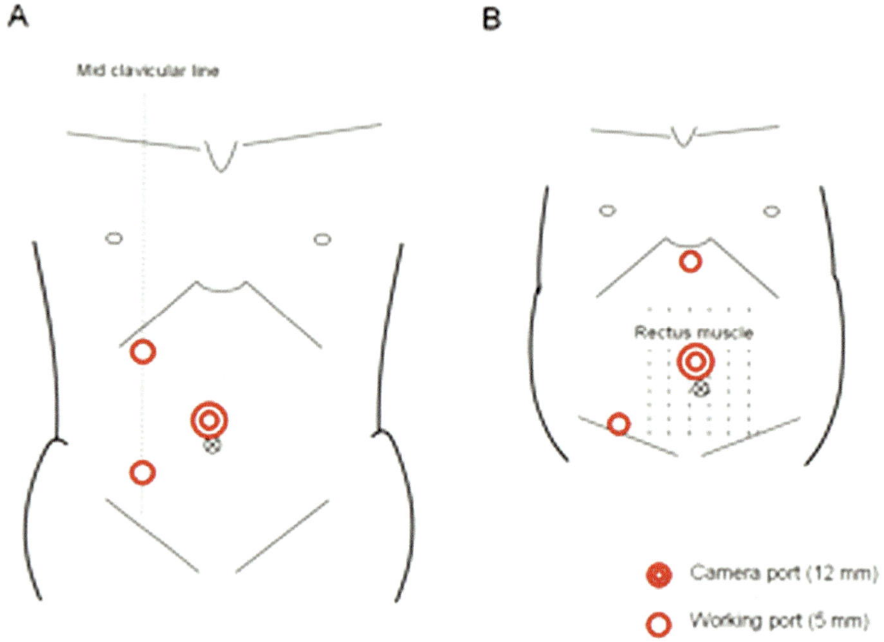

Fig. 9.1 Ports placement of right robotic pyeloplasty in pre-pubertal/teenager (**a**) and infant (**b**)

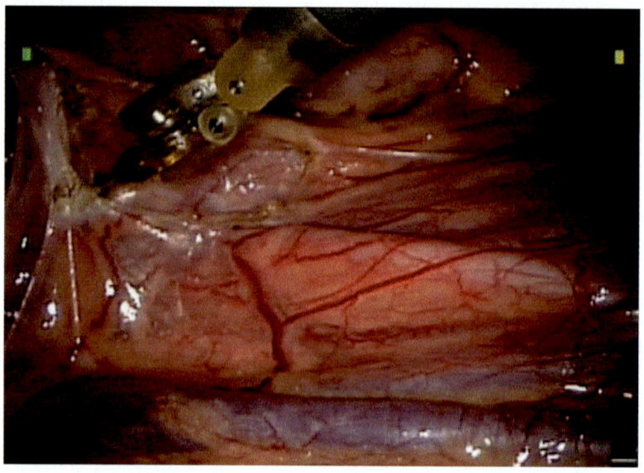

Fig. 9.2 UPJ is exposed transmesenterically on the left. Care should be taken to avoid mesenteric artery or bowel injury

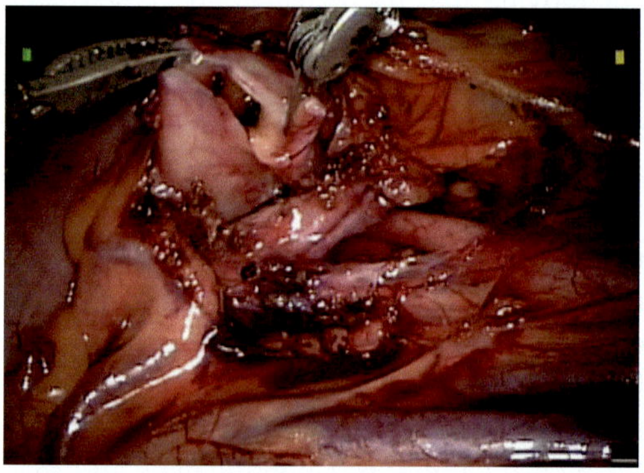

Fig. 9.3 Dismembered pyeloplasty. Incision of renal pelvis, UPJ and ureter, and spatulation of the ureter laterally

experience or the anatomy of the renal pelvis and the ureter such as the presence of crossing vessels.

After the pelvis is incised, the ureter is spatulated laterally and the anastomosis is performed using a running suture (Fig. 9.5). A double-J ureteral stent is placed after the posterior wall closure is complete (Fig. 9.6). This maneuver affords visualization of the anterior wall closure and prevents twisting of the ureter. The double-J ureteral stent placement is performed by placing an 18-gauge angiocatheter through the anterior abdominal wall. A guide wire is then placed in an antegrade fashion. The stent is then passed over the guide wire. We recommend filling the bladder with saline or methylene blue so that one can

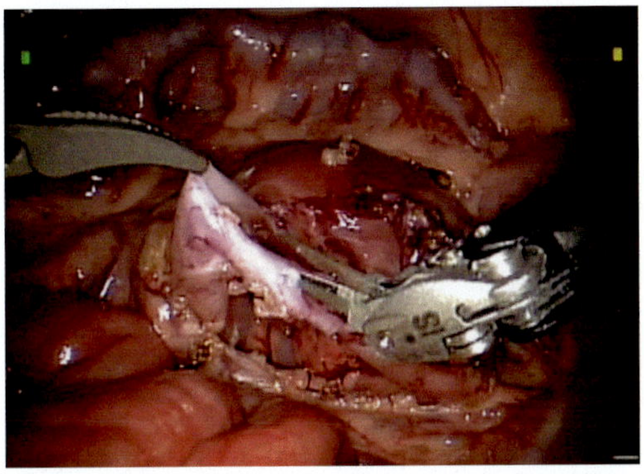

Fig. 9.4 Non-dismembered pyeloplasty (modified bypass plasty). Longitudinal incision on the lateral side from the renal pelvis to the ureter through the stenotic segment of UPJ

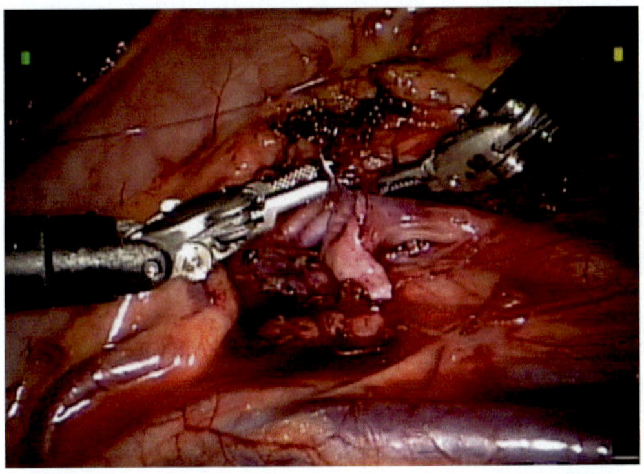

Fig. 9.5 Anastomosis using a running suture (dismembered pyeloplasty)

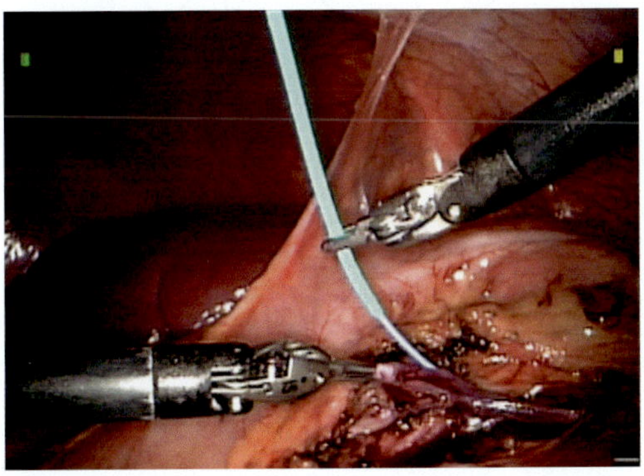

Fig. 9.6 A double pigtail stent placement after the posterior wall closure is complete

observe the efflux of urine when there is access into the bladder by the stent. The stent can also be placed retrograde with a tether left on, facilitating removal as an outpatient.

Approach: Transperitoneal or Retroperitoneal Approach

Open pyeloplasty is performed through the retroperitoneal approach, which has the advantage of less risk of intraperitoneal organ injury, postoperative ileus, and avoidance of potential deleterious effects of peritoneal exposure to blood and urine. Although adhesions may occur with transperitoneal laparoscopic procedures, the incidence appears lower than would be expected with open exploration [15]. Recently, several reports have demonstrated the usefulness of conventional retroperitoneoscopic pyeloplasty for children; however, Canon et al. [16] reported in their comparison study between transperitoneal and retroperitoneal approaches in children that no major difference exists between the two approaches for correcting UPJO, although the average operative time for the retroperitoneoscopic approach was significantly longer than that for the transperitoneal approach. Metzelder et al. [11] concluded that no disadvantage was attributable to a transperitoneal approach in children.

Robotic pyeloplasty can be also performed using a transperitoneal [12, 17–19] or a retroperitoneal approach [19, 20]. There have been no large-scale randomized or prospective studies comparing these different techniques. So as not to limit our working space, we utilize a transperitoneal route. Robotic pyeloplasty via a retroperitoneal approach remains a technically challenging procedure in children because the level of difficulty of manipulation certainly increases in the retroperitoneum [12]. In fact, there are only two reports on the experiences of pediatric robotic pyeloplasty using retroperitoneal approach [19, 20]. Hopefully, such difficulties may be overcome with improvement in operative skill and advancement of robotic technology.

Access: Retrocolic or Transmesenteric Access

Traditionally, a transperitoneal laparoscopic approach to the UPJO has been performed in retrocolic fashion by reflecting the colon and its mesentery medially to expose the renal pelvis and the ureter. A transmesenteric approach to the retroperitoneum may be a better option for left pyeloplasty, allowing direct access to left UPJ with little or no bowel manipulation and shorter operative time [21].

Technique: Dismembered or Non-dismembered Robotic Pyeloplasty

The surgical procedures of robotic dismembered pyeloplasty follow the same steps as the open Anderson–Hynes technique (Fig. 9.7). The stenotic segment is excised and, if necessary, reduction of the renal pelvis accomplished. Position stay sutures should be used with caution to avoid recurrent UPJO since they may leave the renal pelvis and the ureter in an unfavorable position once released and allow to fall back [22].

Non-dismembered pyeloplasty includes the "Fenger-plasty using the Heinicke–Miculicz principle" of a longitudinal incision of the UPJO and vertical suturing, "Y–V plasty" with a V-shaped incision of the renal pelvis, an additional incision of the stenosis including spatulation of the ureter (Y-shaped), and a subsequent closure as a V flap (Fig. 9.8), and "bypass pyeloplasty" with side-to-side anastomosis between the dilated portion of the ureter just distal to the UPJO and the lower and dependent portion of the hydronephrotic renal pelvis [23]. The Fenger-plasty using the Heinicke–Miculicz principle has been abandoned due to inferior long-term success rate. Y–V plasty is better suited for a high insertion of the ureter into the pelvis or for small extrarenal pelvis. Bypass pyeloplasty may be a more physiologic procedure in patients with mid to high insertion of the ureter [23]. We have recently preferred robotic-modified bypass pyeloplasty for children without crossing vessels, which involves an extended longitudinal incision on the lateral side from the renal pelvis to the ureter through the stenotic segment of

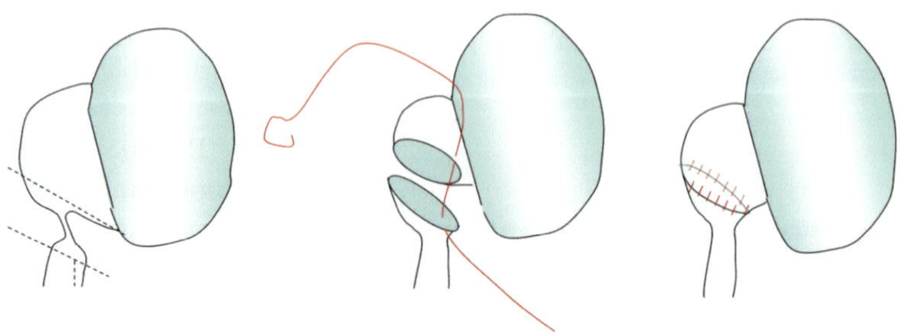

Fig. 9.7 Dismembered pyeloplasty (Anderson–Hynes plasty); the stenotic segment is excised, and the ureter is spatulated along its lateral border to increase the area of the anastomosis which is accomplished with running sutures

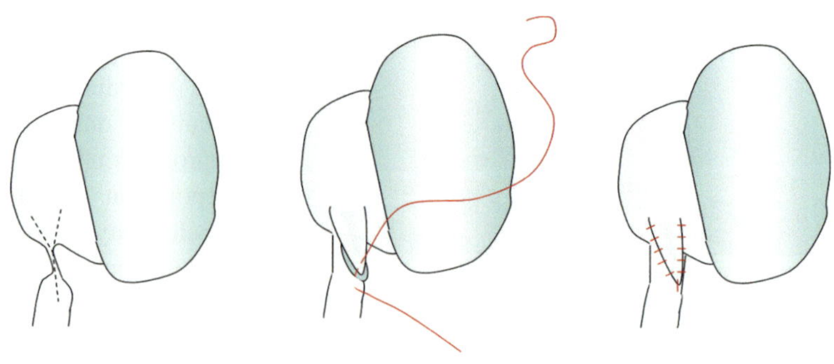

Fig. 9.8 Non-dismembered pyeloplasty (Y–V plasty); creation of a V-shaped incision of the renal pelvis, an additional incision of the stenosis including spatulation of the ureter (Y-shaped) and a closure as a V flap are made

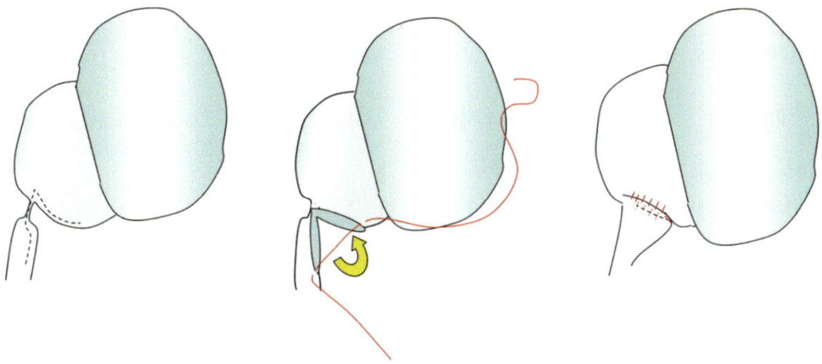

Fig. 9.9 Non-dismembered pyeloplasty (modified bypass plasty): longitudinal incision on the lateral side from the renal pelvis to the ureter through the stenotic segment of UPJ and subsequent side-to-side anastomosis between renal pelvis and ureter with running suture is made

UPJ that is created by side-to-side anastomosis between renal pelvis and ureter with running suture (Fig. 9.9).

In general, the main advantage of dismembered pyeloplasty is the complete excision of stenotic segment of UPJ. On the other hand, non-dismembered pyeloplasty is technically easier because the ureter is not completely transected from the renal pelvis, facilitating tension-free suturing, especially with placement of the first stitch [24], and, as a result, it may enable to reduce suturing time. Comparison study may be required to clarify which procedure is more suitable to robotic performance in children, although the choice between these types of procedures basically depends on the surgeon's experience, the anatomy of the renal pelvis and the ureter, and other intraoperative findings.

Postoperative Management and Follow-up

Postoperative Pain Management

Postoperative pain management for children is always an area for debate, although significant improvements have recently been made. Injection of the port sites does aid in postoperative pain control. An anti-inflammatory such as Ketorolac has also been beneficial to control pain in our experience. For all the patients undergoing robotic procedures at our institution, we utilize intra-thecal opioid injection. We have found that there is decreased length of stay and postoperative pain [25]. There are no intravenous rescues in the first 24 h postoperatively. Ketorolac is our drug of choice for added pain management. On the other hand, Freilich et al. [26] have recently reported that the administration of intraperitoneal aerosolized bupivacaine just prior to incising the perirenal fascia appears to be a simple, effective, and low-cost method to reduce postoperative pain in children undergoing robotic pyeloplasty.

Postoperative Care and Follow-up

Urethral catheter is left overnight for bladder drainage. Double-J ureteral stent is taken out in 2–4 weeks under general anesthesia. If double-J ureteral stent is displaced in the distal ureter, it can be removed using a ureteral basket catheter ureteroscopically.

Postoperative renal ultrasound is usually performed 4 weeks after pyeloplasty with the stent indwelling to document the baseline appearance of the postoperative collecting system. Asymptomatic patients are followed by renal ultrasound at 3 and 6 months postoperatively. Diuretic renogram is performed for symptomatic patients or if the hydronephrosis worsened or did not improve after 3 months. Failure usually occurs within the first year postoperatively.

Outcome

Previous series of robotic pyeloplasties in a pediatric population is shown in Table 9.1. The

Table 9.1 Previous series of robotic assisted pyeloplasties in a pediatric population

References	Atug et al. [17]	Yee et al. [18]	Lee et al. [19]	Kutikov et al. [12]	Olsen et al. [20]
Approach	Transperitoneal	Transperitoneal	Transperitoneal (32) Retroperitoneal (1)	Transperitoneal	Retroperitoneal
No. patients	7	8	33	9	67
Mean age years (range)	13.0 (6–15) years	11.5 (6.4–15.6) years	7.9 (0.2–19.6) years	5.6 (3–8) months	7.9 (1.7–17.1) years
Mean OR time (min) (range)	184 (165–204)	363 (255–522)	219 (133–401)	123	143 (93–300)
Length of stay (days)(range)	1.2 (1.0–1.3)	2.4 (1.0–5.0)	2.3 (0.5–6.0)	1.4	2.0 (1.0–6.0)
Postoperative complications (no.)	1	1	1	0	11
Mean follow (months)	10.9 (2.0–18.0)	14.7 (2–24)	10.0 (0.4–28.0)	–	12.1 (0.9–49.1)
Success rate (%)	100.0	100.0	93.9	100.0	94.0

results described in the literature show similar success as the ''gold standard'' open pyeloplasty of around 95% [12, 17–20, 27, 28]. Atug et al. [17] performed robotic pyeloplasty successfully for seven children and demonstrated that no patient required additional procedures postoperatively. In addition, Olsen et al. [20] performed robotic-assisted retroperitoneoscopic pyeloplasty for 65 children and demonstrated that success rate was 94%. On the other hand, there are two reports comparing an age matched cohort undergoing open pyeloplasty to robotic pyeloplasty in children for safety and efficacy [18, 19]. Yee et al. [18] reported that eight pediatric patients underwent robotic pyeloplasty and were matched by age group with patients undergoing open pyeloplasty, and all robotic procedures were successful as determined by subjective data using pain scales and radiologic data. Additionally, Lee et al. also performed a retrospective case–control study of 33 patients undergoing robotic pyeloplasty and 33 undergoing open pyeloplasties, and reported that robotic pyeloplasty was done at a success rate of 93.9% [19]. These two reports demonstrated that robotic pyeloplasty had advantages of decreased hospital stay and decreased narcotic use in comparison with open pyeloplasty, although mean operative times (363 or 219 min in each report, respectively) were increased relative to open pyeloplasty (248 or 181 min, respectively) [18, 19]. Importantly, increasing experience with robotic pyeloplasty leads to decreased operative times approximating the open experience [19].

Procedure-Related Complications

Complications of the pediatric robotic pyeloplasty series published to date include prolonged drainage [17] and ileus [18], conversion, postoperative nephrectomy, urinary tract infection, hematuria, and displaced double-J ureteral stent [20]. Potential intra- and postoperative complications with robotic pyeloplasty are basically similar to those with conventional laparoscopic pyeloplasty.

Intraoperative Complications

Potential intraoperative complications with robotic pyeloplasty include bleeding requiring transfusion, trocar damage to viscera or vessels, and thermal damage to tissues or organs [8]. Rare but significant possible complication is bowel injury, the risk of which may be higher if a transperitoneal or even a transmesenteric access is used [14]. Diligent inspection of the viscera at the end of every procedure may help identify an injury [8]. In some cases, double-J ureteral stent could not be advanced into the bladder and ureteroscopic reposition of the stent may become necessary [14]. Technical problems in robotic pyeloplasty leading to conversion to conventional laparoscopic procedure may occur.

Postoperative Complications

Potential postoperative complications include hernia at the port site and/or internally, wound infection, persistent urine leakage, and urinary tract infection [14]. Postoperative ileus as a complication to the transperitoneal approach probably may be due to leakage of urine from the anastomosis [18]. Postoperatively, a child should continue to improve hourly in the immediate postoperative period and then dramatically day-by-day over the first week. If this sequence does not occur, then one must be wary of a missed injury or an incomplete or failed anastomosis, and acting quickly to solve it should minimize adverse outcomes [8]. We should not hesitate to do reoperation, even redo open procedure, for the child with significant postoperative complication.

Robotic Procedures for Recurrent UPJO

Although open, laparoscopic, and robotic pyeloplasties have favorable outcome with a success rate exceeding 90%, recurrent UPJO sometimes occurs in all procedures. Factors such as young age at initial surgery (less than 6 months), prolonged urinary diversion (dry anastomosis), missed anatomical findings at the first intervention (crossing vessels or long ureteral segment narrowing), and lack of retrograde pyelogram have been related to open pyeloplasty failure [29, 30]. Second-line therapies have previously been shown to fail at a higher rate than the initial therapeutic procedure [7]. It is a serious complication for which treatment remains challenging because of the extensive scarring and fibrosis from the prior procedure. Patients with recurrent UPJO sometimes present a treatment dilemma to pediatric urologists.

Once recurrent UPJO occurs, redo operation is needed for these cases. The available options for management of recurrent UPJO are balloon dilation, endopyelotomy, open or conventional laparoscopic pyeloplasty. Braga et al. [31] compared retrograde endopyelotomy, which consisted of holmium laser and cautery/balloon dilation, to redo pyeloplasty through a flank incision and by laparoscopy for the treatment of failed pyeloplasty in children and demonstrated that retrograde endopyelotomy had a significantly lower success rate (39%) than redo pyeloplasty (100%) for correction of recurrent UPJO. Piaggio et al. [32] assessed the feasibility of pediatric redo conventional laparoscopic pyeloplasty in comparison to redo open pyeloplasty and demonstrated that success rate was the same in both groups (80%), although surgical time for redo conventional laparoscopic pyeloplasty was longer than that for redo open pyeloplasty. Redo conventional laparoscopic pyeloplasty is technically more challenging than primary conventional laparoscopic pyeloplasty requiring more operative time. Since the most time-consuming part of the operation is the laparoscopic exposure and suturing for recurrent UPJO, robotic procedures such as redo pyeloplasty and ureterocalicostomy for these children can be alternative options.

Redo Robotic Pyeloplasty

Robotic redo pyeloplasty in children with recurrent UPJO after primary pyeloplasty is reported to be a safe and effective option in the treatment of these challenging cases [33, 34]. Basically, the procedure is performed as described for the primary robotic pyeloplasty. Although both dismembered and non-dismembered pyeloplasties are possible, for cases in which scarring prevents extensive mobilization of the renal pelvis and the ureter to allow dismembered pyeloplasty,

Y–V plasty should be selected [33]. Dissection of UPJ area may be technically one of the most difficult parts of performing redo robotic pyeloplasty as well as other procedures in the case of a recurrent UPJO with significant postsurgical adhesion. Because of the presence of scar tissue, care must be taken to avoid injury to the ureter or major vessels [33]. The magnification afforded by the robot may allow for more precise dissection [35]. The degree of adhesion and fibrosis is highly viable, which may be secondary healing factors of the patients as well as to technical problems in the primary operation such as incomplete unfavorable position anastomosis between the renal pelvis and the ureter [36]. The crossing vessels that may be missed during the primary operation must be identified because it can be a cause of recurrent UPJO [37]. The ureter should be free from surrounding structures and spatulated clearly enough to encounter healthy tissue. Passerotti et al. [33] reported redo robotic pyeloplasty for six children with uniform success and no complications. Hemal et al. [34] reported their experience of redo robotic pyeloplasty for five children under 15 years of age as a salvage procedure, and all children had improvement of obstruction; however, although robotic pyeloplasty for children with recurrent UPJO can provide significant advantages such as more precise dissection, faster recovery, and less operative pain over open procedures, more studies will be needed to establish its adequacy.

Robotic Ureterocalicostomy

Robotic ureterocalicostomy is a potential option in not only patients with failed pyeloplasty but also patients with UPJO and significant lower pole calicectasis, and a minimal pelvis, or patients with an exaggerated intrarenal pelvis (Fig. 9.10) [38]. If the pelvis is not readily accessible, robotic ureterocalicostomy will be a better choice than redo robotic pyeloplasty.

The colon is reflected, exposing the massively dilated kidney. The ureters are transected and ligated with absorbable sutures at the level of the renal pelvis or crossing vessels. The ureters are spatulated before transection. The most dependent lower pole calyx is amputated with hot shears. There is a minimal amount of bleeding from the thinned parenchyma of the lower pole system, and the electrocautery of the hot shears easily controlled any bleeding. The posterior anastomosis is performed with 5-0 absorbable suture in a running fashion (Fig. 9.11). The ureteral stent is then placed in the same fashion of robotic pyeloplasty, as described above. The anterior anastomosis is performed in an interrupted manner, allowing visualization and approximation of the renal collecting system to the ureteral mucosa without placing tension on the renal parenchyma. The anterior sutures are then tied in groups so that the last few suture placements are unobstructed and precise. The stent is removed at 6 weeks after surgery with a retrograde ureteropyelogram to visualize the

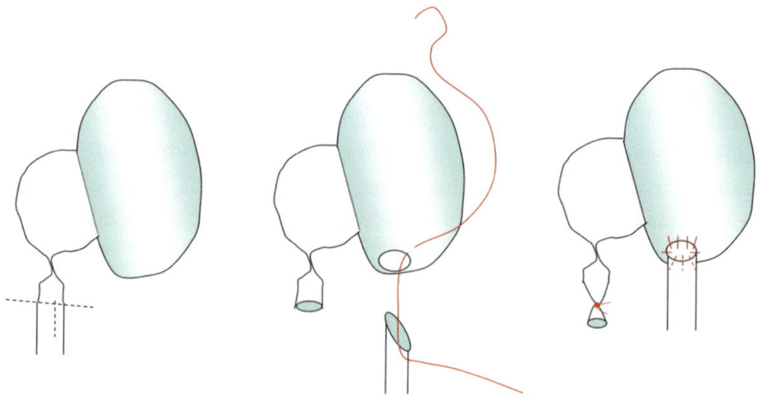

Fig. 9.10 Ureterocalicostomy; spatulation and transection of the ureter, amputation of lower pole calyx, and anastomosis between lower pole calyx and ureter with running suture are made

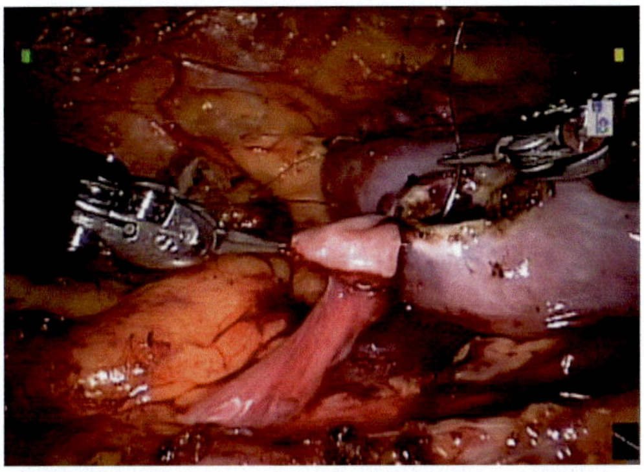

Fig. 9.11 Robotic-assisted laparoscopic ureterocalicostomy; an anastomosis between lower pole calyx and ureter with 5-0 absorbable suture in a running fashion

anastomosis. We performed robotic ureterocalicostomy for nine patients with UPJO (mean age 6.5 years). Mean operative time was 168 min and mean hospital stay was 21 h [38]. There was no evidence of obstruction after operation in any patient.

Conclusions

Robotic surgery enables a revolutionary advance for pediatric urological surgery and provides great benefit for patients and surgeons. Robotic pyeloplasty for adult has been established as one of the most suitable urological operations. Although further outcome studies and prospective randomized comparison studies with open surgery or conventional laparoscopic surgery may be needed, pediatric robotic pyeloplasty will also be established as an alternative minimally invasive surgery in the near future.

Critical Operative Steps

- Positioning: modified flank position with a 60° elevation of the flank
- Port placement
  - (1) Camera port: umbilicus
  - (2) Working port:
    - *Pre-pubertal/teenager:* midline above the umbilicus and mid clavicular line below the umbilicus
    - *Infant:* upper port; sub-xiphoid in the midline/lower port; as lateral a possible to the rectus muscle and close to the inguinal region
- Docking: over the ipsilateral shoulder
- Approach: transperitoneal or retroperitoneal approach depends on the surgeon's experience
- Access: Transmesenterically on the left or by mobilizing the colon on the right
- Procedures: dismembered or non-dismembered pyeloplasty depends on the surgeon's experience or the presence of crossing vessel
- Step 1: UPJO exposure and a hitch stitch placement on the renal pelvis
- Step 2: Incision of renal pelvis, UPJ and ureter, and spatulation of the ureter laterally
- Step 3: Anastomosis using a running suture
- Step 4: A double pigtail stent placement in an antegrade fashion after the posterior wall closure is complete.

Critical Instruments and Supplies

- da Vinci Surgical System® (Intuitive Surgical, Sunnyvale, CA, USA)
- A 12-mm, 0° telescope (Intuitive Surgical)
- Maryland bipolar forceps (Intuitive Surgical)
- Monopolar hook device or curved scissors (Intuitive Surgical)
- Robotic needle driver (Intuitive Surgical)
- PassPort® double-shielded trocars (12 mm; Patton Surgical, Austin, TX, USA): camera port
- PassPort® double-shielded trocars (5 mm; Patton Surgical): working ports
- 5-0, 6-0, or 7-0 MONOCRYL® (monofilament absorbable suture) (ETHICON, Somerville, NJ, USA)

References

1. Peters CA, Schlussel RN, Retik AB. Pediatric laparoscopic dismembered pyeloplasty. J Urol. 1995;153:1962–5.
2. Piaggio LA, Franc-Guimond J, Noh PH, Wehry M, Figueroa TE, Barthold J, González R. Transperitoneal laparoscopic pyeloplasty for primary repair of ureteropelvic junction obstruction in infants and children: comparison with open surgery. J Urol. 2007;178:1579–83.
3. Ravish IR, Nerli RB, Reddy MN, Amarkhed SS. Laparoscopic pyeloplasty compared with open pyeloplasty in children. J Endourol. 2007 21: 897–902.
4. Peters C Laparoscopy in pediatric urology: adoption of innovative technology. BJU Int. 2003;92:52–7.
5. Peters CA. Robotic assisted surgery in pediatric urology. Pediatr Endosurg Innovative Tech. 2003;7: 403–13.
6. Grattan-Smith JD, Jones RA. MR urography: technique and results for the evaluation of urinary obstruction in the pediatric population. Magn Reson Imaging Clin North Am. 2008;16:643–60.
7. Kirsch AJ, McMann LP, Jones RA, Smith EA, Scherz HC, Grattan-Smith JD. Magnetic resonance urography for evaluating outcomes after pediatric pyeloplasty. J Urol. 2006;176:1755-1761.
8. Casale P. A review of pediatric laparoscopic pyeloplasty. UIJ. 2009;2. doi:10.3834/uij.1944-5784. Accessed 09 Dec 2008.
9. Kutikov A, Resnick M, Casale P. Laparoscopic pyeloplasty in the infant younger than 6 months – is it technically possible? J Urol. 2006;175:1477–9.
10. Neheman A, Noh PH, Piaggio L, González R. The role of laparoscopic surgery for urinary tract reconstruction in infants weighing less than 10 kg: a comparison with open surgery. J Pediatr Urol. 2008;4:192–6.
11. Metzelder ML, Schier F, Petersen C, Truss M, Ure BM. Laparoscopic transabdominal pyeloplasty in children is feasible irrespective of age. J Urol. 2006;175: 688–91.
12. Kutikov A, Nguyen M, Guzzo T, Canter D, Casale P. Robot assisted pyeloplasty in the infant-lessons learned. J Urol. 2006;176:2237–9.
13. Thakre AA, Bailly Y, Sun LW, Van Meer F, Yeung CK. Is smaller workspace a limitation for robot performance in laparoscopy? J Urol. 2008;179: 1138–42
14. Rassweiler JJ, Teber D, Frede T. Complications of laparoscopic pyeloplasty. World J Urol. 2008;26:539–47.
15. Moore RG, Kavoussi LR, Bloom DA, Bogaert GA, Jordon GH, Kogan BA, Peters CA. Postoperative adhesion formation after urological laparoscopy in the pediatric population. J Urol. 1995 153: 792–5.
16. Canon SJ, Jayanthi VR, Lowe GJ. Which is better—retroperitoneoscopic or laparoscopic dismembered pyeloplasty in children? J Urol. 2007 178: 1791–5.
17. Atug F, Woods M, Burgess SV, Castle EP, Thomas R Robotic assisted laparoscopic pyeloplasty in children. J Urol. 2005;174:1440–2.
18. Yee DS, Shanberg AM, Duel BP, Rodriguez E, Eichel L, Rajpoot D. Initial comparison of robotic-assisted laparoscopic versus open pyeloplasty in children. Urology. 2006;67:599–602.
19. Lee RS, Retik AB, Borer JG, Peters CA. Pediatric robot assisted laparoscopic dismembered pyeloplasty: comparison with a cohort of open surgery. J Urol. 2006;175:683–7.
20. Olsen LH, Rawashdeh YF, Jorgensen TM. Pediatric robot assisted retroperitoneoscopic pyeloplasty: a 5-year experience. J Urol 2007;178:2137–41
21. Romero FR, Wagner AA, Trapp C, Permpongkosol S, Muntener M, Link RE, Kavoussi LR. Transmesenteric laparoscopic pyeloplasty. J Urol. 2006;176:2526–9.
22. Olsen LH, Rawashdeh YF. Robotics in pediatric urology: pyeloplasty. In: Wilcox DT, Godbole RP, Koyle MA, editors. Pediatric: surgical complication and management. Oxford, UK: Blackwell Publishing; 2008: 145–51.
23. Mesrobian HG. Bypass pyeloplasty: description of a procedure and initial results. J Pediatr Urol. 2009;5:34–6.
24. Casale P, Grady RW, Joyner BD, Zeltser IS, Figueroa TE, Mitchell ME. Comparison of dismembered and nondismembered laparoscopic pyeloplasty in the pediatric patient. J Endourol. 2004;18:875–8.
25. Ganesh A, Kim A, Casale P, Cucchiaro G. Low-dose intrathecal morphine for postoperative analgesia in children. Anesth Analg. 2007;104:271–6.
26. Freilich DA, Houck CS, Meier PM, Passerotti CC, Retik AB, Nguyen HT. The effectiveness of aerosolized intraperitoneal bupivacaine in reducing postoperative pain in children undergoing robotic-assisted laparoscopic pyeloplasty. J Pediatr Urol. 2008;4:337–40.
27. Olsen LH, Jorgensen TM. Computer assisted pyeloplasty in children: the retroperitoneal approach. J Urol. 2004;171:2629–31.
28. Franco I, Dyer LL, Zelkovic P. Laparoscopic pyeloplasty in the pediatric patient: hand sewn anastomosis versus robotic assisted anastomosis—is there a difference? J Urol. 2007;178:1483–6.
29. Thomas JC, DeMarco RT, Donohoe JM, Adams MC, Pope JC 4th, Brock JW 3rd. Management of the failed pyeloplasty: a contemporary review. J Urol. 2005;174:2363–6.
30. Braga LH, Lorenzo AJ, Bägli DJ, Keays M, Farhat WA, Khoury AE, Salle JL. Risk factors for recurrent ureteropelvic junction obstruction after open pyeloplasty in a large pediatric cohort. J Urol. 2008;180:1684–7.

31. Braga LH, Lorenzo AJ, Skeldon S, Dave S, Bagli DJ, Khoury AE, Pippi Salle JL, Farhat WA. Failed pyeloplasty in children: comparative analysis of retrograde endopyelotomy versus redo pyeloplasty. J Urol. 2007;178:2571–5.
32. Piaggio LA, Noh PH, González R. Reoperative laparoscopic pyeloplasty in children: comparison with open surgery. J Urol. 2007;177:1878–82.
33. Passerotti CC, Nguyen HT, Eisner BH, Lee RS, Peters CA. Laparoscopic reoperative pediatric pyeloplasty with robotic assistance. J Endourol. 2007;21:1137–40.
34. Hemal AK, Mishra S, Mukharjee S, Suryavanshi M. Robot assisted laparoscopic pyeloplasty in patients of ureteropelvic junction obstruction with previously failed open surgical repair. Int J Urol. 2008;15:744–6.
35. Atug F, Burgess SV, Castle EP, Thomas R. Role of robotics in the management of secondary ureteropelvic junction obstruction. Int J Clin Pract. 2006;60:9–11.
36. Brito AH, Mitre AI, Srougi M. Laparoscopic pyeloplasty in secondary obstruction. J Endourol. 2007;21:1481–4.
37. Rehman J, Landman J, Sundaram C, Clayman RV. Missed anterior crossing vessels during open retroperitoneal pyeloplasty: laparoscopic transperitoneal discovery and repair. J Urol. 2001;166:593–6.
38. Casale P, Mucksavage P, Resnick M, Kim SS. Robotic ureterocalicostomy in the pediatric population. J Urol. 2008;180:2643–8.

Part IV
Laparoscopic and Robotic Reconstructive Ureteral Surgery

Chapter 10

Laparoscopic Ureteroureterostomy and Correction of Ureteral Defects

Erica J. Traxel and Paul Noh

This chapter contains a video segment which can be found at the URL: http://www.springerimages.com/ost

Abbreviations

IUU ipsilateral ureteroureterostomy
TUU transureteroureterostomy
VUR vesicoureteral reflux

Introduction

Ureteral pathology presents a unique challenge to the surgeon, as it potentially can occur over a considerable distance reaching from the renal fossa down into the pelvis. Consequently, traditional open surgery may require multiple incisions to fully correct the problem, such as the combination of a flank incision with a Pfannenstiel incision. The laparoscopic approach lends itself well to surgery addressing ureteral pathology as it provides ready access to the entire length of the ureter all through the same access points. This chapter will review indications for ureteral surgery, the principles of traditional open ureteral surgery, the laparoscopic approach to ureteral surgery, and potential complications of ureteral surgery.

E.J. Traxel (✉)
Division of Pediatric Urology, Department of Surgery, St. Louis Children's Hospital, Washington University School of Medicine, St. Louis, MO, USA
e-mail: traxele@wudosis.wustl.edu

Indications for Ureteral Surgery

There are a myriad of indications for ureteral surgery. Sometimes the ureteral pathology will call for surgical repair all within the same ureter, that is, ureteroureterostomy of a single ureter to itself, after the intervening diseased segment of ureter has been excised. Additionally, surgical repair could involve ipsilateral ureteroureterostomy (IUU) of one ureter to another within a duplicated collecting system. Other times the ureteral pathology may require operating to involve bilateral renal systems, such as with a transureteroureterostomy (TUU). We will address each of these circumstances individually. Please refer to Table 10.1 for an overview of indications for ureteral surgery.

Indications for Ureteroureterostomy of a Single Ureter to Itself

Disease processes affecting a single ureter include injury (traumatic or iatrogenic), congenital ureteral strictures and/or stenosis, ureteral valves, ureteral diverticula, and retrocaval ureter. Congenital ureteral stricture or stenosis is found at autopsy in 0.6% of children and occurs at points of physiologic narrowing of the ureter, that is, in order of decreasing frequency, the ureterovesicular junction, the ureteropelvic junction, and the midureter at the pelvic brim

M.C. Ost (ed.), *Robotic and Laparoscopic Reconstructive Surgery in Children and Adults*, Current Clinical Urology, DOI 10.1007/978-1-60327-914-7_10,

Table 10.1 Indications for ureteral surgery

- I. Ureteroureterostomy of a single ureter to itself
  - A. Injury (traumatic or iatrogenic)
  - B. Congenital ureteral stricture
  - C. Congenital ureteral valve
  - D. Ureteral diverticula
  - E. Retrocaval ureter
- II. IUU
  - A. Duplication anomalies
    1. VUR into the lower pole ureter
    2. Ureterocele or ectopic insertion obstructing upper pole ureter
- III. TUU
  - A. Primary management of unilateral ureteric pathology
  - B. Undiversion
  - C. Salvage procedure following prior failed ureteral reimplantation
  - D. Bilateral VUR but the bladder is too small for bilateral reimplantation

[1, 2]. Histologic studies reveal a paucity or a disarrangement of ureteral musculature at points of stricture or stenosis, and presumably there was a disturbance in embryogenesis around the 11th or the 12th week of gestation, such as extrinsic compression by a vessel [3, 4]. Of note, such pathology can occur at multiple points along the ureter with intervening normal segments; therefore, it is critical at the time of repair to inspect the entire length of the ureter.

Ureteral valves appear as annular or diaphragmatic lesions with a pinhole opening and with a dilated proximal segment and a distal segment of normal or stenotic caliber. They also can present anywhere along the length of the ureter. The lesion is a transverse fold of redundant mucosa and smooth muscle, occurs in 5% of newborn ureters, and seems to resolve with growth [5]. This lesion may account for the relatively higher incidence of prenatal hydronephrosis that seems to resolve with conservative management. However, in cases of persistent obstruction, surgical intervention is warranted. Ureteral diverticula can be classified as follows: (1) cleavage of the ureteric bud with abortive duplication; (2) true congenital diverticula containing all layers of the ureteral wall; and (3) acquired diverticula with herniation of mucosa through muscle [6]. Single acquired diverticula typically are associated with strictures, calculi, and trauma. Multiple acquired diverticula are often related to infection.

Retrocaval ureter, or preureteral vena cava, occurs with an incidence of 1 in 1,500 and is found more commonly in males [7, 8]. It occurs predominantly on the right side and is related to abnormal fetal vascular development. While the condition does not always lead to obstruction of the collecting system, when it does, it will cause symptoms of renal colic, leading to presentation most commonly during the third or the fourth decade of life [9]. All congenital and acquired causes of ureteral obstruction that persist warrant surgical intervention.

Indications for Ipsilateral Ureteroureterostomy

Since Foley first performed a side-to-side IUU to bypass an impacted stone in 1928 and Kuss applied the approach for an ectopic ureter in 1952, multiple authors have reported their experience with open IUU and proven it to be a viable surgical option when indicated and performed appropriately [10, 11]. In pediatrics, IUU is used to address the pathologies commonly associated with duplication anomaly, those being vesicoureteral reflux (VUR) and/or obstruction.

Duplication of the collecting system occurs in less than 1% of the population [1, 12]. Pathologies commonly associated with duplication include VUR to the lower pole and obstruction of the upper pole, by ureterocele or ectopic insertion. In instances when only one moiety is afflicted, IUU of the diseased ureter to the healthy one is an option. This seems an ideal management approach when the diseased moiety has residual function that warrants salvage, as opposed to partial nephroureterectomy in cases of a nonfunctioning moiety. Even when a moiety would appear to have little function, some may argue that nephron-sparing surgery is still merited, as Smith et al. reported that in 57% of ectopic moieties removed, there was no dysplasia identified histologically, despite appearing grossly abnormal at surgery [13]. VUR occurs in the presence of duplication in 50–60% of cases, and in 97% of duplications it occurs only to the lower pole [14–16]. Ureterocele and ectopic ureteral insertion affects the upper pole system in 90% of duplicated systems [17].

This scenario of ureteral duplication is traditionally managed with common sheath reimplantation; however, in instances when the vesicoureteric junction of one moiety is intact, some might argue that common sheath reimplantation, with an 8% failure rate, will unjustifiably compromise a normal system in order to correct the defect of the diseased moiety and instead propose end-to-side IUU of the diseased segment to the healthy segment [18]. Also, in cases of very young patients, the bladder may be too small to permit common sheath reimplantation and still provide the desired 5:1 ratio of tunnel length to diameter. In these instances, the patient may be better served with IUU. Furthermore, ureteroureterostomy avoids the post-operative morbidity of bladder surgery. Some advocate performing the anastomosis proximally, suggesting even a pyeloureterostomy. This leads to two potential challenges. First, it can be very difficult to anastomose a dilated pelvis to a very delicate ureter. Second, this leaves a long ureteral stump into which the reflux can persist, leading to future infection. Others advocate a lower ureteral approach, performing the IUU close to the bladder. While this avoids the issue of a refluxing ureteral stump, it does pose the theoretical risk of yo-yo reflux between the proximal limbs of each ureter [19].

Indications for Transureteroureterostomy

Boari first described TUU in 1894, while Higgins first used it in patients with success in 1927 [20, 21]. The procedure has three main categories of indications: (1) primary management of unilateral ureteric pathology, such as trauma (both accidental and iatrogenic) and stricture; (2) undiversion, such as following prior cutaneous ureterostomy; (3) salvage procedure following prior attempts to correct reflux that have failed, often in the setting of a neurogenic bladder. It is also suitable in cases of bilateral reflux when the bladder may be too small to permit bilateral reimplantation but would allow unilateral reimplantation and then TUU of the other ureter to the reimplanted ureter.

Not every patient is a candidate for TUU. Cases of aperistaltic ureters, foreshortened ureters which would lead to tension on the anastomosis, and tortuous ureters that would require a great deal of straightening, thereby risking devascularization, may not be the ideal cases for TUU [22]. Contraindications to TUU include prior extensive pelvic irradiation, recurrent nephrolithiasis, and retroperitoneal fibrosis. A relative contraindication is severe size discrepancy between the two ureters. Another relative indication is associated VUR and/or obstruction of the recipient ureter; however, this associated pathology can also be addressed with reimplantation of the recipient ureter in conjunction with TUU.

Principles of the Traditional Open Surgical Approach

In order to understand the laparoscopic approach to ureteral surgery, it is necessary to understand the fundamentals of the traditional open surgical approach. Please refer to Table 10.2 for an overview of key principles of open ureteral surgery. We will address each of the surgical scenarios, including ureteroureterostomy of a single ureter to itself, IUU, and TUU.

Table 10.2 Key principles of open ureteral surgery

I. Pre-operative preparation
   A. Appropriately indicated surgery
   B. Adequate residual renal function to warrant reconstructive surgery
   C. Imaging to localize ureteral pathology
II. Pathology completely excised
   A. Ends of ureter appear viable
   B. Ureter cannulated to ensure no additional proximal/distal lesions
III. Mobilization
   A. Sufficient for a tension-free anastomosis
   B. Preservation of adventitia and vascular supply
IV. Anastomosis performed technically well
   A. Spatulation to ensure wide anastomosis
   B. Alignment to ensure no spiraling or kinking
   C. Mucosa-to-mucosa apposition
   D. Fine absorbable suture
V. Post-operative drainage
   A. Stent across anastomosis
   B. Retroperitoneal drain
   C. Foley catheter

Principles of Open Ureteroureterostomy of a Single Ureter to Itself

Ureteroureterostomy of a single ureter to itself is relatively straightforward, but certain principles should be stressed. Patient selection is critical. Pre-operative nuclear renogram can determine the degree of renal function, and a nonfunctioning or poorly functioning kidney may best be treated with nephroureterectomy. Investigation should be undertaken to precisely determine both the location and the length of the lesion, such as intravenous pyelogram pre-operatively or retrograde pyelogram at the time of surgery. If the ureteral lesion is isolated to the distal one-third of the ureter, the patient may best be served by a ureteroneocystostomy with or without psoas hitch or Boari flap.

Mobilization of the ureter should be limited to only that which is necessary and efforts to preserve the adventitia should be made, in order to prevent devascularization. However, sufficient mobilization must be performed to allow for a tension-free anastomosis once the diseased segment has been excised. Additionally, manipulation of the tissue should be minimized and should be done with delicate instruments. One must ensure that the entirety of the diseased segment has been removed. In cases of trauma or iatrogenic ureteral injury, the ureter must be debrided until the edges bleed. Also, once the ureter has been incised, it should be cannulated to ensure that no additional lesions exist either proximally or distally. Normal ureteral caliber includes 3 Fr at birth, 4 Fr at 1 year, and 6 Fr in adults [23].

The anastomosis should begin with correct orientation of the ends of the ureter to prevent spiraling and kinking. Spatulation is performed on both ends, 180° apart to ensure a wide-mouthed anastomosis. In cases of significant dilation at one end, it is possible to anastomose the obliquely cut end of the dilated segment to the spatulated end of the other segment. Fine absorbable suture is used to sew the apex of one end to the corner of the other end. This is repeated to sew the other corner to the other apex. The intervening anastomosis can be done in either an interrupted or a running fashion. Placement of a stent across the anastomosis, such as a double-J or a nephroureteral stent, and of a retroperitoneal drain should be considered. Also, the repair can be isolated using omentum or retroperitoneal fat. Typically, a Foley catheter is left indwelling postoperatively for a short period of time. When these surgical principles are obeyed, the success rate for ureteroureterostomy approaches 90% [24].

Principles of Open Ipsilateral Ureteroureterostomy

The same key surgical principles apply to IUU as to ureteroureterostomy of a single ureter to itself. Points unique to dealing with ureteral duplication include intra-operative cystoscopy and retrograde pyelogram with placement of ureteral catheter to help distinguish one ureter from another at the time of exploration. Also, extreme caution should be exercised when dissecting the two ureters apart near the bladder, as they are intimately associated at this level and will share a common blood supply for the most distal 2–3 cm. For end-to-side anastomosis, the diseased ureter is sectioned obliquely and a longitudinal incision equal in length to the oblique section is made in the healthy ureter. Again, the anastomosis must be without tension and watertight.

A review of reports from 1965 to 1989 included 124 cases of IUU with a complication rate of only 3.2% [25]. Lashley et al. reported a series of 100 IUU and found an overall 94% success rate. In this series, success was not influenced by pre-operative indication (VUR versus obstruction), nor was it affected by ureteral size discrepancy [26]. Choi et al. compared outcomes of different surgeries used as initial treatment in cases of duplex systems associated with VUR or obstruction. They found that ureterocele incision had the highest failure rate, followed by upper pole partial nephrectomy and ureteric reimplantation (both 22%), while ureteroureterostomy had the lowest failure rate (11%) [27]. When carefully performed in suitable candidates, IUU can successfully address either VUR and/or obstruction associated with a duplex system.

Principles of Open Transureteroureterostomy

Similar principles apply to TUU as to IUU and ureteroureterostomy of a single ureter to itself. In the case of TUU, once the diseased ureter has been identified within the retroperitoneum, it is freed as far distally as possible and as far proximally as is necessary to ensure a smooth, nonangulated course across the midline and also a tension-free anastomosis. Periureteral adventitia should be preserved to avoid devascularization. When very extensive mobilization is necessary, the gonadal vessels can be divided either at the ovary or just above the internal ring and the gonadal vessels are mobilized in continuity with the donor ureter to provide collateral blood supply [28]. A traction suture placed in the end of the diseased ureter can aid in maintaining appropriate orientation when passing the ureter across the midline. It can be passed inferior to the inferior mesenteric artery, but it may be necessary to transpose superior to the inferior mesenteric artery to avoid angulation. Its trajectory should be such that it will meet up with the recipient ureter tangentially rather than perpendicularly. Also, one should bear in mind that a dilated ureter may shorten once its obstruction is removed, so some slack must be afforded in the donor ureter near the anastomosis. If the donor ureter is too short despite mobilization all the way up to the kidney, the kidney itself can be mobilized and the lower pole pexed medially for additional slack [29].

The site of anastomosis on the recipient ureter is ideally 2–4 cm above the pelvic brim as the ureters are closest to each other at this location. An anastomosis near the iliac increases the possibility of stricture due to angulation and increased tension. Minimal mobilization of the recipient ureter helps to avoid its devascularization as well as adhesion of the anastomosis to the lumbar fascia. Also, the recipient ureter should not be mobilized to be brought toward the midline lest it cause angulation of the anastomosis. The donor ureter should be brought to the recipient ureter and not vice versa. The end of the diseased ureter is cut tangentially to maximize the lumen of the anastomosis, and the side of the recipient ureter is incised longitudinally in an area devoid of apparent vessels, a length equivalent to the oblique end of the diseased ureter (at least 1.5 cm). The recipient ureterotomy should be on the anteromedial aspect of the recipient ureter, taking care to avoid spiraling or beveling. Of note, if distal ureteral surgery is to be done to the recipient ureter, such as concomitant reimplantation, this should be done prior to the TUU to prevent kinking and/or tension at the anastomosis.

Ideally, a stent should be left across the anastomosis. If the size of the recipient ureter will permit, two stents can be left in, one across the anastomosis up into the donor kidney and one up into the recipient kidney. A drain should be left in the retroperitoneum to absorb any extravasated urine, as urine left near the anastomosis will contribute to stenosis and stricture of the anastomosis.

With meticulous surgical technique, TUU can be successful. Hendren et al. reported on a series of 75 patients who underwent TUU, resulting in no deaths, anastomotic leaks, or lost kidneys, but there were three patients that required reoperation. Of note, in 59 of 75 patients, the recipient ureter underwent a concomitant procedure altering its drainage, demonstrating that TUU could be successfully performed in conjunction with other procedures such as reimplantation of the recipient ureter [29]. Chilton et al. [30] reported on a series of 55 patients who underwent TUU, resulting in no deaths and only one failure leading to nephroureterectomy. Hodges et al. [31] reported on a series of 100 patients undergoing TUU and found satisfactory results for the donor kidney in 92% of cases and for the recipient kidney in 97% of cases. Pesce et al. reported on a series of 70 patients undergoing TUU, 100% of which had a dilated donor ureter and 4% of which had nondilated and nonrefluxing recipient ureters. After a mean follow-up of 10.8 years, the complication rate was only 1.4%, with one case of anastomotic obstruction requiring stenting and one case of distal obstruction of the reimplanted recipient ureter requiring dilation. There was no deterioration of renal function, and dilation of the donor ureter regressed in 52%, while none of the recipient ureters developed dilation [32]. These reports as well as many others in the literature confirm the viability of TUU as a surgical option in appropriate cases.

Laparoscopic Ureteral Surgery

The same tenets of successful open ureteral surgery must be applied to the laparoscopic approach as well. Laparoscopic ureteral surgery possesses the same advantages as all laparoscopic surgery, those being lessened morbidity with decreased post-operative pain and shortened convalescence with superior cosmesis. Moreover, it provides superior access to the entire length of the ureter all through the same points of entry. We will discuss laparoscopic ureteral surgery as it applies to ureteroureterostomy of a single ureter to itself, IUU, and TUU.

Reports of Laparoscopic Ureteroureterostomy of a Single Ureter to Itself

Originally, laparoscopic ureteroureterostomy was reported to repair cases of iatrogenic ureteral injury, occurring often in the setting of laparoscopic gynecologic procedures. In 1998, Nezhat et al. first described the laparoscopic approach to ureteroureterostomy to repair ureteral injury that had occurred during laparoscopic surgery to treat endometriosis. Laparoscopic ureteroureterostomy was performed in eight patients who had a follow-up of up to 6 years. One patient had a post-operative ureteral stricture that resolved with dilation, and another developed recurrent stricture distal to the original anastomosis, requiring ureteral reimplantation. This original series in an adult gynecologic population demonstrated the feasibility of the laparoscopic approach to ureteroureterostomy [33]. Tulikangas further demonstrated this feasibility when reporting a series of four women who suffered iatrogenic ureteral injuries at the time of laparoscopic pelvic surgery. The repair was performed laparoscopically as well, all through the same initial port sites. Follow-up ranged from 6 to 33 months with stable creatinines and no repeat surgeries being necessary. This report emphasized the placement of a double-J ureteral stent passed retrograde across the injured area and left indwelling for 4–6 weeks [34].

The first report of laparoscopic ureteroureterostomy for congenital stricture was by Bhandarkar et al. in 2005. This was done in a 16-year-old boy presenting with right flank pain and in whom evaluation revealed an area of stenosis in the midureter at the pelvic brim. Follow-up at 18 months showed the patient to be doing well [35]. The first report of robot-assisted laparoscopic ureteroureterostomy was by Passerotti et al. in 2008, including a series of three patients undergoing ureteroureterostomy for midureteral stricture or obstruction. At an average follow-up of 11.6 months, there were no complications and all patients were asymptomatic [36]. Thiel et al. also reported robotic-assisted laparoscopic ureteroureterostomy for congenital midureteral stricture later in 2008. This was done in a 20-year-old woman presenting with pyelonephritis and left flank pain. Again, evaluation revealed a stricture in the midureter at the iliac crest. Follow-up diuretic renogram at 1 year showed no obstruction. The authors stated that the da Vinci robot offers the advantage of precise tissue manipulation, which is critical to the success of ureteral surgery. Additionally, they stated that spatulation with robotic scissors is more precise, as is anastomotic suture placement, owing to the six degrees of freedom afforded by the robot, along with three-dimensional imaging [37].

In order to demonstrate the equivalent efficacy of laparoscopic with open reconstructive surgery for benign ureteral stricture, Simmons et al. compared a group of 34 patients undergoing open surgery (9 ureteroureterostomy, 25 ureteral reimplantation with or without Boari flap) with a group of 12 patients undergoing laparoscopic surgery (5 ureteroureterostomy, 7 ureteral reimplantation with or without Boari flap), with a follow-up of 34 months in the open group versus 23 months in the laparoscopic group. All laparoscopic cases were completed without conversion. They found the laparoscopic group to have significantly less operative blood loss and significantly shorter hospital stays. There was no significant difference in complication rates (14.7% open, 8.3% laparoscopic), and only one stricture occurred in the open group and none in the laparoscopic group. This report shows that laparoscopic ureteral surgery for stricture has at least equivalent if not superior results compared to traditional open surgery [38].

Steps in Laparoscopic Ureteroureterostomy of a Single Ureter to Itself

Prior to surgery, appropriate imaging such as nuclear renogram should be performed to first confirm sufficient residual renal function to warrant reconstructive surgery versus nephrectomy. To maximize potential detectable function, it may first be necessary to place a nephrostomy tube or a ureteral stent. Additionally, imaging such as intravenous pyelogram may help to delineate anatomy pre-operatively.

At the time of surgery, often cystoscopy and retrograde pyelogram are performed to further elucidate anatomy and localize the site of ureteral pathology. It may be possible to pass a ureteral stent retrograde across the area in question, which can later help in identifying the ureter within the retroperitoneum. Additionally, the same double-J stent may be left across the anastomosis postoperatively to aid in healing. Sometimes, the area in question is too narrow or perhaps completely obstructed and will not permit retrograde passage of a stent. In these instances, retrograde passage of a ureteral catheter or wire up to the level of obstruction may aid later in identification of the level of pathology and help to facilitate subsequent passage of a double-J ureteral stent across the anastomosis once the area of pathology has been excised. If a ureteral catheter or a wire is left only up to the level of pathology and the distal end of the catheter or the wire is outside the patient, care must be taken not to dislodge the catheter or the wire at the time of repositioning the patient for the laparoscopic portion of the case.

Patient positioning for the laparoscopic portion of the case is dependent upon location of ureteral pathology. For distal lesions, the patient may be left supine and placed in slight Trendelenburg. For proximal lesions, a lateral decubitus position with the affected side up will help to reflect bowel away from the surgical site (Fig. 10.1). In very small children, a full-body prep up to the nipples may be helpful so that the child can be repositioned throughout the surgery (Fig. 10.2). When a ureteral catheter or a wire is left up to the level of pathology with the distal end of the catheter or the wire outside the body, this must be prepped into the sterile field for later manipulation.

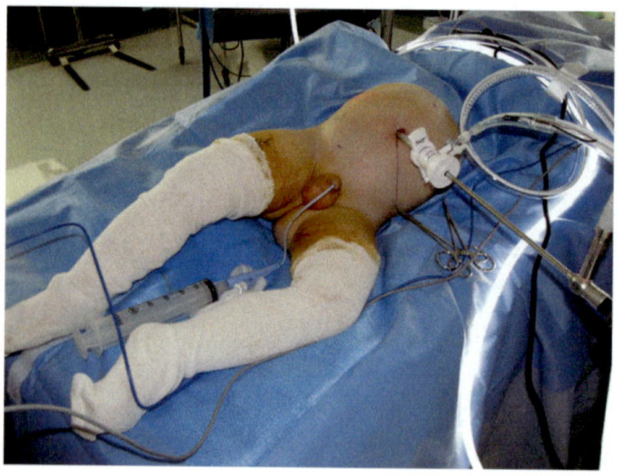

Fig. 10.1 Lateral decubitus position

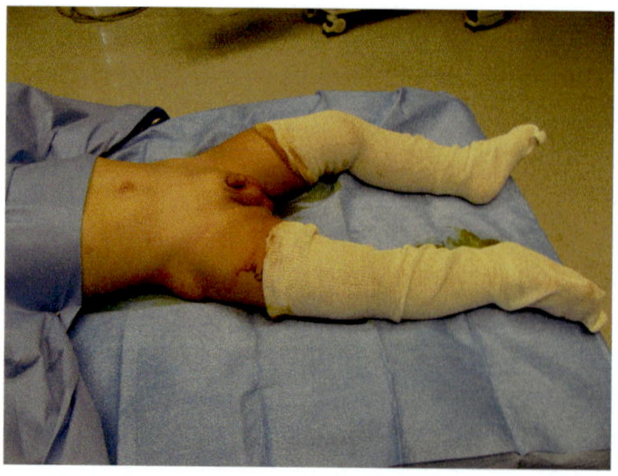

Fig. 10.2 Full-body prep

Port placement will also depend upon the level of ureteral pathology. A periumbilical port is standardly used for camera placement. In adults, this will commonly be a 10-mm port, but in children, this is typically a 5-mm port. For distal lesions, the working ports commonly will be on either side of the abdomen at a level commensurate with the patient size to allow for adequate distance between instruments and to assist in triangulation between instruments and camera. In larger patients, the instrument ports will often be infraumbilical, and as patient size decreases, the ports will move progressively cephalad. For proximal lesions, the working ports often are placed in the upper and lower quadrants on the ipsilateral side of pathology (Fig. 10.3). Instrument port size is dependent upon patient size and whether the robot will be used. In the smallest of patients, it is possible to insert 3-mm laparoscopic instruments directly through the abdominal wall without any trocars (Fig. 10.4). Such instrumentation allows for very satisfactory post-operative cosmesis, as insertion sites are almost undetectable (Fig. 10.5).

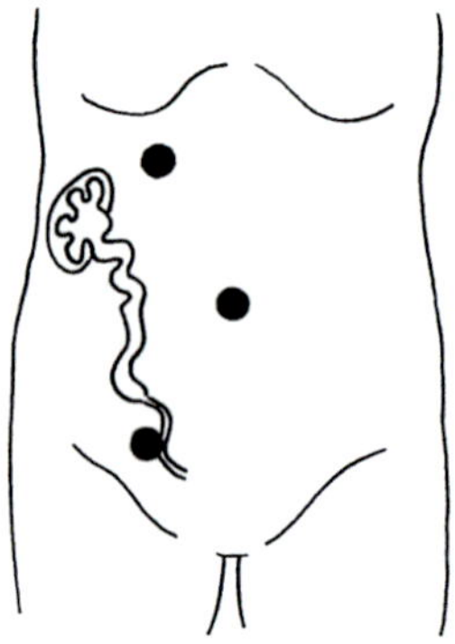

Fig. 10.3 Trocar placement for ureteroureterostomy

The colon is reflected and efforts are made to identify the ureter, which is often most apparent at the level of the iliacs. The level of pathology is identified (Fig. 10.6). This can be made clear sometimes by noting the level of demarcation between a dilated proximal ureter and a

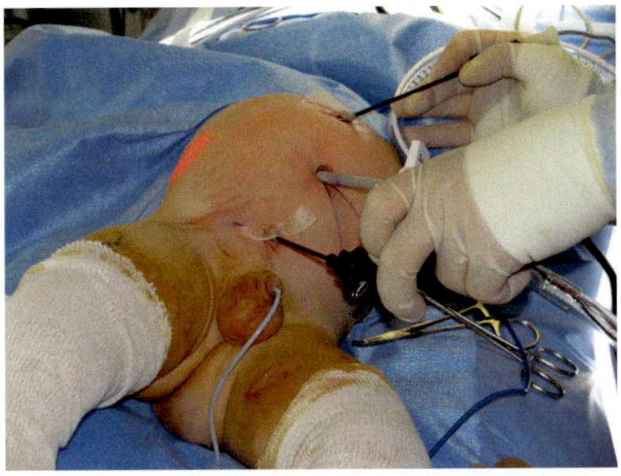

Fig. 10.4 Laparoscopy without trocars for instruments

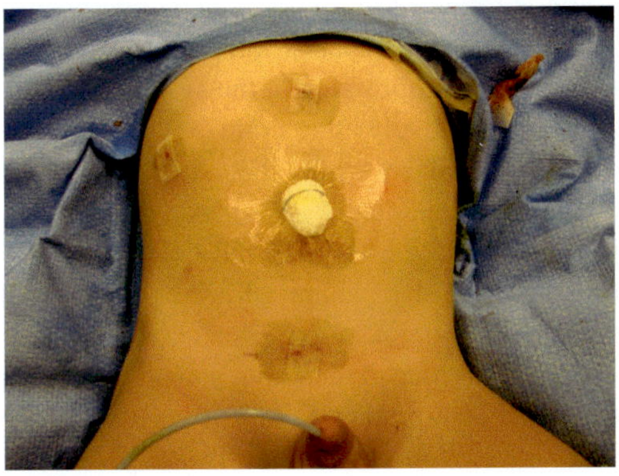

Fig. 10.5 Immediate post-operative appearance with dressings in place

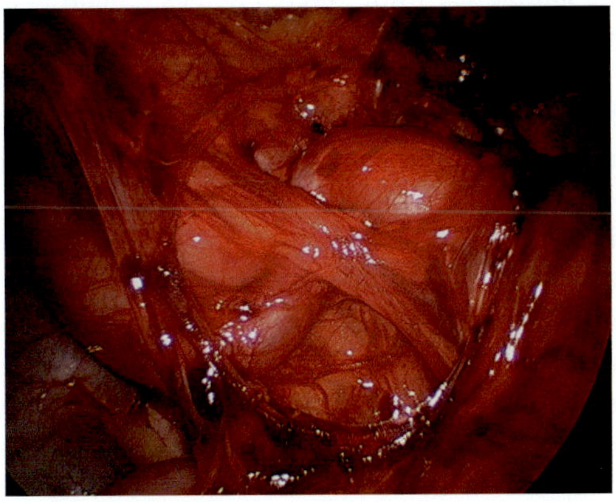

Fig. 10.6 Congenital midureteral stricture

normal caliber distal ureter. Also, if a ureteral catheter or a wire was placed up to the level of pathology previously, this may help. Abaza and Zafar also described a technique of intra-operative ureteroscopy with the ureteroscope directed by one surgeon up to the level of the narrowing, while the other surgeon laparoscopically visualizes the ureter and looks to see where the light from the ureteroscope transilluminates and then incises the ureter at this point. While this may be possible in adults, the pediatric ureter usually is too small to allow passage of a ureteroscope. Additionally, Abaza and Zafar describe cystoscopic retrograde placement of a ureteral occlusion balloon catheter that is passed proximal to the area of narrowing, the balloon inflated, and then pulled snug against the narrowing. This could potentially be dislodged and migrate proximally when repositioning the patient for the laparoscopic portion of surgery and may require cinching the ureteral balloon catheter back against the narrowing. The balloon can then be seen and/or palpated laparoscopically [39]. The ureter is mobilized sufficiently such that once the diseased segment has been excised, there will not be tension on the anastomosis. As with open surgery, care must be taken not to excessively mobilize the ureter and not to devascularize the ureter. The diseased segment is sharply excised and retrieved. Of note, if a double-J ureteral stent has already been placed cystoscopically, care must be taken not to incise it accidentally.

Each end of the ureter may have a stay suture placed through it, which helps in tissue manipulation and in ensuring proper alignment of the ends to prevent spiraling. Then each end of the ureter is spatulated. Again, care must be taken not to spiral the spatulation. If the proximal end is quite dilated, it may not be necessary to spatulate it. The ends are aligned using absorbable sutures placed between the spatulated apices and corners. While some have reported using 4-0 Vicryl, we feel that a monofilament suture such as PDS or Monocryl is superior as it does not drag the tissue. Additionally, in children, we prefer to use smaller suture material, like 6-0, as this better replicates the open surgery. As the corner sutures are tied down, one must be certain that there is not too much tension on the anastomosis, and if so, further mobilization is required. After placement of apical sutures, one can either run the anastomosis or place interrupted sutures (Fig. 10.7).

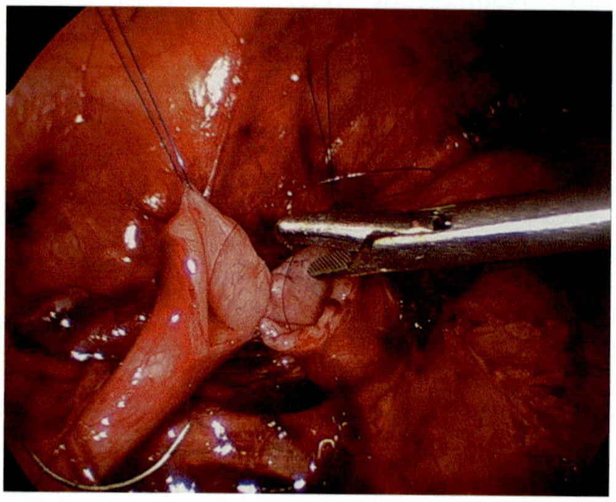

Fig. 10.7 Anastomosis for repair of midureteral stricture

Once one side of the anastomosis is complete, a stent may be passed across it. This can be done in a number of ways. If a double-J stent was placed cystoscopically at the beginning and has not been injured, the proximal end can be guided up into the pelvis. If a ureteral catheter was placed at the beginning, a guidewire can be passed through it, the catheter removed, and a double-J stent passed over the guidewire up into the renal pelvis. If no stent or catheter or wire was placed previously, a stent can later be introduced transabdominally. An angiocatheter can be seen laparoscopically to enter the abdominal wall. Its trajectory should be such that it is in line with the ureter. A guidewire is then placed through the angiocatheter and directed through the anastomosis distally down the ureter into the bladder, and the angiocatheter is removed. A double-J stent is then passed over the wire into the bladder. The guidewire is removed and the proximal end of the stent is guided up into the renal pelvis. Alternatively, if the ureterovesicular junction is too small to allow passage of a double-J stent, as in infants, a nephroureteral stent may be placed and the distal end guided laparoscopically across the anastomosis.

Once the stent is placed, the anastomosis is completed. Traction sutures are removed and the anastomosis inspected again to ensure that it is without tension and without spiraling. Additionally, with a stent in the bladder, the anastomosis can be inspected to look for evidence of leakage. If there is no stent in the bladder, intravenous indigo carmine can be administered and the anastomosis examined for evidence of leakage. Once satisfied with the anastomosis, a drain may be left near but not on the anastomosis to evaluate post-operatively for urinary leakage. The colon is replaced in a normal anatomic position. Also, a Foley catheter is left in the bladder for maximal decompression of the system.

Post-operatively, the drain and the catheter are left in place while the patient's diet and activity are gradually advanced. Typically on post-operative day 1 or 2, the Foley catheter is removed and the patient allowed to void spontaneously. If drain output remains undetectable, it can be removed and the patient discharged to home. If a double-J stent is in place, it can be removed 4–6 weeks later. If a nephroureteral stent is left in place, an antegrade nephrostogram can be performed 1–2 weeks later and if there is no extravasation, the nephroureteral stent can be removed. Of note, the patient should remain on antibiotics while foreign bodies remain in the urinary tract.

Once stents have been removed, the patient should have a follow-up study approximately 1 month later. This can be an ultrasound to look for evidence of hydroureteronephrosis. Additionally, it can be a diuretic renogram to rule out obstruction. The patient should return for further evaluation 1 year after surgery, as stricture recurrence typically occurs in the first year after surgery. However, extensive long-term follow-up is not mandated, as Selzman and Spirnak [40] demonstrated only an 11% recurrence rate after 1 year with an average follow-up of 8.5 years.

Reports of Laparoscopic Ipsilateral Ureteroureterostomy

Gonzalez and Piaggio reported the first series of laparoscopic IUU in 2007. This included eight laparoscopic IUU in four patients, four with ectopic ureter, and two with bilateral lower pole vesicoureteral reflux, all done without intraoperative complication. Of note, in the two patients with bilateral VUR, bilateral IUU was performed in the same operative setting. Postoperatively, the only complications were two cases of pyelonephritis, and at a mean follow-up of 10.7 months, all patients were doing well with decreasing or no residual hydronephrosis [41].

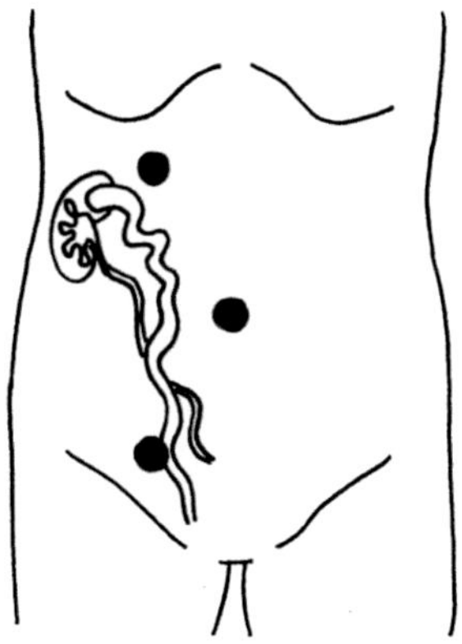

Fig. 10.8 Trocar placement for duplication anomaly ureteroureterostomy

Steps in Laparoscopic Ipsilateral Ureteroureterostomy

Prior to performing a laparoscopic IUU, investigations should be completed to ensure that there is sufficient function of the diseased pole to warrant reconstructive surgery rather than partial nephroureterectomy and to ascertain that the recipient ureter of the ipsilateral pole is without abnormality that would endanger the repair. At the time of surgery, cystoscopy and retrograde ureteral stent or catheter placement into the recipient ureter should be done. This will aid in distinguishing the donor and recipient ureters at the time of exploration. The stent can also be left post-operatively to aid in healing.

When performing the IUU low in the pelvis, the patient can be left in the supine position. The camera port is periumbilical and two instrument ports are positioned so as to maximize triangulation with a comfortable distance between working ports (Fig. 10.8). If necessary, the colon is reflected, and the ureters are identified at the pelvic brim. The donor ureter is mobilized as far distally as possible and transected, then spatulated if not already dilated. Care must be taken when approaching the common sheath not to injure the vascular supply to the recipient ureter. If the donor ureter is known to be refluxing, then the stump should be tied off. By taking the donor ureter as far distally as feasible, there is little chance for subsequent complications related to a residual stump. The laparoscopic approach makes it possible to essentially take a donor ureter all the way to its site of insertion, whether that is into the bladder or an ectopic location.

The recipient ureter is left in situ, to minimize potential for vascular injury, and incised longitudinally to match the diameter of the end of the donor ureter. While it is desirable to have some laxity in the donor ureter so as to prevent tension on the anastomosis, too much slack may lead to future kinking, and excess donor ureter may need to be excised prior to anastomosis. Once the ureters are properly aligned without spiraling, the anastomosis can be done using a fine monofilament suture in either a running or an interrupted fashion. Having a stent already present within the recipient ureter helps to prevent back-walling at the time of anastomosis. If preferred, the stent can be advanced across the anastomosis up into the donor renal pelvis after half of the anastomosis is complete; however, just leaving the stent within the recipient ureter seems to provide satisfactory results.

A retroperitoneal drain is left near the anastomosis and a Foley catheter is left in the bladder.

Post-operatively, the patient's diet and activity are advanced, and typically on post-operative day 1 or 2, the Foley catheter is removed and the patient allowed to void. Provided drain output is minimal, it can be removed prior to discharge. Ureteral stents are left indwelling and removed cystoscopically 4–6 weeks later. Once the stent is removed, the patient should be followed clinically as well as with imaging, such as ultrasound and nuclear renogram.

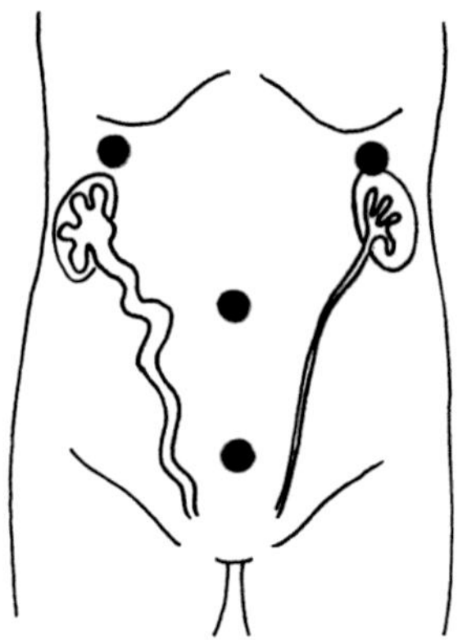

Fig. 10.9 Trocar placement for transureteroureterostomy

Reports of Laparoscopic Transureteroureterostomy

Dechet et al. [42] first demonstrated feasibility of laparoscopic TUU in 1999 when they described a side-to-side approach in a series of nine porcine models. Piaggio and Gonzalez in 2007 reported the first series of laparoscopic TUU in humans when they described their experience with the procedure in three patients with diagnoses of unilateral refluxing megaureter, unilateral obstruction following trans-trigonal reimplantation for VUR, and ureteral injury following bladder diverticulectomy. All three were completed without conversion or complication, and at a mean follow-up of 6 months, all had normal kidney function with improvement in hydronephrosis [43].

Steps in Laparoscopic Transureteroureterostomy

As with other ureteral surgeries, pre-operative investigation to confirm adequate renal function warranting salvage and a normal recipient ureter should be done. At the time of surgery, the patient should first undergo cystoscopy and retrograde placement of a ureteral stent or a catheter or a wire in the recipient ureter. The patient is then placed in the supine position and access is gained first with insertion of a periumbilical camera port. Working ports are placed on either side of the abdomen, and the younger and smaller the patient is, the more cephalad these ports must be placed (Fig. 10.9). Once port position is complete, the table is tilted in Trendelenburg position and angled with the diseased side elevated 30–45°.

The donor ureter can typically be identified at the pelvic brim, and the overlying peritoneum incised. The donor ureter is then mobilized as far distally as possible, taking care not to damage other structures in the area, such as the vas deferens in the male and the ovary and fallopian tube in the female. The ureter is transected and the stump tied off. Proximal mobilization of the donor ureter is then performed, preserving the periureteral adventitia and vascular supply. A stay suture can be placed through the end of the donor ureter for tissue handling.

The table is then angled with the recipient side elevated 30–45° and the recipient ureter is identified and overlying peritoneum incised. The recipient ureter should not be mobilized in an effort to preserve all collateral blood supply. A tunnel is created under the rectosigmoid mesentery and the stay suture on the donor ureter is grasped and brought under the rectosigmoid. If there is any tension on the donor ureter, further proximal mobilization is necessary. If there is excess donor ureter that would create kinking at the anastomosis, the redundant ureter can be excised.

A longitudinal incision is made on the medial aspect of the recipient ureter at a level that will permit a tangential anastomosis, rather than a perpendicular one, and for a length that will match the diameter of the donor ureter. Stay sutures can be placed between the ureters at the apices of the anastomosis and then the sutures can be placed in either a running or an interrupted fashion to complete the anastomosis. If the recipient ureter is of sufficient caliber, it may be possible to place a stent across the anastomosis up into the donor pelvis in addition to the stent up into the recipient pelvis. Otherwise, only a stent left in the recipient ureter is sufficient. Again, a drain should be left near the anastomosis to monitor for leakage post-operatively, and a Foley catheter should be left in the bladder. The Foley catheter can be removed on post-operative day 1 or 2 and drain output monitored while the patient voids spontaneously. Provided drain output remains minimal, it can be removed prior to discharge. Ureteral stents are removed 4–6 weeks post-operatively and the patient is followed both clinically and radiologically with ultrasounds and nuclear renograms.

Management of Complications

As with open ureteral surgery, when proper patient selection and surgical techniques are adhered to, the complication rate is extremely low. One of the most common complications seems to be urinary extravasation. If a drain is left in the retroperitoneum, the urine leak can be identified early and dealt with. Usually conservative management, with Foley catheter placement and leaving the drain in place until the leak has resolved, is satisfactory. If a ureteral stent was not already left indwelling at the time of initial repair, either a retrograde ureteral stent or a percutaneous nephrostomy tube can be placed to decompress the system.

Another potential complication is stricture of the anastomosis. This can be detected early prior to deleterious effect on renal function by close post-operative surveillance with ultrasonography. Mild stricture can be managed via minimally invasive approaches, like balloon dilation. More severe stricture may require repeat surgery with excision of the stricture and repeat anastomosis.

Conclusion

Ureteral surgery is indicated to treat a myriad of pathology, particularly in the pediatric population. It lends itself well to the laparoscopic approach, which permits access to the entire length of the ureter. The laparoscopic approach has been reported with satisfactory results for ureteroureterostomy of a single ureter to itself, IUU within a duplicated system, and TUU. This success is due to strict adherence to the principles of open ureteral surgery and is perhaps enhanced by the magnification of laparoscopy. Complications are infrequent and can usually be managed conservatively.

Critical Operative Steps

1. Identify recipient ureter with ureteral catheter (duplication anomalies).
2. Recipient ureter remains in situ (duplication anomalies).
3. Align anastomosis with fixation sutures.
4. Limit dissection to preserve blood supply.
5. Use fine suture in infants and small children.
6. Stent the reconstruction.

Critical Instruments and Supplies

1. Atraumatic graspers
2. Sharpened fine tissue scissors
3. Needle drivers (according to surgeon's preference)
4. Monitors in close proximity to both surgeon and camera driver
5. Heated insufflation for infants and small children

References

1. Campbell M. Anomalies of the ureter. In: Campbell MF, Harrison JH, editors. Urology. 3rd ed. Philadelphia, PA: W.B. Saunders; 1970. p. 1515.
2. Campbell MF. Anomalies of the upper urinary tract. In: Bauer S, Perlmutter A, Retik A, editors. Urology. Philadelphia, PA: W.B. Saunders; 1979. p. 1317.
3. Allen TD. Congenital ureteral strictures. J Urol. Jul 1970;104(1):196–204.
4. Tanagho EA, Smith DR, Guthrie TH. Pathophysiology of functional ureteral obstruction. J Urol. Jul 1970;104(1):73–88.
5. Wall B, Wachter E. Congenital ureteral valve: its role as a primary obstructive lesion: classification of the literature and report of an authentic case. J Urol. Oct 1952;68(4):684–90.
6. Gray S, Skandalakis J. Embryology for surgeons: the embryological basis for the treatment of congenital defects. Philadelphia, PA: W.B. Saunders; 1972.
7. Heslin JE, Mamonas C. Retrocaval ureter: report of four cases and review of literature. J Urol. Feb 1951;65(2):212–22.
8. Zhang XD, Hou SK, Zhu JH, Wang XF, Meng GD, Qu XK. Diagnosis and treatment of retrocaval ureter. Eur Urol. 1990;18(3):207–10.
9. Kenawi MM, Williams DI. Circumcaval ureter: a report of four cases in children with a review of the literature and a new classification. Br J Urol. Jun 1976;48(3):183–92.
10. Foley F. Uretero-ureterostomy. As applied to obstruction of the duplicated upper urinary tract. J Urol. 1928;20:109.
11. Küss RR. Chirurgie plastique et réparatrice de la voie excrétrice du rein; indications et techniques opératoires. Paris: Masson; 1954.
12. Nation E. Duplication of the kidney and ureter: a statistical study of 230 new cases. J Urol. 1944; 51:456–65.
13. Smith FL, Ritchie EL, Maizels M, et al. Surgery for duplex kidneys with ectopic ureters: ipsilateral ureteroureterostomy versus polar nephrectomy. J Urol. Aug 1989;142(2 Pt 2):532–4; discussion 542–3.
14. Amar AD. Reimplantation of completely duplicated ureters. J Urol. Feb 1972;107(2):230–2.
15. Johnston JH, Heal MR. Reflux in complete duplicated ureters in children: management and techniques. J Urol. Jun 1971;105(6):881–7.
16. Barrett DM, Malek RS, Kelalis PP. Problems and solutions in surgical treatment of 100 consecutive ureteral duplications in children. J Urol. Jul 1975;114(1):126–30.
17. Diaz-Ball FL, Fink A, Moore CA, Gangai MP. Pyeloureterostomy and ureteroureterostomy: alternative procedures to partial nephrectomy for duplication of the ureter with only one pathological segment. J Urol. Nov 1969;102(5):621–6.
18. Huisman TK, Kaplan GW, Brock WA, Packer MG. Ipsilateral ureteroureterostomy and pyeloureterostomy: a review of 15 years of experience with 25 patients. J Urol. Nov 1987;138(5):1207–10.
19. O'Reilly PH, Shields RA, Testa HJ, Lawson RS, Edwards EC. Ureteroureteric reflux. Pathological entity or physiological phenomenon? Br J Urol. Apr 1984;56(2):159–64.
20. Casati E, Boari A. Contributo sperimentale alla plastica dell'urretere. Atti Acad Med Natl. 1894;14:149.
21. Higgins C. Transuretero-ureteral anastomosis: report of a clinical case. J Urol. 1935;34:349–55.
22. Halpern GN, King LR, Belman AB. Transureteroureterostomy in children. J Urol. Mar 1973;109(3):504–9.
23. Ayyat FM, Adams G. Congenital midureteral strictures. Urology. Aug 1985;26(2):170–2.
24. Carlton CE Jr., Guthrie AG, Scott R Jr.. Surgical correction of ureteral injury. J Trauma. Jun 1969;9(6):457–64.
25. Jelloul L, Valayer J. Ureteroureteral anastomosis in the treatment of reflux associated with ureteral duplication. J Urol. May 1997;157(5):1863–5.
26. Lashley DB, McAleer IM, Kaplan GW. Ipsilateral ureteroureterostomy for the treatment of vesicoureteral reflux or obstruction associated with complete ureteral duplication. J Urol. Feb 2001;165(2):552–4.
27. Choi H, Oh SJ. The management of children with complete ureteric duplication: selective use of uretero-ureterostomy as a primary and salvage procedure. BJU Int. Sep 2000;86(4):508–12.
28. Young JD Jr., Aledia FT. Further observations on flank ureterostomy and cutaneous transureteroureterostomy. J Urol. Mar 1966;95(3):327–33.
29. Hendren WH, Hensle TW. Transureteroureterostomy: experience with 75 cases. J Urol. Jun 1980;123(6):826–33.
30. Chilton CP, Vordermark JS, Ransley PG. Transuretero-ureterostomy – a review of its use in modern paediatric urology. Br J Urol. Dec 1984;56(6):604–08.
31. Hodges CV, Barry JM, Fuchs EF, Pearse HD, Tank ES. Transureteroureterostomy: 25-year experience with 100 patients. J Urol. Jun 1980;123(6):834–8.
32. Pesce C, Costa L, Campobasso P, Fabbro MA, Musi L. Successful use of transureteroureterostomy in children: a clinical study. Eur J Pediatr Surg. Dec 2001;11(6):395–8.
33. Nezhat CH, Nezhat F, Seidman D, Nezhat C. Laparoscopic ureteroureterostomy: a prospective follow-up of 9 patients. Prim Care Update Ob Gyns. 1 Jul 1998;5(4):200.
34. Tulikangas PK, Gill IS, Falcone T. Laparoscopic repair of ureteral injuries. J Am Assoc Gynecol Laparosc. May 2001;8(2):259–62.
35. Bhandarkar DS, Lalmalani JG, Shah VJ. Laparoscopic resection and ureteroureterostomy for congenital midureteral stricture. J Endourol. Mar 2005;19(2):140–2.

36. Passerotti CC, Diamond DA, Borer JG, Eisner BH, Barrisford G, Nguyen HT. Robot-assisted laparoscopic ureteroureterostomy: description of technique. J Endourol. Apr 2008;22(4):581–4; discussion 585.
37. Thiel DD, Badger WJ, Winfield HN. Robot-assisted laparoscopic excision and ureteroureterostomy for congenital midureteral stricture. J Endourol. Dec 2008;22(12):2667–9.
38. Simmons MN, Gill IS, Fergany AF, Kaouk JH, Desai MM. Laparoscopic ureteral reconstruction for benign stricture disease. Urology. Feb 2007;69(2):280–4.
39. Abaza R, Zafar SS. Techniques for laparoscopic and robotic localization of intraluminal ureteral pathology. Urology. Mar 2009;73(3):582–5.
40. Selzman AA, Spirnak JP. Iatrogenic ureteral injuries: a 20-year experience in treating 165 injuries. J Urol. Mar 1996;155(3):878–81.
41. Gonzalez R, Piaggio L. Initial experience with laparoscopic ipsilateral ureteroureterostomy in infants and children for duplication anomalies of the urinary tract. J Urol. Jun 2007;177(6):2315–8.
42. Dechet CB, Young MM, Segura JW. Laparoscopic transureteroureterostomy: demonstration of its feasibility in swine. J Endourol. Sep 1999;13(7):487–93.
43. Piaggio LA, Gonzalez R. Laparoscopic transureteroureterostomy: a novel approach. J Urol. Jun 2007;177(6):2311–4.

Chapter 11

Robotic Ureteroureterostomy and Correction of Ureteral Defects

Patricio C. Gargollo and Hiep T. Nguyen

This chapter contains a video segment which can be found at the URL: http://www.springerimages.com/ost

Introduction

The first reports of laparoscopy were published in the early twentieth century [1]. The introduction of improved instrumentation and advances in optical systems has led to not only increased use of minimally invasive surgery but also an expansion of the types of procedures that can be done laparoscopically. With the increasing use of minimally invasive techniques in urology over the past decade, the feasibility of pediatric laparoscopic reconstructive urologic surgery with and without robot assistance has been demonstrated [2, 3]. The da Vinci® surgical robot has now become widely utilized in adult and pediatric urology. In adults, radical prostatectomy and pyeloplasty are the most popular robotic procedures, although virtually all major urologic procedures involving the genitourinary tract have been performed with the robot. In the realm of pediatric urology, robotic pyeloplasty and ureteral reimplantation for vesicoureteral reflux (VUR) are now the most commonly performed robotic procedures. Similar to the adult population, essentially all intra-abdominal urologic procedures in the pediatric population have been performed laparoscopically with and without robotic assistance.

P.C. Gargollo (✉)
Pediatric Urology, Childrens Medical Center, UT Southwestern Medical Center, Dallas, TX, USA
e-mail: patricio.gargollo@childrens.com

Ureteral obstruction can occur anywhere from the kidney to the bladder, with the two most common locations being the ureteropelvic and the ureterovesical junctions. Obstruction at the mid-ureteral level is unusual, accounting for approximately 4% of all cases, and can have a varied etiology [4]. The ureteroureterostomy (UU) was first described by Foley in 1928 [5] and has been a valuable procedure to treat most cases of ureteral obstruction, which may be secondary to congenital anatomic abnormalities, calculus disease, or even iatrogenic events. The approaches for performing a UU range from open procedures to endoscopic treatment with the primary goal being reconstitution of a normal ureteral lumen using healthy tissue.

Early laparoscopic efforts to reconstruct ureteral segments via UU were mainly after iatrogenic injuries acquired during gynecological surgery [6]. Over the last few decades, however, there have been published reports of laparoscopic ureteroureterostomy (LAU) in adults and children [7]. The advantages of the da Vinci Robotic system over traditional laparoscopy for performing a UU include improved optics and ease of the intricate suturing required for creating a watertight anastomosis. Over time it has become evident that LAU is an invaluable technique both for ureteral reconstruction secondary to injury and for the management of congenital and acquired conditions of the ureter.

This chapter will cover LAU for the correction of ureteral obstruction, ureteral duplication with

M.C. Ost (ed.), *Robotic and Laparoscopic Reconstructive Surgery in Children and Adults*, Current Clinical Urology, DOI 10.1007/978-1-60327-914-7_11, © Springer Science+Business Media, LLC 2011

reflux or obstruction, and ureteral injury in children. The techniques described herein can also be applied to robotic-assisted LAU. The corrections of ureteropelvic and ureterovesical obstructions are covered elsewhere in this text.

Indications

The decision to approach ureteral abnormalities via a laparoscopic or an open approach is multifactorial. A laparoscopic or a robotic-assisted approach should be attempted only by experienced laparoscopic surgeons with the appropriate equipment easily accessible.

The etiologies for which a LAU may be considered as a reconstructive technique are listed in Table 11.1. Congenital ureteral anomalies include duplication anomalies, ureteral valves, and retrocaval ureters. Duplication anomalies can further be sub-divided into obstructing and refluxing. The former include ureteral ectopia and ureteroceles which almost exclusively affect the upper pole of duplex systems. The latter usually affect the lower pole moiety. Whether a UU is the optimal modality for these duplication anomalies is controversial. However, in open series, several authors have shown that this is a viable treatment option for these conditions yielding excellent results [8–10].

Other congenital causes of ureteral obstruction that may be amenable to treatment by LAU include ureteral valves and retrocaval ureters. Both are exceedingly rare. There are fewer than 50 cases of congenital ureteral valves reported in the literature. These structures can occur at any point along the ureter. Leading theories as to their origin cite abnormal embryogenesis of the ureter and possibly persistence of Chawalla's membrane [11]. The feasibility of employing laparoscopic techniques for the reconstruction of retrocaval ureters has been established [12].

Pathologic obstruction can occur intrinsic or extrinsic to the ureter. Intrinsic lesions include iatrogenic or acquired ureteral strictures (usually from prolonged endoscopy, vascular injury, or recurrent calculus disease), ureterolithiasis, and fibroepithelial polyps. LAU is particularly useful in cases of ureterolithiasis when previous endoscopic therapy has failed [13]. Extrinsic lesions are also rare and include retroperitoneal fibrosis and retroperitoneal tumors. Lastly iatrogenic or traumatic injury (usually penetrating trauma) could be approached by LAU.

The only case series of robotic-assisted UU was published by Passerotti et al. in 2008 [14]. In that series, three patients were treated for ureteral obstruction at the mid-ureter. All patients had a non-eventful post-operative course without complications. The mean operative time was 244 min, and the mean length of stay was 3.5 days. Both the operative times and total analgesic use in this series were similar to those reported in the two largest series of pediatric robot-assisted laparoscopic pyeloplasties [3, 15]. Published series of open UU show a shorter LOS and mean operative time [16]. However, from the experience in robotic-assisted pyeloplasty in children, it is feasible to predict that increased familiarity with this procedure will decrease both operative times and LOS [3].

Table 11.1 Indications for laparoscopic UU

Congenital ureteral anomalies
Duplication anomalies
Ureteral ectopia
Ureterocele
Vesicoureteral reflux
Ureteral valves
Retrocaval ureter
Pathologic obstruction
Intrinsic
Ureteral strictures
Polyarteritis nodosa (PAN)
Prolonged endoscopy
Recurrent ureterolithiasis
Vascular injury
Ureterolithiasis
Fibroepithelial polyps
Extrinsic
Retroperitoneal fibrosis
Tumor
Iatrogenic injury
Penetrating trauma

Surgical Technique

Pre-operative Preparation

Many of the below steps are surgeon dependent. These are the preparative steps we follow at Children's Hospital Boston and Children's Medical Center Dallas. Patients receive a clear liquid diet for 24 h and a rectal suppository the night before the procedure. Upon arrival to the operating room, they receive a dose of antibiotics, usually cefazolin (unless they have a documented allergy). Depending on surgeon's preference, cystoscopy, retrograde pyelogram, and double-J stent placement are performed at the start of the procedure. In cases of duplication anomalies and ureteral ectopia where there may not be proximal dilation of the obstructed ureter, we strongly recommend ureteral stent placement in order to aid in ureteral identification. This also avoids potentially cumbersome ureteral stent placement from the mid-ureter during the procedure. A Foley catheter and an orogastric tube are placed prior to trocar placement.

Patient Positioning

The procedure is performed under general endotracheal anesthesia. After induction, the patient is positioned supine in low lithotomy using padded stirrups. The arms are tucked at the sides. A 30° wedge is placed under the patient, elevating the affected side. In cases of duplication anomalies, the ureter is approached lower in the pelvis and thus no wedge is necessary. Figure 11.1 shows the appropriate room and surgical team setup. All pressure points are carefully padded. The patient

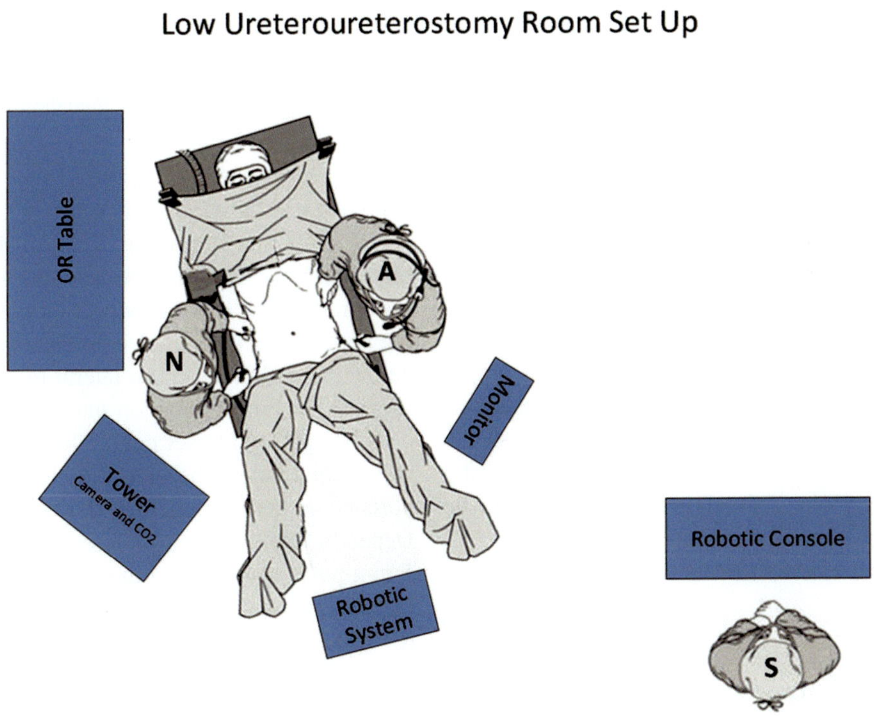

Fig. 11.1 The figure shows the appropriate setup of the surgical team for a low robotic UU. The patient is placed in a low dorsal lithotomy and the table is placed in Trendelenburg. In cases of mid-ureteral anomalies where a mid-ureter UU is necessary, the affected side is raised on a wedge and the port setup as well as the robotic system is arranged as depicted in Fig. 11.2. N, nurse; A, surgical assistant; S, console surgeon

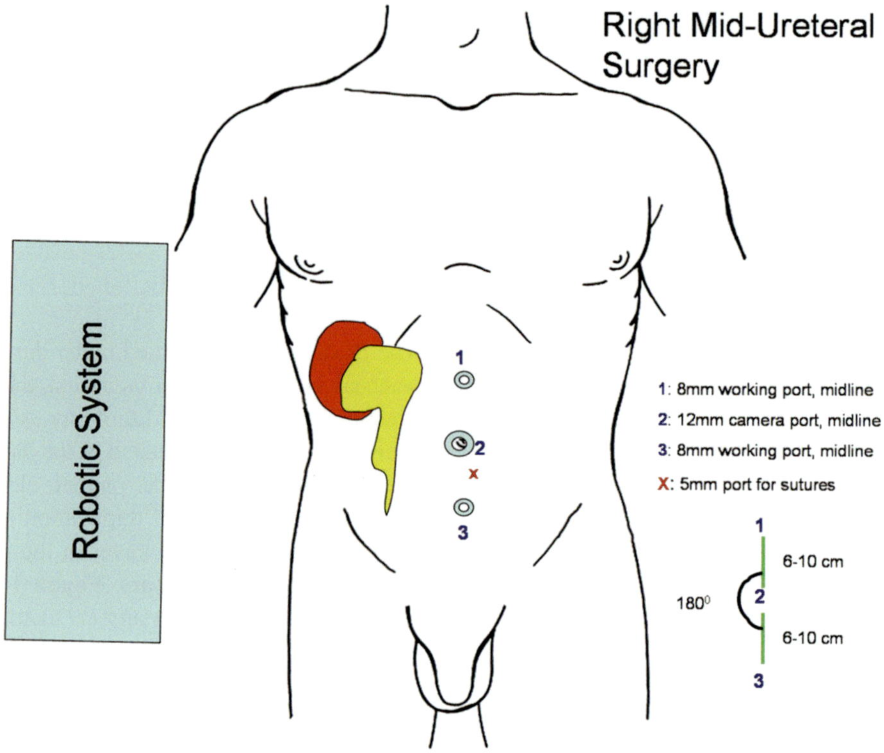

Fig. 11.2 Depicted are the port placements necessary for a mid-ureteral UU. Depending on the available equipment, smaller camera and working ports may be used. Alternatively a fourth, 5-mm assistant port can be placed slightly off the midline and away from the affected site

is then secured to the operating table and a sterile prep and draping proceeds as standard. An alternative is to use a vacuum bean bag under the patient. A wedge can then be placed under the bean bag under the site of interest. The shoulder extensions are placed over the patient's shoulders prior to deflating it. The shoulder extensions are then taped in a crossed fashion across the patient's chest and the tape is secured to the operating table. This allows for the table to be placed in steep Trendelenburg without fear that the patient will not remain securely in position.

Port Placement

The table is rotated to place the patient in a flat supine position in order for the ports to be placed safely. Either a Hasson or a Veress needle approach can be used for first access. A 12-mm port (or 10 mm depending on availability) for the camera is first inserted into the umbilicus. For mid-ureteral lesions, two 5- or 8-mm working ports are then inserted, equidistant above and below the umbilicus, 1 cm lateral to the midline (Fig. 11.3). For duplication anomalies (ureterocele, ectopia, and lower pole reflux), the ureter is approached below the iliac vessels and thus the ports could be positioned as shown in Fig. 11.4. Depending on surgeon's preference, an additional 5-mm port can be placed in the midline between the superior working port and the camera port to help with suctioning, passing sutures, and holding the tissues. Of importance, radiographic images of the obstruction should be reviewed prior to placing the ports; the positions of the working ports may have to be adjusted laterally or medially in order to place the instruments at the optimal distance and location. For mid-ureteral

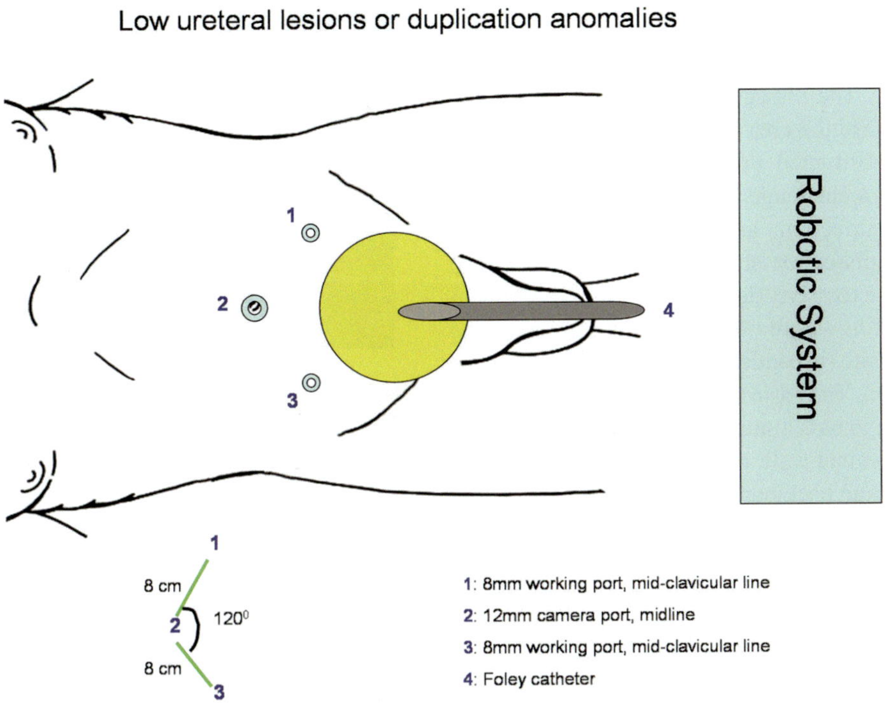

Fig. 11.3 Depicted are the port placements necessary for a low UU. This setup is particularly useful for duplication anomalies or bilateral processes. Depending on the available equipment, smaller camera and working ports may be used. Alternatively a fourth, 5-mm assistant port can be placed slightly off the midline and away from the affected site

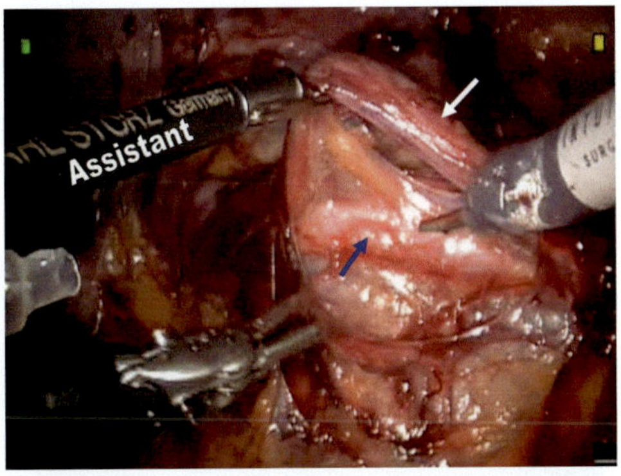

Fig. 11.4 Identification and dissection of the ureter(s). The figure depicts the initial step in performing a UU for a duplication anomaly. In this case the patient had an ectopic right upper pole ureter (*blue arrow*). The lower pole ureter (*white arrow*) is reflected superiorly by an assistant and the ureters are separated by the robotic surgeon

lesions (Fig. 11.2) the patient is rotated maximally in the opposite direction and the robot is engaged coming over the affected side. For low approaches to the ureter (Fig. 11.3), the robot is engaged between the patient's legs.

Approach and Identification of the Ureteral Obstruction

Access to the ureter can be through a transmesenteric or retroperitoneal approach. In the latter the colon is reflected medially by incising along the white line of Toldt, exposing the retroperitoneum. The transmesenteric approach is particularly feasible in younger children where mesenteric adiposity does not obscure the vascular tributaries to the colon. If a UU is to be performed below the femoral vessels, the retroperitoneum is opened and the ureters can easily be identified coursing along their normal path (Fig. 11.4).

In cases of ureteral obstruction, because the ureter is dilated proximal to the area of the obstruction, it can be identified more easily by first dissecting near the lower pole of the kidney. Caution should be exercised not to injure the gonadal vessels, which lie close to the ureter in this area. The dissection is then carried out distally toward the area of the obstruction. Isolation of the obstructed ureteral segment may sometimes be a challenge because of previous inflammation, infection, and scarring. The extent of ureteral dissection should be limited in order to prevent excessive devascularization. Placement of a holding suture often is helpful in keeping the surgical site suspended above the pooling of urine and blood. The easiest method of placing a "hitch stitch" is to pass a suture from the outside through the abdominal wall, then through the structure to be held, and back out of the abdomen (Fig. 11.5). This allows the tension on the hitch stitch to be adjusted as needed. The ureter is then incised above and below the area of obstruction. In the case involves ureterolithiasis, the stone can be removed at this time [17]. The proximal segment of the ureter is spatulated medially and the distal segment laterally. Depending on surgeon's preference, the anastomosis can be performed in an interrupted or a running fashion with 6-0 Vicryl with the posterior wall being approximated first. A fourth port may be helpful to allow the tissues to be moved and retracted to facilitate suturing. As stated above, a double-J stent can be placed either prior to the start of or during the procedure although the former method tends to be easier. The stent is placed retrograde up to the stenotic site, and after the obstructed segment is removed, the stent is pulled out of the distal ureter and inserted into the upper ureter.

In cases of ureteral duplication and ectopia, the ureters are approached below the pelvic brim and the trocar positions are shifted (Fig. 11.3). The obstructed upper pole ureter can usually be identified because it is more dilated than the lower pole ureter. Again, placement of a stent into the intravesical, lower pole ureter, simplifies ureteral identification during the robotic portion of the procedure. If a lower pole to upper pole UU is to be performed for VUR, a stent is placed into the upper pole ureter. In these unique situations, the upper pole ureter (ectopia, ureterocele) or the lower pole ureter (reflux) is transected and anastomosed in an end-to-side fashion to the recipient ureter after spatulation of the donor ureter (Figs. 11.6 and 11.7). The ureterotomy in the recipient ureter should be of approximately the same size as the spatulated segment of donor ureter.

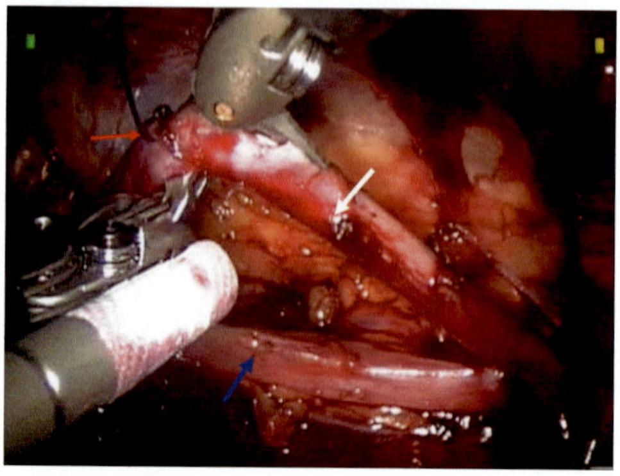

Fig. 11.5 Placement of the "hitch stitch." The figure depicts placement of the hitch stitch (*red arrow*). The hitch stitch is placed in the recipient ureter (*white arrow*). In this case the recipient ureter is the lower pole in the case of ureteral duplication with upper pole ureteral (*blue arrow*) ectopia. However, in cases of vesicoureteral reflux, the upper pole may be the recipient ureter

After the completion of the anastomosis (Fig. 11.8), the retroperitoneal wall can be reconstituted using a running 4-0 Vicryl suture. The robot is disengaged and the ports are removed under vision. We close all fascia with a single interrupted 2-0 Vicryl suture on a UR-6 needle. A

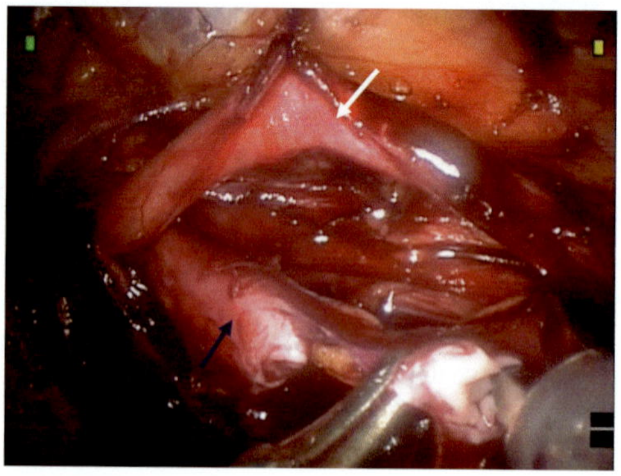

Fig. 11.6 Donor ureter transection. The figure depicts transection of the upper pole (*blue arrow*) donor ureter. The recipient lower pole ureter is shown by the *white arrow*

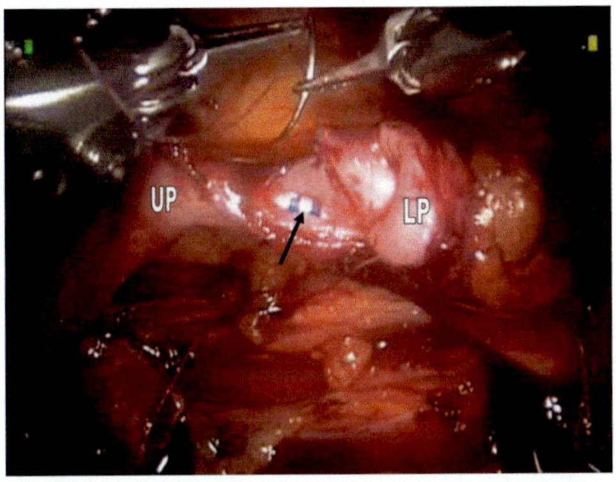

Fig. 11.7 Anastomosis. The anastomosis of the donor ureter (*upper pole*, UP) to the recipient ureter (*lower pole*, LP) is completed in an end-to-side fashion. A ureteral stent (*black arrow*) is ideally placed as the initial step in the case and left in place after the anastomosis is complete

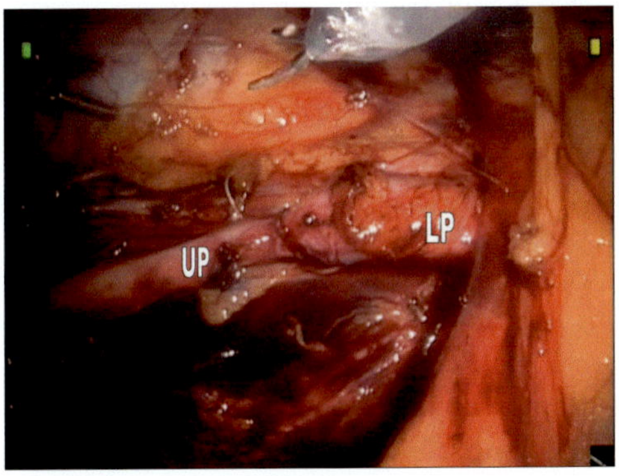

Fig. 11.8 Completed anastomosis. This figure shows the completed UU. The *upper pole* (UP) has been anastomosed to the *lower pole* (LP)

drain is not routinely used since we prefer to leave a ureteral stent. The skin can enclosed with a 5-0 Monocryl subcuticular stitch. Patients are admitted overnight. The Foley catheter is removed on post-operative day 1 and the patient is sent home if stable. Ureteral stents are removed 3–4 weeks post-operatively.

Follow-up

The exact timing and modality for radiographic follow-up is the subject of debate and is usually surgeon dependent [16]. We advocate a renal ultrasound 2 weeks after stent removal or at 6 weeks post-operatively if a stent is not used. In cases of a ureterocele or a VUR, we advocate a cystogram 3 months post-operatively.

Surgical Considerations

Several points require discussion when the treatment of ureteral pathology (obstruction or reflux) in duplication anomalies is considered. Concerns have been raised about performing this procedure when significant ureteral size disparity is present [18, 19]. In these cases, several authors have suggested that if the recipient ureterotomy length is equal to the diameter of the larger donor ureter, then ureteral size disparity has no influence on surgical outcome [10]. This has been our experience as well.

It is not clear if the function of the upper pole moiety in cases of ectopia or ureterocele has any bearing on operative success of UU. There is a theoretical risk in these cases of either jeopardizing the lower pole if an anastomotic complication ensues or creating "yo-yo" reflux [20]. This entity has not been observed in over 200 patients undergoing UU [9, 10, 16, 21]. Furthermore, concerns that a retained poorly functioning moiety will lead to hypertension, proteinuria, or malignancy have not been substantiated [22].

Operative Complications

There are complications related to the technique of laparoscopy regardless of the type of surgery being performed. A thorough review of these is beyond the scope of this chapter but any surgeon who performs laparoscopic surgery should be very familiar with the potential physiologic complications of pneumoperitoneum, access injuries (including bowel and vascular injuries), thermal injuries from cautery devices, and peripheral nerve injuries from inappropriate patient positioning [23–25].

Post-operative Complications

Complication rates are not available for LAU since there is only one series in the pediatric literature involving three patients [26]. The complication rates below are therefore for published series of open UU. Urine leak from the ureter-oureteral anastomosis can be observed as an early or a late complication and is the most common published complication of UU affecting up to 14% of patients [10]. For this reason, and to aid in intraoperative identification of the ureters, we advocate ureteral stent placement into the recipient ureter as well as a running anastomosis. Other reported complications include urinary tract infections, urinoma, inadvertent transaction of the recipient ureter, ileus, anastomotic stricture, bleeding, persistent or de novo vesicoureteral reflux, and persistent hydronephrosis. Infection of retained ureteral segments has been reported [10, 27]. We advocate complete excision of the donor ureteral stump as far distal as possible to attempt to prevent this.

The theoretical complication of "yo-yo" reflux [28] has not been reported in any pediatric series where UU was employed as a treatment modality for the conditions outlined in Table 11.1 [8–10, 16, 18, 21, 29–33]. If there is concern for "yo-yo" reflux, the LAU could be performed closer to the kidney with excision of the remaining ureteral stump.

Conclusions

Similar to the adult population, essentially all intra-abdominal urologic procedures in the pediatric population including upper pole heminephrectomy, orchidopexy for undescended testis, and ureterocalicostomy have been performed using laparoscopy with and without robotic assistance. In fact, virtually any major urologic procedure can be performed in a minimally invasive fashion. Robotic-assisted laparoscopic ureteroureterostomy has been shown to be safe, feasible, and effective in pediatric patients. This method can be employed in the management of congenital and acquired ureteral anomalies at all anatomic levels of the ureter and is an important laparoscopic technique in the pediatric urologist's armamentarium.

Critical Instruments and Supplies

- Cystoscopic equipment
- Open-ended ureteral catheters
- Double-J stent
- Veress needle
- VersaStep™ bladeless trocars (Covidien, Mansfield, MA)
  - A 12- or 10-mm camera port
  - Optional 5-mm port to be used as fourth "assistant port"
- Laparoscopic instrumentation
  - Bipolar cautery grasper
  - Monopolar scissors or monopolar hook dissector
  - Laparoscopic Potts scissors
  - Laparoscopic needle drivers
  - Laparoscopic microforceps
- Sutures
  - 6-0 Vicryl for anastomosis
  - 2-0 PDS for "hitch stitch"
  - 4-0 Vicryl to re-approximate retroperitoneal layer
  - 5-0 Monocryl suture for subcuticular skin closure
- Intraoperative ultrasound with laparoscopic transducer (optional) if a case of ureterolithiasis

Critical Operative Steps

- Placement of Foley catheter and orogastric tube after induction.

- Cystoscopic placement of ureteral stent into the affected ureter if single system or into the recipient ureter if duplicated system (optional).
- Appropriate patient positioning depending on the ureteral level of interest (Figs. 11.2 and 11.3) taking care to pad all pressure points and ensuring that the patient is secured to the OR table.
- Appropriate port placement for ureteral level of interest (Figs. 11.2 and 11.3).
- Docking of robotic system if robotic-assisted laparoscopy is to be performed.
- Dissection and exposure of ureter (Fig. 11.4).
- Transection of ureter and excision of stricture segment if appropriate (Fig. 11.6).
- Ureteral spatulation and ureterotomy of recipient ureter if duplicated system.
- End-to-end (single system) or end-to-side (duplicated system) anastomosis. We prefer a running technique using two suture lines one on the posterior aspect and one on the anterior aspect of the anastomosis (Figs. 11.7 and 11.8).
- Antegrade ureteral stent placement according to surgeon's preference.
- Closure of the peritoneal or mesenteric defect
- Port removal, fascial and skin closure

References

1. Lau W, Leow CK, Li AK. History of endoscopic and laparoscopic surgery. World J Surg. 1997;21: 444–53.
2. Passerotti C, Cendron M, Gargollo P, et al. Minimally invasive surgical approaches to retrovesical structures. Int J Med Robot. Dec 2007;3(4): 307–11.
3. Lee RS, Retik AB, Borer JG, Peters CA. Pediatric robot assisted laparoscopic dismembered pyeloplasty: comparison with a cohort of open surgery. J Urol. Feb 2006;175(2):683–7; discussion 687.
4. Kim EK, Song TB. A study on fetal urinary tract anomaly: antenatal ultrasonographic diagnosis and postnatal follow-up. J Obstet Gynaecol Res. Dec 1996;22(6):569–73.
5. Foley F. Uretero-ureterostomy: as applied to obstructions of the duplicated urinary tract. J Urol. 1928;20:109.
6. Gomel V, James C. Intraoperative management of ureteral injury during operative laparoscopy. Fertil Steril. Feb 1991;55(2):416–9.
7. Bhandarkar DS, Lalmalani JG, Shivde S. Laparoscopic ureterolysis and reconstruction of a retrocaval ureter. Surg Endosc. Nov 2003;17(11):1851–2.
8. Huisman TK, Kaplan GW, Brock WA, Packer MG. Ipsilateral ureteroureterostomy and pyeloureterostomy: a review of 15 years of experience with 25 patients. J Urol. Nov 1987;138(5):1207–10.
9. Chacko JK, Koyle MA, Mingin GC, Furness PD 3rd. Ipsilateral ureteroureterostomy in the surgical management of the severely dilated ureter in ureteral duplication. J Urol. Oct 2007;178(4 Pt 2): 1689–92.
10. Lashley DB, McAleer IM, Kaplan GW. Ipsilateral ureteroureterostomy for the treatment of vesicoureteral reflux or obstruction associated with complete ureteral duplication. J Urol. Feb 2001;165(2):552–4.
11. Rabinowitz R, Kingston TE, Wesselhoeft C, Caldamone AA. Ureteral valves in children. Urology. May 1998;51(5A Suppl):7–11.
12. Ameda K, Kakizaki H, Harabayashi T, Watarai Y, Nonomura K, Koyanagi T. Laparoscopic ureteroureterostomy for retrocaval ureter. Int J Urol. Feb 2001;8(2):71–4.
13. Bove P, Micali S, Miano R, et al. Laparoscopic ureterolithotomy: a comparison between the transperitoneal and the retroperitoneal approach during the learning curve. J Endourol. Jun 2009;23(6):953–7.
14. Passerotti CC, Nguyen HT, Lais A, et al. Robot-assisted laparoscopic ileal bladder augmentation: defining techniques and potential pitfalls. J Endourol. Feb 2008;22(2):355–60.
15. Yee DS, Shanberg AM, Duel BP, Rodriguez E, Eichel L, Rajpoot D. Initial comparison of robotic-assisted laparoscopic versus open pyeloplasty in children. Urology. Mar 2006;67(3):599–602.
16. Prieto J, Ziada A, Baker L, Snodgrass W. Ureteroureterostomy via inguinal incision for ectopic ureters and ureteroceles without ipsilateral lower pole reflux. J Urol. Apr 2009;181(4):1844–8; discussion 1848–50.
17. Williams SK, Leveillee RJ. Expanding the horizons: robot-assisted reconstructive surgery of the distal ureter. J Endourol. Mar 2009;23(3):457–61.
18. Jelloul L, Valayer J. Ureteroureteral anastomosis in the treatment of reflux associated with ureteral duplication. J Urol. May 1997;157(5):1863–5.
19. Belman AB, Filmer RB, King LR. Surgical management of duplication of the collecting system. J Urol. Sep 1974;112(3):316–21.
20. Lenaghan D. Bifid ureters in children: an anatomical, physiological and clinical study. J Urol. 1962;87:808.
21. Gonzalez R, Piaggio L. Initial experience with laparoscopic ipsilateral ureteroureterostomy in

infants and children for duplication anomalies of the urinary tract. J Urol. Jun 2007;177(6): 2315–8.
22. Husmann DA. Renal dysplasia: the risks and consequences of leaving dysplastic tissue in situ. Urology. Oct 1998;52(4):533–6.
23. Chandler JG, Corson SL, Way LW. Three spectra of laparoscopic entry access injuries. J Am Coll Surg. Apr 2001;192(4):478–90; discussion 490–1.
24. Penfield AJ. How to prevent complications of open laparoscopy. J Reprod Med. Sep 1985;30(9): 660–3.
25. Bishoff JT, Allaf ME, Kirkels W, Moore RG, Kavoussi LR, Schroder F. Laparoscopic bowel injury: incidence and clinical presentation. J Urol. Mar 1999;161(3):887–90.
26. Passerotti CC, Diamond DA, Borer JG, Eisner BH, Barrisford G, Nguyen HT. Robot-assisted laparoscopic ureteroureterostomy: description of technique. J Endourol. Apr 2008;22(4):581–4; discussion 585.
27. De Caluwe D, Chertin B, Puri P. Fate of the retained ureteral stump after upper pole heminephrectomy in duplex kidneys. J Urol. Aug 2002;168(2): 679–80.
28. Stephens FD, Lenaghan D. The anatomical basis and dynamics of vesicoureteral reflux. J Urol. May 1962;87:669–80.
29. Peng HC, Chen HC. Surgical management of complete ureteric duplication abnormalities in children. Zhonghua Yi Xue Za Zhi (Taipei). Mar 2000;63(3):182–8.
30. Gran CD, Kropp BP, Cheng EY, Kropp KA. Primary lower urinary tract reconstruction for nonfunctioning renal moieties associated with obstructing ureteroceles. J Urol. Jan 2005;173(1): 198–201.
31. Choi H, Oh SJ. The management of children with complete ureteric duplication: selective use of uretero-ureterostomy as a primary and salvage procedure. BJU Int. Sep 2000;86(4): 508–12.
32. Bieri M, Smith CK, Smith AY, Borden TA. Ipsilateral ureteroureterostomy for single ureteral reflux or obstruction in a duplicate system. J Urol. Mar 1998;159(3):1016–8.
33. Bockrath JM, Maizels M, Firlit CF. The use of lower ipsilateral ureteroureterostomy to treat vesicoureteral reflux or obstruction in children with duplex ureters. J Urol. Mar 1983;129(3):543–4.

Part V
Laparoscopic and Robotic Reconstructive Bladder Surgery

Chapter 12

Robotic Radical Cystectomy and Use of Intestinal Segments for Reconstruction in the Adult Patient

Nikhil Waingankar, Mostafa A. Sadek, Michael J. Schwartz, Douglas S. Scherr, and Lee Richstone

Introduction

Perioperative advantages of minimally invasive techniques are well documented for a broad range of surgeries, both for benign and malignant pathology. These include decreased analgesic requirement, shorter hospital stay and convalescence, decreased morbidity, and improved cosmetic outcomes. Equivalence in oncologic outcomes between open and laparoscopic or robotic approaches has led to minimally invasive techniques becoming the standard of care for a number of different malignancies.

Traditionally carried out using an open approach, radical cystectomy remains the surgical standard of care for muscle-invasive bladder cancer. While radical cystectomy has been demonstrated to provide long-term survival or cure in many cases [1], it is also associated with high complication rates, with a reported range between 28 and 64% [1, 2]. For this reason, a number of surgeons have turned to minimally invasive approaches in an effort to decrease morbidity. In this chapter, we review the techniques and outcomes of laparoscopic and robotic radical and partial cystectomy and urinary diversions.

N. Waingankar (✉)
North Shore-Long Island Jewish Health System, Arthur D. Smith Institute for Urology, New Hyde Park, NY, USA
e-mail: nwaingankar@nshs.edu

Robotic-Assisted Radical Cystoprostatectomy

Minimally invasive approaches for the treatment of invasive bladder cancer were initiated in 1992 with laparoscopic cystectomy [3]. However, over the next 10 years, little was reported on minimally invasive bladder surgery. As experience with laparoscopic techniques increased, particularly with prostatectomy, reports of laparoscopic radical cystectomy began to re-emerge. Laparoscopic intracorporeally created diversions, including both ileal conduit and orthotopic neobladder, were also described [4, 5].

Growing experience with robotic surgery has also precipitated a large amount of interest in the performance of radical cystectomy using a robotic-assisted laparoscopic technique [6–11], with either intra- or extracorporeally created urinary diversion. Several institutions have explored feasibility and perioperative outcomes of minimally invasive extirpative surgery for the treatment of bladder cancer (Table 12.1). Questions of long-term oncologic efficacy in comparison to open surgery are beginning to be explored as institutions are examining their initial experiences with short-term oncologic outcomes.

Indications and Contraindications

Open radical cystectomy is the gold-standard treatment for patients with muscle-invasive bladder cancer [12]. However, a number of

M.C. Ost (ed.), *Robotic and Laparoscopic Reconstructive Surgery in Children and Adults*, Current Clinical Urology, DOI 10.1007/978-1-60327-914-7_12, © Springer Science+Business Media, LLC 2011

Table 12.1 Perioperative data

Author	Technique	N	Age	ASA	BMI	ORT	EBL	LOS	Complication rate
Pruthi and Wallen [6]	RRC	20	62.3			366	313	4.35	30%
Wang et al. [7]	RRC	33	70	2	26.7	390	400	5	9% major, 12% minor
	Open	21	66	2	27.1	300	750	8	19% major, 5% minor
Murphy et al. [8]	RRC	23	64.8	2.2	28.9	397	278	11.6	26%
Ng et al. [16]	RRC	83	71	57% were 1–2	26.3	375	460	5.5	41 (9.6% major)
	Open	104	67	52% were 1–2	27.2	358	1172	8	58.7 (29.8% major)
Nix et al. [18]	RRC	21	67.4	2.7	27.5	252	258	5.1	33%
	Open	20	69.2	2.7	28.4	210	575	6	50%
Ha et al. [19]	LRC	36	67.5		23.2	428	420	10.9	
	Open	34	55.9		22.7	358	942	17	
Haber and Gill [20]	LRC	37	66	1.9	26	498	608		46%
Menon et al. [22]	RRC	17				308	<150		
Yuh et al. [23]	RRC	54	67	2.3	27.7	318	557	9.1	
Butt et al. [24]	RRC	51	67	2.3	28	366	546	9.4	27%
Cathelineau et al. [25]	LRC	84	61	1.9		280	550	12	18%
Hemal et al. [26]	LRC	48	59	2.1	25	310	456	10.2	27%
Huang et al. [27]	LRC	85	62.4	2.3	21.8	320	280	17	14.10%
Guillotreau et al. [28]	LRC	38	67.9	2.1	25.9	382	430	12.7	8% major, 26% minor
	Open	30	64.9	2.4	26.1	334	923	15.6	23% major, 60% minor

ASA, American Society of Anesthesiologists score; BMI, body-mass index; ORT, operating room time; EBL, Estimated blood loss; LOS, length of stay.

reports have demonstrated that robotic surgery has perioperative equivalence or superiority to the open approach, with equivalent pathologic outcomes (Tables 12.1 and 12.2). As with open surgery, the primary indication for performing laparoscopic or robotic-assisted radical cystectomy is the presence of muscle-invasive bladder cancer. Patients with high grade T1 disease or carcinoma in situ may also be considered candidates for radical surgery, with age and medical comorbidities taken into account when making treatment recommendations. A consultation with the patient's medical oncologist should take place prior to surgery to discuss neoadjuvant chemotherapy, particularly in patients with $\geq$ T2 disease. Morbid obesity and history of prior pelvic surgery or radiation therapy may increase the technical difficulty of the case and are considered relative contraindications. However, patient selection may be tempered by surgeon's experience and the only absolute contraindication for robotic-assisted radical cystectomy is uncorrected coagulopathy.

Operating Room Setup

The authors' preferred operating room configuration, although determined in part by the layout of the operating room and available assistants, includes two assistants, one at each side of the table. The scrub nurse stands on the side closest to the assistant using the 12-mm assistant port (see Fig. 12.1 for port placement) to allow for easier exchange of instruments and specimens. The primary surgeon sits at the console, which is placed in a location that provides convenient access to the operating table.

In the case that only one assistant is scrubbed in, this person should stand on the left side of the bed. A fourth robotic arm can then be equipped with a grasper and employed on the right side.

Patient Preparation and Positioning

Patients are asked to avoid anti-platelet agents or other anti-coagulants for 7 days prior to surgery.

Table 12.2 Oncologic data

Author	Technique	Nodes	Pos margins	≤ T2 (%)	≥ T2 (%)	Follow-up	Recurrence (%)	Mets (%)	Survival
Pruthi and Wallen [6]	RRC	19	0	70	20				
Wang et al. [7]	RRC	17	6	71	29				
	Open	20	14	44	56				
Murphy et al. [8]	RRC	16	7	74	17	17 month		4.3	91% DFS
Ng et al. [16]	RRC	17.9	9	61	39				
	Open	15.7	0	58	42				
Nix et al. [18]	RRC	19	0	66	14				
	Open	18	0	40	25				
Ha et al. [19]	LRC	14.2	0	23	13	22 month	0	19.4	73% DSS, 71% DFS
	Open	15.7		19	15	67 month	3	29.40	75% DSS, 73% DFS
Haber and Gill [20]	LRC	14	50	62	38	31 month	0	5	92% DSS, 92% DFS
Pruthi [21]	RRC	19	0	66	14	13.2 month	14		94% DFS
Yuh et al. [23]	RRC	16.8	13	44	56				
Butt et al. [24]	RRC	17	12	43	57				
Cathelineau et al. [25]	LRC			86	14	18 month	2	13	83% DFS
Hemal et al. [26]	LRC	14	2	39	61	38 month	0	19	73% DFS
Huang [27]	LRC	12	0	68	32	21.3 month	4	7	85% DFS
Gullotreau et al. [28]	LRC	11.9	11	60	40				
	Open	11.5	23	37	63				

DFS, disease-free survival; DSS, disease specific survive.

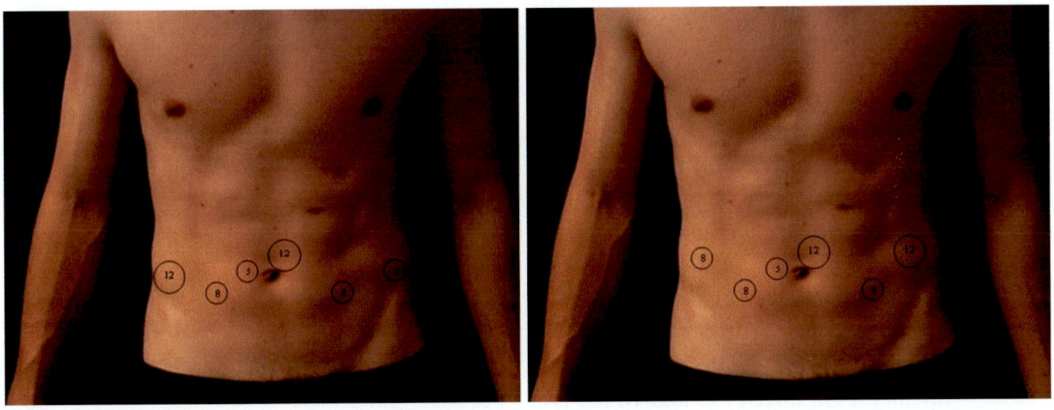

Fig. 12.1 Port placement for robotic-assisted radical cystoprostatectomy with two assistants (*left*) and robotic-assisted radical cystoprostatectomy employing a fourth robotic arm (*right*); trocar size noted in millimeters

In addition to a clear liquid diet for 24 h prior to surgery, a bottle of magnesium citrate is administered for mechanical bowel preparation. An antibiotic bowel preparation is not routinely used. While no difference in wound infections, anastomotic leakage, intra-abdominal abscess formation, or reoperation rate has been demonstrated in a large meta-analysis of patients receiving mechanical bowel prep versus no mechanical bowel prep [13], our experience is that the main advantage in mechanical prep lies in improved intra-abdominal working space afforded by the decompressed bowel. The disadvantages are potential electrolyte imbalance, induction of a pre-renal state secondary to volume depletion, and selection of pathogenic intestinal flora.

Following induction of anesthesia and intubation, the patient is placed in dorsal lithotomy position with the arms tucked. An X-shaped harness is fashioned from egg crate foam and is placed across the patient's shoulders with the inferior end of the harness positioned just above the costal margin in order to avoid interference with port placement. The harness is then secured to the bed with wide cloth tape. The table is then positioned in 30° steep Trendelenburg position, and a Foley catheter is placed on the operative field. Deep venous thrombosis (DVT) prophylaxis is recommended, typically including sequential compression stockings and 5,000 units of subcutaneous heparin administered just after anesthesia induction.

Port Placement

A midline incision is marked that allows enough space for specimen extraction. This incision may be periumbilical if an ileal conduit will be used for urinary diversion or low midline if an extracorporeal orthotopic neobladder will be constructed. A Veress needle is inserted and the abdomen is insufflated to 15 mmHg. A 10–12-mm trocar is placed 5 cm superior to the umbilicus; used as the camera port, this location allows for maximal visualization of the aortic bifurcation during extended lymphadenectomy and also facilitates cranial dissection of the ureters. The following ports are placed under direct vision (Fig. 12.1): 8-mm robotic ports are placed bilaterally 4 cm inferior to and 10 cm lateral to the camera port. If two bedside assistants are utilized, a 12-mm trocar is placed two fingerbreadths above the right anterior-super iliac spine (ASIS) in the mid-axillary line; this port will be used by the primary bedside assistant. A 5-mm port is placed in the same location above the left ASIS and is used by the second assistant. Alternatively, if a fourth robotic arm is employed, it is inserted through an 8-mm trocar above the right ASIS, and the bedside assistant will work from a 12-mm trocar placed in the same location above the left ASIS. A 5-mm trocar is then placed at the level of the umbilicus between the camera port and the robotic port ipsilateral to the primary assistant; this will be used primarily for suction, irrigation, and retraction.

The description of the procedure below is for that of robotic-assisted radical cystoprostatectomy. Purely laparoscopic cystectomy follows essentially the same procedure but with different instrumentation.

Identification and Transection of the Ureters

Surgery begins with incision of the white line of Toldt lateral and inferior to the descending colon. The bedside assistant or the robotic fourth arm retracts the colon medially using a ProGrasp™ (Intuitive Surgical, Sunnyvale, CA). The posterior peritoneum overlying the iliac bifurcation is incised, allowing for identification of the ureter. The assistant or the robotic fourth arm then grasps just beneath the ureter, retracting it anteriorly to facilitate further dissection, both cranially and caudally. Ureteral dissection should be carried out proximally to the level of the upper common iliac artery and distally to the level of the ureteral hiatus (Fig. 12.2). Extent of dissection may depend to some degree on body habitus. Dissection is carried out in a similar fashion bilaterally.

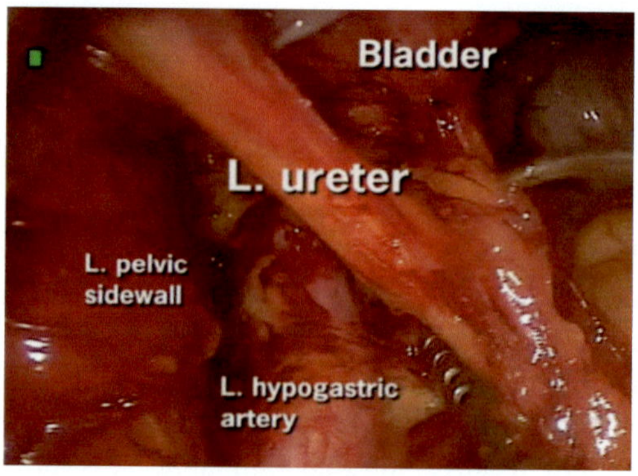

Fig. 12.2 Identification of the ureter

Division of the Anterior Pedicle

The avascular plane between the external iliac vessels and the lateral aspect of the bladder is entered next (Fig. 12.3). The superior vesical artery, which lies in the posterior aspect of this plane and forms part of the anterior pedicle, is clipped and divided. In nerve-sparing surgery, the remainder of the pedicle is clipped and divided as well in order to avoid thermal injury to the neurovascular bundles; otherwise, in non nerve-sparing surgery, a 10-mm LigaSure^{TM} (Valley Lab, Boulder, CO) may be used to divide the remainder of the anterior pedicle.

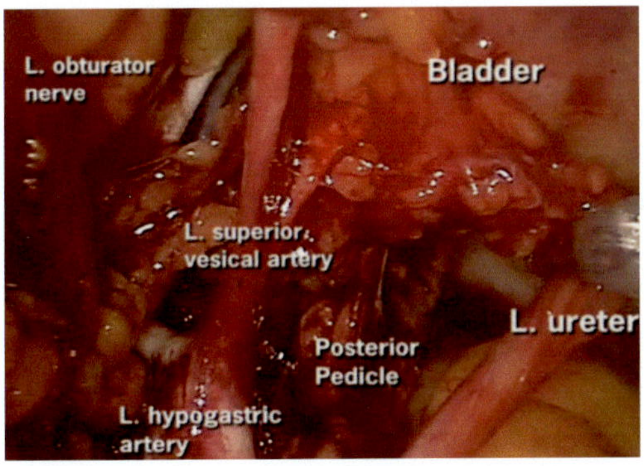

Fig. 12.3 Development of the anterior pedicle

The vasa deferentia and ureters can now be clipped and divided. A suture may be tied to the proximal ureteral clip to facilitate identification and transposition later in the case.

Development of the Posterior Plane

The posterior plane consists of the space between the bladder and the rectum. To develop this plane, the left assistant lifts the bladder anteriorly, while the right assistant retracts the posterior peritoneal edge. Monopolar scissors are then used in a broad, sweeping motion to divide the posterior peritoneal reflection. Dissection is carried out distally to the prostatic apex and should be done beneath the posterior leaflet of Denonvillers' fascia in order to obtain an adequate posterior margin.

Division of the Posterior Bladder and Prostatic Pedicles

Once development of the posterior plane is complete, the posterior pedicle can be visualized just distal to the previously clipped anterior pedicle. Further exposure of the pedicle is gained with the primary assistant (or fourth robotic arm) retracting the bladder superomedially and the second assistant retracting the rectum posteriorly. Pedicles are then divided bilaterally as distally as possible using a 10-mm LigaSure^{TM} (Valley Lab, Boulder CO) device. In a nerve-sparing procedure, a reticulating laparoscopic stapler with 2.5-mm vascular staple loads or clips can be used instead in order to prevent thermal transmission injury. Next, the endopelvic fascia is divided bilaterally using robotic shears, exposing the prostatic pedicles, which are then divided using the LigaSure^{TM} (or Hem-o-lock^{TM} clips in nerve-sparing surgery). Dissection should be carried out as caudally as possible, as the next step in the surgery—anterior release of the bladder—will limit exposure of the posterior plane.

Anterior Bladder Release

The urachus is first divided below the level of the umbilicus. The medial umbilical ligament is then grasped and retracted medially by the robotic fourth arm or the contralateral assistant. Monopolar scissors are used to incise the anterior peritoneum, taking a wide margin throughout the dissection as the surgeon proceeds inferiorly toward the pubic bone. The median umbilical ligaments are divided, and any remaining endopelvic fascia is opened. If orthotopic urinary diversion is planned, the puboprostatic ligaments are spared; otherwise, they are divided.

Division of the Dorsal Venous Complex

The prostatic dissection continues with the division of the dorsal venous complex. To start, a

0-polyglactin suture is passed beneath the DVC distal to the prostatic apex. In nerve-sparing surgery, the DVC is clipped and divided; otherwise, thermal modalities can be used. The bladder is then retracted superiorly, putting traction on the now-exposed urethra. The anterior half of the urethra is divided distal to the prostatic apex; electrocautery should not be used if an orthotopic neobladder is planned. The Foley catheter is then clipped with a large Hem-o-lock^{TM} clip to prevent tumor spillage and divided distal to the clip. The left-side assistant grasps the cut end of the Foley catheter and retracts the bladder and prostate superiorly, and the posterior half of the urethra is then divided. Any remaining attachments are released. The bladder, prostate, and seminal vesicles are all placed in a 15-mm endocatch bag (Fig. 12.4).

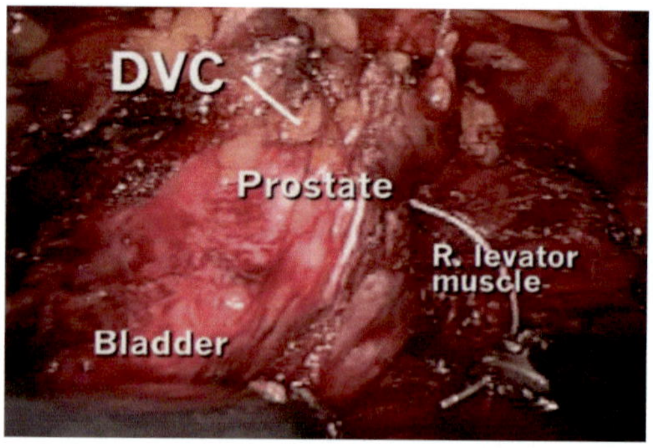

Fig. 12.4 Controlling the dorsal venous complex

Extended Pelvic Lymph Node Dissection

Adequate dissection of lymph nodes involves removal of all lymph tissue between the aortic bifurcation superiorly and the Cooper's ligament inferiorly, and between the genitofemoral nerve laterally and the sacral promontory medially. Dissection begins at the external iliac nodes and then proceeds to the internal iliac and obturator groups (Fig. 12.5). Next, the left and right colon are retracted medially to allow for dissection of the pre-sacral nodes bilaterally. All

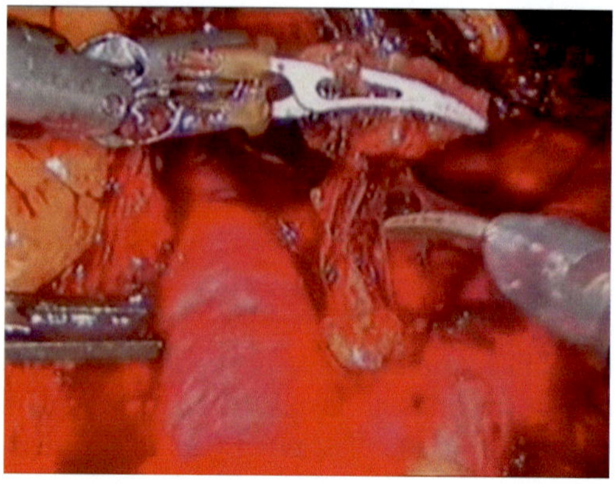

Fig. 12.5 Lymph node dissection at aortic bifurcation

groups are removed en bloc and are placed in a 10-mm Endocatch^{TM} bag. Dissection should be done bilaterally, and nodes from each side are extracted and labeled separately.

Transposition of the Left Ureter to the Right Side

The first step in transposing the left ureter to the right side is the development of a plane posterior to the sigmoid colon and anterior to the aorta, superior to the level of the common iliac takeoff. A suction device is passed from left to right along the plane until it can be visualized on the right side. The right assistant then places a Maryland grasper into the tip of the suction device, and together the instruments are moved along the plane back to the patient's left side. The Maryland grasper is then used to grab the suture attached to the left ureter. The left ureter is pulled by its suture along the plane behind the sigmoid mesentery to the patient's right side. Alternatively, the ureter may be passed beneath the sigmoid colon once the open urinary diversion is initiated; however, this may necessitate a larger incision, particularly with ileal conduit creation.

Radical Cystectomy and Anterior Pelvic Exenteration

While radical cystoprostatectomy is the standard treatment for men with invasive bladder cancer, women have traditionally been treated using radical cystectomy with anterior pelvic exenteration. The steps of this surgery briefly [14] are the following:

(1) Identification and division of ovarian pedicles
(2) Identification of ureters
(3) Superior vesical pedicles and uterine vessels divided
(4) Plane between bladder and vagina developed (vagina-sparing) or vagina entered at junction with bladder and incision extended beyond the urethra
(5) Urachus divided and bladder released from abdominal wall
(6) Endopelvic fascia opened
(7) DVC cauterized
(8) Ileal conduit: vagina divided distally to urethra. Orthotopic neobladder: Urethra divided just distal to bladder neck
(9) Hysterectomy, en bloc or separate (if not sparing uterus)
(10) Vagina entered posteriorly with fourth arm and divided distal to cervix
(11) Specimen extracted, vagina closed

Alternatively, a vaginal- and uterine-sparing posterior approach has been described [15]:

(1) Using posterior approach through cul-de-sac, an inverted U-shaped incision made in the peritoneum of cul-de-sac between bladder and uterus. Vertical limbs of "U" follow the course of the lower ureters from the iliac bifurcation to the ureteral hiatus, whereas the horizontal portion of the "U" is made anterior to the ovaries and uterine corpus.
(2) Plane between uterus and bladder developed as far inferiorly as possible.
(3) Ureters dissected from ureterovesical junction (UVJ) to iliac bifurcation
(4) Inferior vesical pedicle divided
(5) Ureter transected
(6) Lymphadenectomy
(7) Uterine artery clipped
(8) Anterior bladder released
(9) Endopelvic fascia opened lateral to urethra
(10) Dorsal venous complex secured
(11) Urethral apex dissected free from anterior vaginal wall and superior vesical pedicle divided
(12) Plane between lateral vaginal sulci and lateral wall of urethra dissected
(13) Urethra transected, specimen extracted

Urinary Diversion

Orthotopic Neobladder

In cases performed with a periumbilical incision, the robot is undocked and the neobladder is created and anastomosed to the ureters extracorporeally. A Foley catheter is inserted through the urethra and is passed into the neobladder, and the balloon is inflated with 15 cm^3 sterile water. The neobladder is then pulled back down into the abdomen and the catheter is placed on gentle traction. The fascia is closed except for the superior-most 1 cm, which is left open for re-insertion of a 10–12 mm camera port. The robot is then re-docked, and the patient is placed back in 30° Trendelenburg position. For the urethral anastomosis, a double-arm suture is created from a 10–in. segment of undyed 2-0 Biosyn on a GU-46 needle tied to a 10–in. segment of dyed 2-0 Monocryl on a UR-6 needle. The anastomosis starts with the dyed Monocryl suture at the 6 o'clock position, with the needle being driven from outside to inside on the neobladder and then inside to outside on the urethra. This is repeated in a running fashion five times in the clockwise direction, at which point the left assistant grasps the dyed suture and places it on gentle traction to control the posterior portion of the anastomosis.

Suturing with the undyed Biosyn is then started at the 5 o'clock position with the needle being driven from outside to inside on the urethra and then inside to outside on the neobladder. This is repeated in a running fashion until the surgeon reaches the 2 o'clock position, at which point the right assistant grasps the undyed Biosyn and places it on gentle traction. The dyed Monocryl is re-loaded and running of the suture continues as described above until it is outside the urethra at the 12 o'clock position. Both needles are cut from the sutures, and the two ends are then tied. The case concludes with placement of a Jackson–Pratt drain through the 5-mm left port, undocking of the robot, and irrigation and closure of all wounds.

Alternatively, anastomosis of the orthotopic neobladder to the urethra may be accomplished through a low-midline incision. This offers the advantages of removing the specimen and creating the neobladder and ureteral anastomoses through the same incision, then completing the urethral anastomosis in standard open fashion. This maneuver saves time versus the periumbilical approach described above by eliminating the need to undock and then redock the robot.

Ileal Conduit Urinary Diversion

Following robotic cystoprostatectomy, the robot is undocked and an ileal conduit is created via the periumbilical incision in standard open fashion, albeit through a smaller incision. Ureteral stents are placed along with a 24-Fr stomal catheter, which is advanced beyond the abdominal wall fascia. The stents and stomal catheter are removed prior to hospital discharge.

Continent Cutaneous Urinary Diversion

To create a right colon pouch, standard laparoscopic equipment is used at the beginning of the case to reflect the right and transverse colon. Following cystectomy, the diversion is created through a periumbilical incision.

Outcomes

Radical cystectomy has traditionally carried a high degree of morbidity relative to other urological procedures. Complications commonly reported in the minimally invasive literature include bleeding, urinary tract infection, ileus, cellulitis, thromboembolism, and abdominal abscess. Although there are relatively few case series on robotic radical cystoprostatectomy compared to open series, there is sufficient short-term data to suggest that robotic surgery can reduce the number and severity of postoperative complications associated with radical cystectomy (Table 12.1).

In a prospective study comparing open versus robotic surgery, Ng et al. found that open cystectomy carried a significantly higher complication rate than robotic surgery (58.7 and 41%, respectively) and a higher rate of major complications (29.8 and 9.6%, respectively). Furthermore, robotic surgery was found to be an independent predictor of fewer overall and major (grades III–V on the modified Clavien classification system) complications at 30 and 90 days versus open surgery [16], and that major complications generally occur after postoperative day 30 [17]. In the only reported prospective, randomized study comparing open versus robotic surgery, Nix et al. [18] found that the robotic cohort not only had a significantly longer operative time but also had a significantly lower EBL, faster return of bowel function, and lower postoperative analgesic requirement. In addition to having equivalent or improved perioperative outcomes compared to open surgery, short-term oncologic data for minimally invasive surgery appear to be equivalent to open surgery (Table 12.2). Ha et al. [19] compared oncologic outcomes between laparoscopic and open cases and found no significant difference in overall, cancer-specific, and recurrence-free survival at 3 years. Haber and Gill [20] have also evaluated oncologic efficacy of laparoscopic radical cystectomy. Outcomes appear comparable to contemporary series of open radical cystectomy with a mean follow-up of 31 months.

These early studies show promising results for perioperative, pathologic, and short-term oncologic outcomes. However, the definitive test lies in long-term follow-up data which is not yet available to draw conclusions regarding the long-term oncologic efficacy of minimally invasive cystoprostatectomy. Nevertheless, early comparative data show that minimally invasive approaches can duplicate oncologic results of open surgery while decreasing perioperative morbidity.

Minimally Invasive Partial Cystectomy

While minimally invasive approaches for many urologic procedures have been demonstrated to offer equivalent or superior outcomes when compared with open surgery, there is relatively limited experience with minimally invasive partial cystectomy (MIPC). Partial cystectomy, which involves removing the full thickness of a selected part of the bladder wall, has been described for benign tumors such as pelvic paragangliomas [29], bladder leiomyomas, infected urachal cysts, and endometriomas [30, 31]. While shown to be a feasible procedure, outcome data for its use in malignant disease are limited to small series [32–37]. Part of the explanation is that most patients with invasive bladder cancer require radical cystectomy due to multifocality, presence of carcinoma in situ, or location of the lesion, even when unifocal. Therefore, the number of patients considered candidates for a bladder-sparing approach for urothelial malignancy is small. However, in appropriately selected patients, partial cystectomy for malignancy can provide oncologic outcomes equivalent to radical surgery while sparing the patients significant morbidity [38, 39]. Herein, we describe the technique of MIPC for the treatment of both benign and malignant pathologies.

Indications

In an attempt to spare the functioning normal segments of the bladder, preserve erectile function, and avoid the potential metabolic complications and lifestyle impact of urinary diversion, partial cystectomy may be performed for both benign and malignant bladder conditions in appropriately selected patients. A spectrum of benign indications is presented in Table 12.3.

Table 12.3 Benign indications for partial cystectomy

Bladder diverticula
Cavernous hemangioma
Ulcerative interstitial cystitis
Colovesical fistulas
Vesicovaginal fistulas
Endometriosis involving the bladder
Infected/recurrent urachal cysts
Bladder pheochromocytoma

Cancer patients considered for partial cystectomy must be carefully selected [40]. Patients with solitary lesions at the bladder dome or contained in a bladder diverticulum may be offered a bladder-sparing approach. Patients with multifocal disease, carcinoma in situ, or those with prior history of urothelial carcinoma are not candidates for partial cystectomy, mandating thorough cystoscopic evaluation with random bladder and prostatic urethral biopsies to confirm the absence of carcinoma in situ or unsuspected multifocality. Urachal adenocarcinoma is a rare tumor accounting for less than 1% of all bladder tumors, but their typical location at the bladder dome makes patients potential candidates for partial cystectomy [32].

Positioning and Trocar Placement

For laparoscopic and robotic-assisted partial cystectomy, patients are positioned in the dorsal lithotomy position with steep Trendelenburg position, similar to that described for radical cystectomy. A five-port configuration is used, as depicted in Fig. 12.6. When performing MIPC

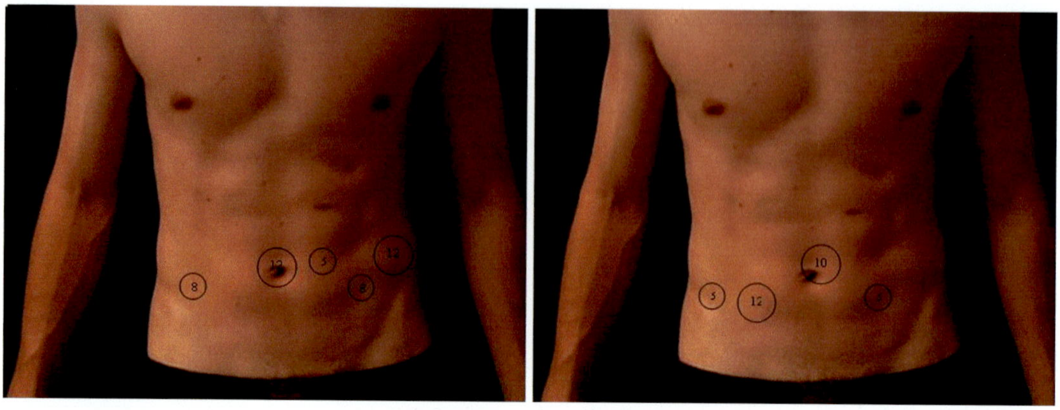

Fig. 12.6 Port placement for robotic partial cystectomy (*left*) and laparoscopic partial cystectomy (*right*); trocar size noted in millimeters

Critical Operative Steps

1) Cystoscopy performed to localize lesion
2) Electrocautery used to delineate tumor and dissect bladder sparing mucosa
3) Bladder lesion excised circumferentially with 2 cm margin
4) Specimen placed in retrieval bag, margins analyzed by frozen section
5) Bladder closed in two layers
6) Extended pelvic lymph node dissection
7) Perivesical drains placed

Instruments

- Curved monopolar scissors
- Laparoscopic Needle driver
- MicroFrance grasper
- Valley Lab™ 10mm LigaSure™ Atlas
- Large/Small Hem-o-lock™ clip applier
- 10mm clip applier
- 10mm and 15mm retrieval device
- Flexible cystoscope set

for urachal carcinoma, the camera port should be positioned at least 5 cm above the umbilicus to facilitate adequate mobilization of the urachal remnant.

Cystoscopy

Once the patient is positioned and the ports are placed, a cystoscope is introduced to concurrently visualize the interior of the bladder. This facilitates tumor localization and delineation of margins, promoting a more accurate excision with an increased likelihood of attaining negative margins. Electrocautery is utilized to outline the area of resection on the external aspect of the bladder. Once this is complete, the cystoscope is removed and a Foley catheter is placed.

Technique

The MIPC technique described here is specific to malignant indications, although the general technique is similar for both malignant and benign conditions. The bladder is irrigated with 200–300 ml sterile water to better define the anatomy. Using electrocautery, the surgeon dissects through the layers of the bladder, leaving the mucosa intact. Prior to dividing the bladder mucosa, the bladder should be emptied to avoid any spillage of bladder contents into the abdominal cavity. Alternatively, a laparoscopic stapling device may be placed under cystoscopic guidance and used to exclude and excise the lesion. Suture closure of the bladder under the staples allows for the subsequent excision of the staple line. Care should be taken to ensure adequate margins of 2 cm around the tumor, and the perivesical fat overlying the tumor should be removed en bloc with the specimen [41]. For urachal adenocarcinoma, the urachus is dissected with wide peritoneal wings to the level of the umbilicus. With the urachus free, a cystostomy is performed and the bladder lesion is excised circumferentially, also with a margin of at least 2 cm. A frozen section analysis is performed on the bladder margin to ensure complete resection. If negative margins are not achievable, then a radical cystoprostatectomy is performed. If, on the other hand, margins are free of disease, the bladder is closed with polyglactin suture in two layers. The surgeon should then proceed to do an extended pelvic lymph node dissection, as described above. A Foley catheter and perivesical drain are placed. The specimens are extracted within an impermeable specimen-retrieval bag and all ports are removed and closed in standard fashion. The drain is routinely removed 24 h postoperatively and the Foley catheter is left in place for 7–10 days. Performance of a cystogram prior to catheter removal is at the surgeon's discretion.

Specific technical precautions should be observed in MIPC. A tension-free closure is necessary and may require bladder mobilization, as previously described. Techniques of intracorporeal suturing and ureteric reanastomosis should be mastered by the surgeon as they are utilized when concurrent distal ureterectomy is required or if ureteric injury occurs.

Outcomes and Complications

Complications of MIPC follow those of most published series in laparoscopic urological procedures, including bleeding, viscous injury, urosepsis, and wound infection; no increased incidence of partial cystectomy-specific complications have been reported [34].

MIPC is an effective treatment option for benign bladder conditions, offering patients the advantages of less analgesic requirement and shorter hospital stay and convalescence. Outcomes of MIPC in patients with bladder cancer are limited to date. The largest urologic case series of MIPC in the treatment of malignancy detailed the perioperative and follow-up care of six patients, including three with urachal carcinoma and three with transitional cell carcinoma. There were no intraoperative or postoperative complications, and at a mean follow-up of 28.5 months, all patients remained disease free [32]. Additional small series and case reports have demonstrated the feasibility of laparoscopic and robotic partial cystectomy for urachal carcinoma [32, 33, 36, 37]. Given this limited experience, no definitive conclusions can be drawn regarding the oncologic efficacy of MIPC for malignancy. Nevertheless, studies to date demonstrate the feasibility and safety of laparoscopic and robotic partial cystectomy. Careful attention to oncologic principles should allow for oncologic outcomes equivalent to those of open surgery.

Conclusion

Minimally invasive surgery of the bladder is safe and technically feasible, with excellent outcomes for the treatment of benign bladder pathology. As the technology of surgical instruments and operative techniques continue to improve, morbidity is expected to continue to decline. Outcomes for malignancy have thus far been promising, but long-term oncologic data are needed to determine whether laparoscopic and robotic-assisted approaches can provide oncologically sound minimally invasive alternatives to open surgery.

Critical Operative Steps

(1) Identification and distal transection of ureters
(2) Division of anterior pedicle
(3) Development of posterior plane
(4) Division of the posterior bladder and prostatic pedicles
(5) Anterior bladder release

(6) Division of the dorsal venous complex
(7) Specimen placed in retrieval bag
(8) Extended pelvic lymph node dissection
(9) Transposition of ureter
(10) Urinary diversion

Critical Instruments

- Valley Lab™ 10-mm LigaSure™ Atlas
- Curved monopolar scissors
- Laparoscopic Scissors
- Laparoscopic needle driver
- Laparoscopic Maryland grasper
- Precise™ bipolar grasper
- MicroFrance grasper
- ProGrasp™ grasper
- Suction irrigator
- Large/small Hem-o-lock™ clip applier
- Clip applier (10 mm)
- Laparoscopic stapler with 2.5-mm vascular staple loads
- Retrieval device (10 and 15 mm)

References

1. Stein JP, Lieskovsky G, Cote R, et al. Radical cystectomy in the treatment of invasive bladder cancer: long-term results in 1,054 patients. J Clin Oncol. 2001;19:666–75.
2. Shabsigh A, Kurtas R, Vora KC, et al. Defining early morbidity of radical cystectomy for patients with bladder cancer using a standardized reporting methodology. Eur Urol. 2008;55:164–76.
3. Parra RO, Andrus CH, Jones JP, Boullier JA. Laparoscopic cystectomy: initial report on a new treatment for the retained bladder. J Urol. 1992;148:1140–4.
4. Gill IS, Fergany A, Klein EA, et al. Laparoscopic radical cystoprostatectomy with ileal conduit performed completely intracorporeally: the initial 2 cases. Urology. 2000;56:26–9. discussion 9–30.
5. Gill IS, Kaouk JH, Meraney AM, et al. Laparoscopic radical cystectomy and continent orthotopic ileal neobladder performed completely intracorporeally: the initial experience. J Urol. 2002;168:13.
6. Pruthi RS, Wallen EM. Robotic assisted laparoscopic radical cystoprostatectomy: operative and pathological outcomes. J Urol. 2007;178:814–8.
7. Wang GJ, Barocas DA, Raman JD, Scherr DS. Robotic vs. open radical cystectomy: prospective comparison of perioperative outcomes and pathological measures of early oncological efficacy. BJU Int. 2007;101:89–93.
8. Murphy DG, Challacombe BJ, Elhage O, O'Brien TS, Rimington P, Khan SS, Dasgupta P. Robotic-assisted laparoscopic radical cystectomy with extracorporeal urinary diversion: initial experience. Eur Urol. 2008;54:570–80.
9. Beecken WD, Wolfram M, Engl T, et al. Robotic-assisted laparoscopic radical cystectomy and intra-abdominal formation of an orthotopic ileal neobladder. Eur Urol. 2003;44:337.
10. Balaji KC, Yohannes P, McBride CL, et al. Feasibility of robot-assisted totally intracorporeal laparoscopic ileal conduit urinary diversion: initial results of a single institutional pilot study. Urology. 2004;63:51–5.
11. Menon M, Hemal AK, Tewari A, et al. Nerve-sparing robot-assisted radical cystoprostatectomy and urinary diversion. BJU Int. 2003;92:232.\
12. Stein JP, Lieskovsky G, Cote R, Groshen S, Feng AC, Boyd S, Skinner E, Bochner B, Thangathurai D, Mikhail M, Raghavan D, Skinner DG. Radical cystectomy in the treatment of invasive bladder cancer: long-term results in 1,054 patients. J Clin Oncol. 2001 Feb 1;19(3):666–75.
13. Guenaga KF, Matos D, Castro AA, Atallah AN, Wille-Jorgensen P. Mechanical bowel preparation for elective colorectal surgery (Cochrane Review). Oxford: Cochrane Library; 2003.
14. Guru KA, Kim HL, Piacente PM, Mohler JL. Robot-assisted radical cystectomy and pelvic lymph node dissection: initial experience at Roswell Park Cancer Institute. Urology. 2007 Mar;69(3):469–74.
15. Menon M, Hemal AK, Tewari A, Shrivastava A, Shoma AM, Abol-Ein H, Ghoneim MA. Robot-assisted radical cystectomy and urinary diversion in female patients: technique with preservation of the uterus and vagina. J Am Coll Surg. Mar 2004;198(3):386–93.
16. Ng CK, Kauffman EC, Lee MM, Otto BJ, Portnoff A, Ehrlich JR, Schwartz MJ, Wang GJ, Scherr DSA. Comparison of postoperative complications in open versus robotic cystectomy. Eur Urol. 10 Jun 2009;Epub ahead of print.
17. Kauffman EC, Ng CK, Lee MM, Otto BJ, Portnoff A, Wang GJ, Scherr DS. Critical analysis of complications after robotic-assisted radical cystectomy with identification of preoperative and operative risk factors. BJU Int. 4 Sep 2009;Epub ahead of print.
18. Nix J, Smith A, Kurpad R, Nielsen ME, Wallen EM, Pruthi RS. Prospective randomized controlled trial of robotic versus open radical cystectomy for bladder cancer: perioperative and pathologic results. Eur Urol. 20 Oct 2009;Epub ahead of print.
19. Ha US, Kim SI, Kim SJ, Cho HJ, Hong SH, Lee JY, Kim JC, Kim SW, Hwang TK. Laparoscopic versus open radical cystectomy for the management of bladder cancer: mid-term oncological outcome. Int J Urol. 23 Nov 2009;Epub ahead of print.

20. Haber GP, Gill IS. Laparoscopic radical cystectomy for cancer: oncological outcomes at up to 5 years. BJU Int. 2007 Jul;100(1):137–42.
21. Pruthi RS, Wallen EM. Is robotic radical cystectomy an appropriate treatment for bladder cancer? Short term oncological and clinical follow-up in 50 consecutive patients. Urology. 2008;72(3):617–20.
22. Menon M, Hemal AK, Tewari A, Shrivastava A, Shoma AM, El-Tabey NA, Shaaban A, Abol-Enein H, Ghoneim MA. Nerve-sparing robot-assisted radical cystoprostatectomy and urinary diversion. BJU Int. 2003 Aug;92(3):232–6.
23. Yuh B, Padalino J, Butt ZM, Tan W, Wilding GE, Kim HL, Mohler JL, Guru KA. Impact of tumour volume on surgical and pathological outcomes after robotic-assisted radical cystectomy. BJU Int. 2008;102:840–3.
24. Butt ZM, Perlmutter AE, Piacente PM, Wilding G, Tan W, Kim HL, Mohler JL, Guru KA. Impact of body mass index on robot-assisted radical cystectomy. JSLS. Jul–Sep 2008;12(3):241–5.
25. Cathelineau X, Arroyo C, Rozet F, Barret E, Vallancien G. Laparoscopic assisted radical cystectomy: the Montsouris experience after 84 cases. Eur Urol. Jun 2005;47(6):780–4. Epub 11 Apr 2005.
26. Hemal AK, Kolla SB, Wadhwa P, Dogra PN, Gupta NP. Laparoscopic radical cystectomy and extracorporeal urinary diversion: a single center experience of 48 cases with three years of follow-up. Urology. Jan 2008;71(1):41–6.
27. Huang J, Lin T, Xu K, Huang H, Jiang C, Han J, Yao Y, Guo Z, Xie W, Yin X, Zhang C. Laparoscopic radical cystectomy with orthotopic ileal neobladder: a report of 85 cases. J Endourol. May 2008; 22(5):939–46.
28. Guillotreau J, Gamé X, Mouzin M, Doumerc N, Mallet R, Sallusto F, Malavaud B, Rischmann P. Radical cystectomy for bladder cancer: morbidity of laparoscopic versus open surgery. J Urol. Feb 2009;181(2):554–9.
29. Huang Y, Tian XJ, Ma LL. Pre-peritoneal laparoscopic partial cystectomy of the bladder pheochromocytoma. Chin Med J (Engl). 20 May 2009;122(10):1234–7.
30. Seracchioli R, Mabrouk M, Montanari G, Manuzzi L, Concetti S, Venturoli S. Conservative laparoscopic management of urinary tract endometriosis (UTE): surgical outcome and long-term follow-up. Fertil Steril. 29 May 2009;[Epub ahead of print] PMID: 19481740.
31. Ferzli G, Wenof M, Giannakakos A, Raboy A, Albert P. Laparoscopic partial cystectomy for vesical endometrioma. J Laparoendosc Surg. Apr 1993;3(2):161–5.
32. Colombo JR, Desai M, Canes D, Frota R, Georges-Pascal H, Moinzadeh A, Tuerk I, Desai M, Gill IS. Laparoscopic partial cystectomy for urachal and bladder cancer. Clinics. 2008;63(6):731–4.
33. Wadhwa P, Kolla SB, Hemal AK. Laparoscopic en bloc partial cystectomy with bilateral pelvic lymphadenectomy for urachal adenocarcinoma. Urology. 2006;67(4):837–43.
34. Mariano MB, Tefilli MV. Laparoscopic partial cystectomy in bladder cancer – initial experience. Int Braz J Urol. May–Jun 2004;30(3):192–8.
35. Nerli RB, Reddy M, Koura AC, Prabha V, Ravish IR, Amarkhed S. Cystoscopy-assisted laparoscopic partial cystectomy. J Endourol. 2008 Jan;22(1):83–6.
36. Spiess PE, Correa JJ. Robotic assisted laparoscopic partial cystectomy and urachal resection for urachal adenocarcinoma. Int Braz J Urol. Sep–Oct 2009;35(5):609.
37. Milhoua PM, Knoll A, Bleustein CB, Ghavamian R. Laparoscopic partial cystectomy for treatment of adenocarcinoma of the urachus. Urology. Feb 2006;67(2):423.e15–7.
38. Kassouf W, Swanson D, Kamat AM, Leibovici D, Siefker-Radtke A, Munsell MF, Grossman HB, Dinney CP. Partial cystectomy for muscle invasive urothelial carcinoma of the bladder: a contemporary review of the M. D. Anderson Cancer Center experience. J Urol. Jun 2006;175(6):2058–62.
39. Capitanio U, Isbarn H, Shariat SF, Jeldres C, Zini L, Saad F, Graefen M, Montorsi F, Perrotte P, Karakiewicz PI. Partial cystectomy does not undermine cancer control in appropriately selected patients with urothelial carcinoma of the bladder: a population-based matched analysist. Urology. Oct 2009;74(4):858–64. Epub 22 Jul 2009.
40. Holzbeierlein JM, Lopez-Corona E, Bochner BH, Herr HW, Donat SM, Russo P, Dalbagni G, Sogani PC. Partial cystectomy: a contemporary review of the Memorial Sloan-Kettering Cancer Center experience and recommendations for patient selection. J Urol. Sep 2004;172(3):878–81.
41. Dandekar NP, Tongaonkar HB, Dalal AV, Kulkami JM, Kamat MR. Partial cystectomy for invasive bladder cancer. J Surg Oncol. 1995; 60:24.

Chapter 13

Laparoscopic Bladder Augmentation and Creation of Continent-Catheterizable Stomas in the Pediatric Patient

Kristin A. Kozakowski and Walid A. Farhat

This chapter contains a video segment which can be found at the URL: http://www.springerimages.com/ost

Introduction

The need for creation of a suitable urinary reservoir that provides a socially acceptable degree of both continence and independence arises in a wide variety of conditions in children. These conditions include spina bifida, posterior urethral valves, bladder exstrophy, and severe dysfunctional voiding. Augmentation cystoplasty with bowel segments along with the creation of a continent-catheterizable stoma is a well-described procedure that results in reducing the storage pressure of the native bladder and increasing the overall capacity to store urine while maintaining continence. Bladder augmentation is considered only after conservative medical management with anticholinergic medications and intermittent catheterization fails.

Traditionally, bladder augmentation and creation of a continent-catheterizable stoma has been a major abdominal operation with large abdominal scars, long post-operative stays, and significant analgesic requirements. Despite the widespread introduction of laparoscopic procedures in pediatric urology, augmentation cystoplasty is still mainly performed as an open procedure due to the intricacy of the surgical technique and bowel reconstruction. Recently, multiple groups have introduced techniques for both laparoscopic-assisted and complete laparoscopic bladder augmentation and creation of a continent catheterizable stoma that have proven to be a safe, feasible minimally alternative approach that offers better post-operative recovery, reduced analgesia requirements, and improved cosmesis [1–8].

Indications

Bladder augmentation is used to increase bladder capacity and reduce bladder pressure in an effort to protect the upper tracts from progressive deterioration and to achieve urinary continence. Patients who are being considered for bladder augmentation must be thoroughly evaluated with urodynamic studies to determine bladder pressure, compliance, and capacity. They must also be committed to lifelong intermittent catheterization, either per urethra or through a continent-catheterizable stoma, since normal voiding will no longer be possible. Due to the risk of development of future malignancy which has recently been reported, bladder augmentation is reserved

K.A. Kozakowski (✉)
Urology, The Hospital for Sick Children, Toronto, ON, USA
e-mail: kkoz99@gmail.com

M.C. Ost (ed.), *Robotic and Laparoscopic Reconstructive Surgery in Children and Adults*, Current Clinical Urology, DOI 10.1007/978-1-60327-914-7_13, © Springer Science+Business Media, LLC 2011

as a final step after anticholinergics and intermittent catheterization alone have failed. The laparoscopic approach to bladder reconstruction can be considered in any patient by a surgeon who is technically competent in laparoscopy. As with other forms of minimally invasive surgery, a major advantage of laparoscopic bladder augmentation is smaller surgical scars, improved analgesia, and quicker return to ambulation. In a selected group of patients, particularly ambulatory patients with intact sensation, these advantages become more desirable.

Contraindications

In general, bladder augmentation with bowel segments is contraindicated in patients with compromised renal function, renal tubular acidosis, hepatic failure, inflammatory bowel disease, short gut syndrome, and poor compliance with intermittent catheterization. With the laparoscopic approach, the ileum is the only intestinal segment that can be used in the current technique.

Although the laparoscopic approach can be considered in any patient, there are several situations which would be unsuitable. Many patients who require bladder augmentation, particularly the population with neurogenic bladders secondary to spina bifida, have a body habitus that does not ideally lend itself to insufflation that would allow enough room for adequate exposure. Thus, patients who have a very small torso with limited intraabdominal area may not be suitable candidates for the laparoscopic approach. Due to adhesions, a history of prior major abdominal or pelvic surgery may also pose a contraindication. This may not become apparent until laparoscopy has been attempted and the insufflated peritoneal cavity has been inspected. Most of the spina bifida patients also have a history of ventriculoperitoneal shunt placements. While not an absolute contraindication to laparoscopy, the surgical team must be aware of possible complications from ventriculoperitoneal shunt failure secondary to obstruction caused by peritoneal insufflation [9].

Thus, as with all laparoscopic procedures, patients and their families must be informed that an open conversion may be needed due to unfavorable operative conditions. In addition, the surgery team, both the primary surgeon and the assistant, must be proficient in advanced laparoscopy as this is a complex reconstructive procedure. Improved cosmesis and quicker recovery time should not compromise surgical success.

Surgical Technique

Pre-operative Considerations

Since the bowel segment is irrigated and opened in situ, there is increased risk for intraperitoneal spill of poorly prepared bowel segments with potentially serious complications. Thus, a full mechanical and antibiotic bowel prep to decrease the bacterial load is recommended when using the laparoscopic approach. This is despite recent reports that suggest bowel preparation is unnecessary for enterocystoplasty in children [10]. In addition, the surgical team must be prepared for open conversion at any point in the case, particularly when insurmountable difficulties are encountered with exposure or operating space or if prolonged anesthesia time becomes unsafe for the patient.

Surgical Procedure

Introduction

Since the first reported case of laparoscopic bladder augmentation using stomach in a 17-year-old girl by Docimo in 1995 [1], there have been only a few published reports of the laparoscopic approach [2–8]. In 2000, Sung et al. reported their initial experience with laparoscopic augmentation cystoplasty in three patients, ages 32–45, for interstitial cystitis, multiple sclerosis, and neurogenic bladder secondary to cervical

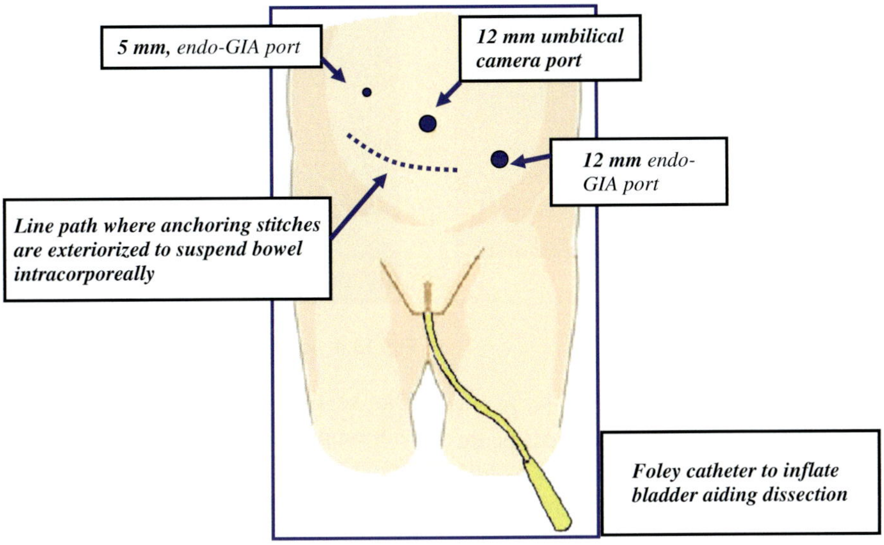

Fig. 13.1 Placement of laparoscopic trocars and sutures

spine injury; only one patient had concomitant creation of a continent-catheterizable stoma [2]. The bowel reconstruction was performed extracorporeally. Their operative times ranged from 5 to 8 h but had no significant intraoperative complications. Their results showed a trend toward earlier return of bowel function and decreased needs for post-operative analgesia, although one patient had a prolonged post-operative ileus. In 2002, Meng et al. [3] reported complete laparoscopic ileal cystoplasty with an operative time of 9 h and successful outcome of bladder capacity of 550 ml and continence between catheterizations at 8 months post-operatively. Recently, Abdel-Hakim et al. published their series of 23 patients, mean age 27 years, with extracorporeal creation of the ileal pouch [8]. They reported a mean operative time of 202 min, mean hospital stay of 5 days, and two long-term complications in a 39-month follow-up.

Augmentation Enterocystoplasty

Access

The patient is placed supine with the legs slightly apart and a Foley catheter is inserted per urethra. Earlier techniques included a cystoscopy and placement of ureteral stents to aid in identifying the ureters, but this has not been carried out in the more recent cases. A total of three ports are placed with the configuration shown in Fig. 13.1. A 12-mm trocar is inserted at the umbilicus. In cases in which a Mitrofanoff appendicovesicostomy is considered, this umbilical location is later used to create the stoma for the catheterizable channel. After achieving adequate intraperitoneal pressure, a 5-mm trocar is inserted in the right upper quadrant and a 12-mm trocar in the left lower quadrant. The peritoneum is then carefully inspected and lysis of adhesions is performed if necessary.

Isolation of Bowel Segment

Attention is then directed toward isolation of the bowel segment and appendix. A premeasured 15-cm vessel loop segment is used for measurement of an appropriate section of bowel and is inserted through one of the trocars (Fig. 13.2). To select the segment of bowel, attention is paid to the distance of the loop from the ileocecal valve and the mobility of the mesentery. The bowel segment must have sufficient mobility to allow

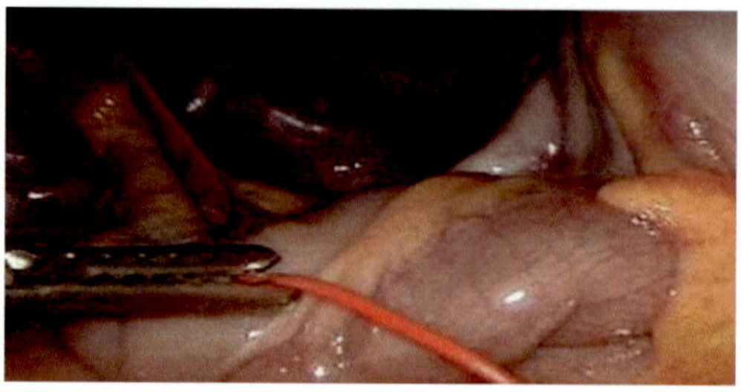

Fig. 13.2 Vessel loop used to identify correct length of bowel

for tension-free advancement toward the pelvis. Once the intestine segment is identified, percutaneous transabdominal fixating sutures using a Keith needle can be done (Fig. 13.3). These transabdominal fixating sutures provide an easy visual aid to help identify these points; two different sutures can be used to differentiate between the proximal and the distal end of the bowel segment.

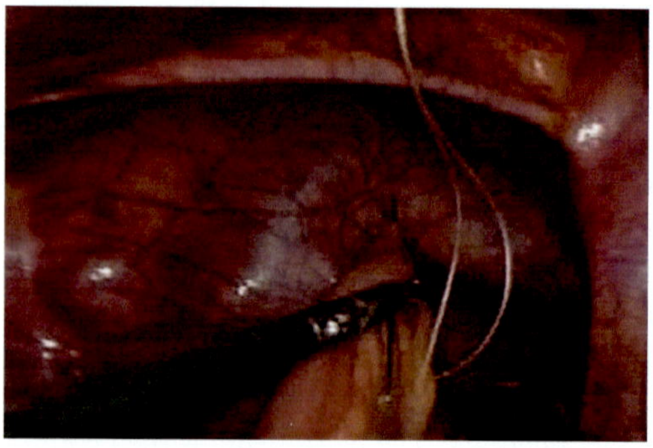

Fig. 13.3 Transabdominal traction sutures

They also provide tension, secure the structure of interest in proper orientation, decrease the number of ports needed, and can be easily relocated depending upon the angle of dissection.

Bowel Anastomosis

The mesenteric vessels can be identified by holding the mesentery against the laparoscopic light as in open surgery (Fig. 13.4). The mesenteric window is then developed with the assistance of the laparoscopic hemostatic cutting devices.

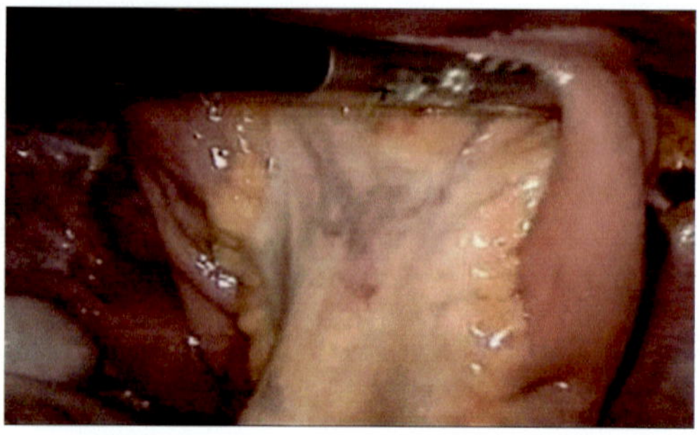

Fig. 13.4 Identification of the mesenteric vessels

The segments of bowel are transected with endoscopic gastrointestinal anastomosis staplers (Endo-GIA), and subsequently bowel continuity is restored with a side-to-side anastomosis using the stapler device (Fig. 13.5) and intracorporeal free-hand sutures in two layers (Fig. 13.6). The direction of the stapler is crucial, aiming toward the antimesenteric border with parallel alignment of the anastomotic ends. The mesenteric defect is then approximated with intracorporeal free-hand sutures.

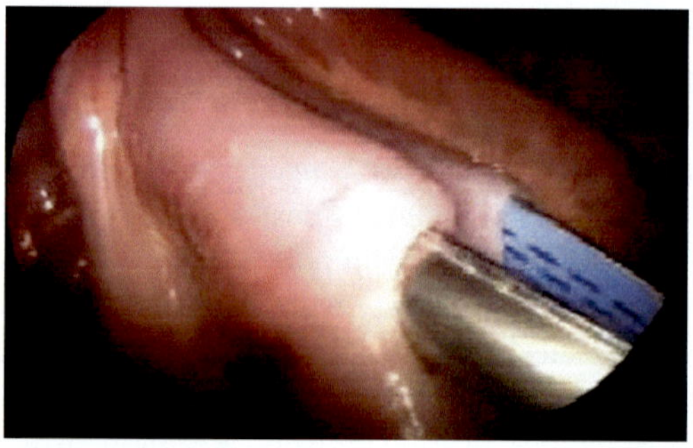

Fig. 13.5 Side-to-side bowel anastomosis using the Endo-GIA stapler

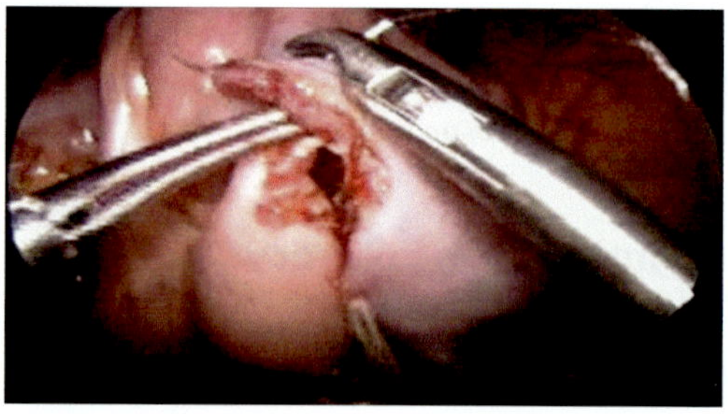

Fig. 13.6 Intracorporeal sutures to close the bowel in two layers

Detubularization

The isolated ileal loop is opened at one end and irrigated in situ with the laparoscopic suction irrigator, using antibiotic solution. This is repeated several times to attempt to clean the bowel of particulate matter and minimize the bacterial load. Once the mechanical cleansing is completed to an acceptable degree, the staple lines are sharply resected, and the bowel is opened on its antimesenteric border, using a laparoscopic hemostatic cutting device (Fig. 13.7). The U-shaped reconfiguration of the detubularized patch is achieved by securing the apex to the anterior abdominal wall and expedited by intracorporeal free-hand sutures or the use of the Endo-Stitch Autosuture device.

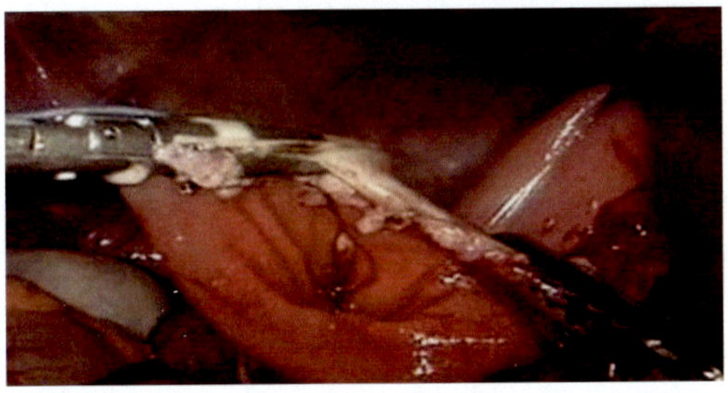

Fig. 13.7 Detubularization of the bowel

Bladder Incision and Cystoplasty

The bladder is prepared by opening the peritoneal reflection and dissecting around the perivesical space until enough exposure is gained. As in the open procedure, the detrusor muscle is subsequently opened in a longitudinal or a transverse fashion, mindful of the need for a generous cystotomy to avoid an hourglass configuration (Fig. 13.8). The bladder mucosa is then exposed using careful dissection (Fig. 13.9).

A running anastomosis with the bladder and detubularized ileal patch can be achieved by either intracorporeal free-hand sutures or the use of the Endo-Stitch Autosuture device under direct visualization. A watertight closure is then verified by irrigating the bladder with sterile saline through the Foley catheter. Either port can then be used to advance a closed suction drain near the anastomosis.

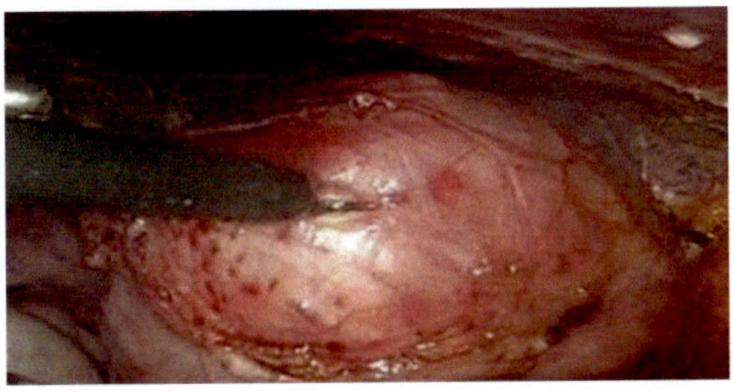

Fig. 13.8 Opening of the detrusor muscle in longitudinal direction

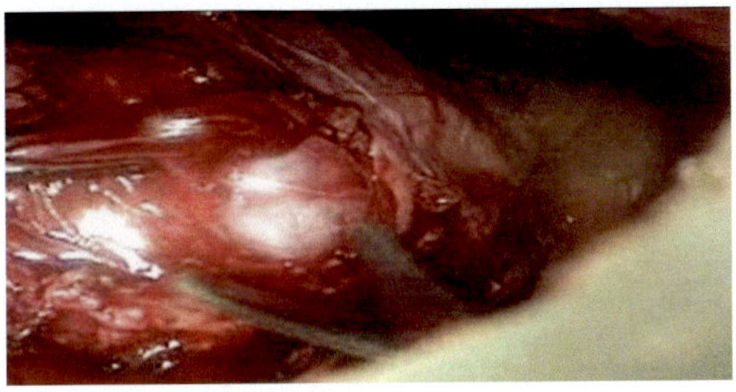

Fig. 13.9 Exposure of the mucosa

Creation of Continent-Catheterizable Stoma

Introduction

The feasibility of laparoscopic-assisted appendicovesicostomy was first reported in 1999 by Van Savage and Slaughenhoupt [11] in their series of three obese female patients; they had no intraoperative laparoscopic complications, and at 1 year of follow-up, all three had patent catheterizable channels. In 2004, Casale et al. [12] reported their initial case of completely intracorporeal, laparoscopic appendicovesicostomy in a 4-year old with the VATER malformation. Their operative time was 198 min, there were no complications, and the patient was discharged home on postoperative day 3. At 8 months of follow-up, the channel remained patent and continent. Shortliffe and Hsu [13] also reported their initial case of fully laparoscopic Mitrofanoff appendicovesicostomy in a 11-year-old girl with spina bifida in 2004. Laparoscopic operative time was 360 min, hospital stay was 7 days, and the stoma was patent and continent at 9 months of follow-up.

Access

The patient is placed supine with the legs slightly apart and a Foley catheter is inserted per urethra. Earlier techniques included a cystoscopy and placement of ureteral stents to aid in identifying the ureters, but this has not been carried out in the more recent cases. A total of three ports are placed with the configuration shown in Fig. 13.1. A 12-mm trocar is inserted at the umbilicus. In cases in which a Mitrofanoff appendicovesicostomy is considered, this umbilical location is later used to create the stoma for the catheterizable channel. After achieving adequate intraperitoneal pressure, a 5-mm trocar is inserted in the right upper quadrant and a 12-mm trocar in the left lower quadrant. The peritoneum is then carefully inspected and lysis of adhesions is performed if necessary.

Isolation and Harvest of the Appendix

After appropriate lysis of adhesions and identification of the ileocecal valve, the appendix will be identified. Note that in patients with significant kyphosis, the appendix may be located in the right upper quadrant, not necessarily the right lower quadrant. Furthermore, in some patients with previous spinal surgery or ventriculoperitoneal shunt placement, the bowel can be relocated into different quadrants to facilitate medialization of the appendix. The right colon is mobilized medially. After sufficient mobilization, the appendix should be brought toward the bladder to ensure that it has an adequate length without tension to reach the skin. The blood supply to the appendix, often fragile, is also carefully identified by holding the mesentery against the laparoscopic light as in open surgery. To facilitate appendiceal vessels dissection, percutaneous traction anchoring stitches can be used along the lower abdominal quadrant (Fig. 13.1). The appendix is then harvested using the Endo-GIA stapler, leaving an approximately 5-mm cuff of cecum to ensure adequate closure of the bowel defect and preserving adequate vascular supply. Using intracorporeal free-hand suturing, the cecal staple line is then oversewn in two layers with 2-0 silk suture.

Appendicovesicostomy

The native bladder is identified and dissected free from the peritoneum if not already adequately mobilized during the augment section of the operation. An approximately 4-cm detrusor muscle trough is created along the identified section of the posterior bladder. At the distal end of the trough, a small cystotomy is created for anastomosis of the appendix. To aid in this part of the operation, the bladder may either be filled with normal saline as in the open procedure, or inflated with separate CO_2 insufflator.

Attention is then turned to prepare the appendix. The distal 5 mm of the appendix is excised sharply and spatulated. The lumen should be irrigated in situ to clear any fecaliths and to ensure an adequately patent lumen. The appendix is then brought to the cystotomy and the anastomosis is sewn circumferentially with interrupted 4-0 Vicryl sutures using intracorporeal technique. The detrusor tunnel is then created by placement of the appendix into the detrusor trough. The two edges of the detrusor muscle are brought together over the appendix and imbricated using interrupted 4-0 Vicryl suture taking care not to strangulate the appendix or to place too much tension on the mesenteric vessels. The channel and the cecum are fixed to the abdominal wall with 3-0 Vicryl sutures to prevent internal herniation. At the conclusion of the laparoscopic segment of the case, the proximal cuff of the appendix is then brought out through the umbilical port and matured into a catheterizable stoma.

Results

In our experience with laparoscopic Mitrofanoff creation without concomitant bladder augmentation, we identified a total of 11 patients with an average age of 12 years (range 2–18). Six patients had a VP shunt in place, and no patients had previous major abdominal surgeries. A concomitant laparoscopic c-tube placement was performed in three children. A complete laparoscopic procedure was achieved in four patients (mean operative time 361 min/mean hospital stay 5.5 days). A laparoscopic-assisted procedure was performed in four patients (mean operative time 242 min/mean hospital stay 5.7 days). An open conversion was necessary due to peritoneal adhesions or inability to maintain an adequate pneumoperitoneum in three patients (mean operative time 257 min/mean hospital stay 8 days). No intraoperative complications were identified. In a mean follow-up time of 18 months, two patients in the purely laparoscopic group required stoma revision due to stomal stenosis.

Complications

Laparoscopic enterocystoplasty is a technically demanding procedure that requires a high level of laparoscopic skill and an experienced surgical team. As with any laparoscopic procedure, there is always the risk of vascular or organ injury from the Veress needle or trocar insertion, port-site hernia, and thromboembolic events. At any point in the procedure, conversion to an open operation may be required because of both failure to progress and a complication that cannot be repaired with laparoscopy. It is also important to stress that conversion to open procedure should be performed if it becomes apparent that the laparoscopic technique will compromise the surgical outcome.

With laparoscopic enterocystoplasty, there is a risk of inadvertent bowel injury during the initial lysis of adhesions, mobilization of the bowel segment, and intracorporeal suturing. It is important to recognize bowel injury early and to repair it as soon as it is discovered. This procedure is routinely performed on spina bifida patients who have ventriculoperitoneal shunts in place which also need to be considered during the surgery. Potential complications which are specific to the bowel harvest and reanastomosis are ileus, bowel obstruction, anastomotic stricture, and peritonitis. Care must be taken to achieve a bowel anastomosis that is as precise as with the open procedure. Because there are smaller incisions and potentially less manipulation of the bowel during laparoscopy, the post-operative ileus may be shorter than with the open procedure.

During the augmentation cystoplasty, if ureteral catheters are not placed in the beginning of the case, it is important to identify the ureters and ensure that they are not inadvertently injured. During the incision in the bladder, care must also be taken to avoid accidentally damage the ureteral orifices. As in open surgery, care must be taken during intracorporeal suturing of the bladder and bowel to ensure precise tissue approximation to avoid leakage from the bladder, particularly since we do not place a suprapubic tube unless deemed necessary.

Post-operative complications are the same as with the open procedure. They include prolonged ileus, leakage from the bladder, leakage from the bowel, sepsis, metabolic disarray, wound infection, catheter blockage from mucus production, and ventriculoperitoneal shunt malfunction. Long-term complications include bladder stones, urinary tract infections, bladder perforation, stomal stenosis, inadequate bladder volume, and metabolic abnormalities.

Post-operative Management

A Foley is left in the Mitrofanoff, accompanied by a urethral catheter. A Penrose drain is placed through a port site. Antibiotic coverage is also continued post-operatively to protect from sepsis secondary to bowel spillage. The main advantages of the laparoscopic approach are decreased post-operative analgesia requirements and quicker return to normal levels of activity. Post-operatively, a nasogastric tube is not left in place, and clears can be started on POD#1 with diet advancement based on return of bowel function. The patient can be managed with minimal narcotics that can be discontinued earlier than with the open approach. Due to decreased pain levels, patients can be moved out of bed and returned to their pre-operative activity level sooner.

Critical Surgical Instruments

- Trocars (2–12 mm)
- A 1–5-mm trocar
- A 30° laparoscope
- Bowel grasper
- L hook
- Bioplar
- Maryland grasper
- Scissors
- Roticulating GIA
- Suction
- Irrigation (bacitracin solution)
- 5-0 Prolene sutures
- 4-0 Vicryl sutures
- Keith needles

References

1. Docimo SG, Moore RG, Adams J, et al. Laparoscopic bladder augmentation using stomach. Urology. 1995;46:565–9.
2. Gill IS, Rackley R, Meraney AM, Marcello PW, Sung GT. Laparoscopic enterocystoplasty. Urology. 2000;55:178–81.
3. Elliotte SP, Meng MV, Anwar HP, Stoller ML. Complete laparoscopic ileal cystoplasty. Urology. 2002;59:939–43.
4. Chung SY, Meldrum K, Docimo SG. Laparoscopic assisted reconstructive surgery: a 7-year experience. J Urol. 2004;171:372–5.
5. Hsu TH, Shortliffe LD. Laparoscopic Mitrofanoff appendicovesicostomy. Urology. 2004;64:802–4.
6. Casale P, Fend WC, Grady RW, Joyner BD, Lee RS, Mitchell ME. Intracorporeal laparoscopic appendicovesicostomy: a case report of a novel approach. J Urol. 2004;171:1899.
7. Lorenzo AJ, Cerveira J, Farhat WA. Pediatric laparoscopic ileal cystoplasty: complete intracorporeal surgical technique. Urology. 2007;69:977–81.
8. El-feel A, Adel-Hakim MA, Aboeul-Fettouh H, Abdel-Hakim AM. Laparoscopic augmentation ileocystoplasty: results and outcome. Eur Urol. 2009;55:721–8.
9. Baskin JJ, Vishteh AG, Wesche DE, Rekate HL, Carrion CA. Ventriculoperitoneal shunt failure as a complication of laparoscopic surgery. JSLS. 1998;2:177–80.
10. Gundeti MS, Godble PP, Wilcox DT. Is bowel preparation required before cystoplasty in children? J Urol. 2002;167:1574–7.
11. Van Savage JG, Slaughenhoupt BL. Laparoscopic-assisted continent urinary diversion in obese patients. J Endourol. 1999;13:571.
12. Casale P, Feng WC, Grady RW, Joyner BD, Lee RS, Mitchell ME. Intracorporeal laparoscopic appendicovesicostomy: a case report of a novel approach. J Urol. 2004;171:1899.
13. Hsu THS, Shortliffe LD. Laparoscopic Mitrofanoff appendicovesicostomy. Urology. 2004;64:802–4.

Chapter 14

Laparoscopic Ureteral Reimplant Surgery to Correct Reflux Disease

Bekir Aras, Levent Gurkan, Ali Serdar Gözen, Dogu Teber, and Jens Rassweiler

Introduction

Vesicoureteral reflux (VUR) is considered as a significant factor for the development of urinary tract infection, progressive renal damage or scarring, and end-stage renal failure [1]. Mild cases of VUR are likely to resolve spontaneously, but high-grade VUR may require surgical correction. Open ureteral reimplantation surgery has been extremely successful, with success rates of 95–98% in children [2]. However, open surgical repair involves in-splitting of the abdominal wall, forced retraction of the bladder and long postoperative need for indwelling catheter causing pain, bladder spasms, and longer hospital stay [3–5]. Laparoscopy is proposed to overcome these advantages of the traditional open surgery in the treatment of VUR, reflecting the advance in other fields of urologic surgery. Despite initial description in 1994, standard laparoscopic ureteral reconstructive surgery has lagged behind because of its complexity and requirement of advanced laparoscopic skills [6].

Historical Evolution

Minimally invasive ureterovesical reimplantation techniques have evolved over time. Following initial attempts described in pig models [7], laparoscopic extravesical reimplantation akin to the Lich–Gregoir technique was reported in 1994 [8, 9]. Early reports of this transperitoneal technique were met with some skepticism. After performing this procedure in six children, Janetschek and colleagues concluded that it was not a feasible approach. They described intraperitoneal dissection as too time consuming and without real advantage over open procedure [10]. Later reports have cited modifications to make it an appealing option in the hands of a skilled laparoscopist.

In 1995, Okamura et al. described first transvesical technique for the correction of VUR. Due to the difficulty in suturing laparoscopically in a small space, initial intravesical procedures utilized a modification of the Gil Vernet trigonoplasty procedure [11, 12]. The success rates of these procedures' preliminary series (62–79%) did not match those for open surgery, and splitting of the trigone proved to be a significant problem 1 year postoperatively [5, 11, 13]. With further modification of this technique by the same group, namely endoscopic trigonoplasty II, in which a reliable muscular backing and elongation of the intramural ureter were made, success rate of 86% was achieved [14].

Open transvesical approach with high success rates was first transcribed to laparoscopy by Gill et al. in 2001 [15]. In 2005, Yeung presented a series of patients undergoing cross-trigonal ureteral reimplantation using carbon dioxide pneumovesicum with success rates (96%) nearly identical to standard open repair [3]. Further studies focusing on vesicoscopic reimplantation

J. Rassweiler (✉)
Department of Urology, SLK-Klinikum Heilbronn, University of Heidelberg, Heilbronn, Germany
e-mail: jens.rassweiler@slk-kliniken.de

M.C. Ost (ed.), *Robotic and Laparoscopic Reconstructive Surgery in Children and Adults*, Current Clinical Urology, DOI 10.1007/978-1-60327-914-7_14, © Springer Science+Business Media, LLC 2011

for both primary reflux and megaureter repair demonstrated decreased pain in patients undergoing a vesicoscopic approach compared to open surgical Cohen repair with similar success rates [5, 16–18].

Starting in year 2005, robotic-assisted laparoscopic techniques using the da Vinci (Intuitive Surgical, Mountain View, CA) Surgical System for the treatment of VUR were reported, adding yet another approach to this rapidly expanding field of minimal invasive treatment options [19, 20]. They made good use of the experience gained with conventional laparoscopy, adding potential advantages of robotics: enhanced dexterity of the instruments, absence of tremor, and 3D vision. The evolution parallels the one seen in conventional laparoscopy, experience reported with the extravesical as well as intravesical approach [3, 21].

Surgical Techniques for Laparoscopic Treatment of VUR

Patient and Surgeon Position

The patient is positioned in Trendelenburg position, legs spread apart, and the arms tucked in at the side. The abdomen, pelvis, and perineum are prepared from the xiphoid process to midthigh. Adhesive drapes are used to isolate the anorectal region from the operative field. A standard laparoscopy drape covers the abdomen, slit down the middle inferiorly to allow perineal access [22]. Careful positioning and padding of the legs is needed to prevent nerve palsy. A right-handed surgeon stands on the left side of the patients to perform surgery. The assistant stands on the right side. Two video columns are placed over the patient's legs at both sides.

Extravesical Procedure

Trocar Placement

Using the Hasson technique, a small incision is made in the infraumbilical fold and a pneumoperitoneumis created. In standard three-port setting, first trocar is placed infraumbilically and two further trocars are placed along a Pfannenstiel incision outline, in case an open conversion is required [2]. If an additional trocar is needed, it is placed on midline at the level of anterior–superior iliac spine, forming an arc with the two other trocars placed on either lateral edge of rectus muscle. All ports are 5 mm except for the 3-mm inferior midline port. A telescope is introduced through the supraumbilical port.

Ureterovesical Junction Exposure

The peritoneal reflection is incised and the posterior bladder visualized. In female patients, the initial dissection is made in the peritoneal fold between the bladder and the uterus. The ureter is identified as it crosses through the uterine and vaginal vessels lateral to the uterus and cervix and then takes a course medially to reach the trigone anterior to the vagina. In males, the ureter can be identified as it crosses posterior to the vas deferens [23]. A peritoneal window is created, and the ureter is freed from adjacent connective tissue. The ureter is elevated inferior to the vas deferens using a large Babcock forceps or an umbilical tape [2].

Detrusor Tunnel Dissection

Meticulous dissection of the posterior bladder wall is advised and a hitch stitch through the posterior wall can be used to improve exposure and stabilize bladder. The detrusor muscle is incised without puncturing the bladder mucosa. A full-thickness detrusor trough is created such that the mucosa bulges out [22] (Fig. 14.1). Newly created detrusor tunnel should course slightly laterally to avoid kinking of the ureter. In most cases, a 3-cm tunnel is adequate to obtain a 5:1 ratio of length to width [2].

Tunnel Suturing

The ureter is placed in the new tunnel, and the detrusor muscle is approximated with interrupted

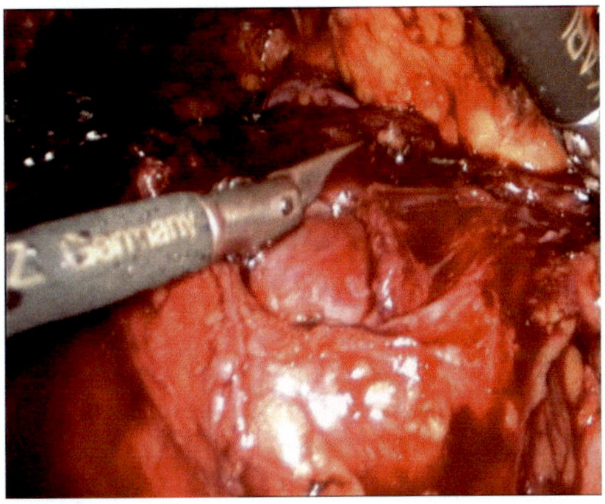

Fig. 14.1 Dissection of the submucosal tunnel and mucosal bulging

4-0 synthetic absorbable sutures in 0.5 cm intervals. The last detrusor stitch is placed sufficiently far from the ureter to avoid kinking or strangulating the ureter (Fig. 14.2).

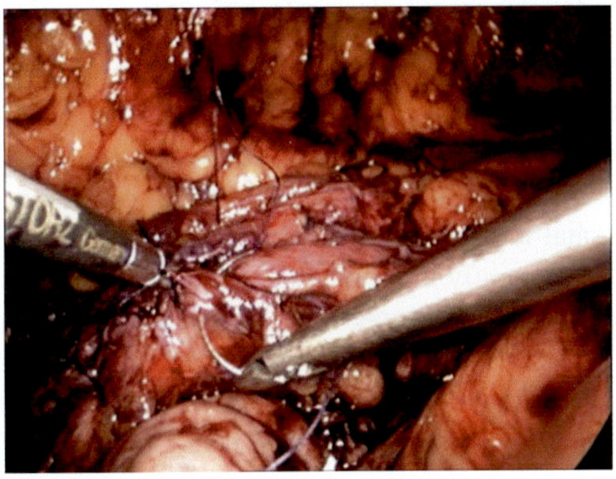

Fig. 14.2 Detrusor tunnel is closed over ureter

After the surgery is complete, instruments and trocars are removed under endoscopic vision and the trocar sites are checked for bleeding and visceral injury. The fascial defects of 5-mm ports and skin of each port are closed with absorbable sutures. Bladder catheters are retained for 12–24 h, until 4–6 h prior to the expected time of discharge from the hospital. Satisfactory bladder emptying is confirmed by ultrasonographic bladder scans before discharge [22].

Intravesical Procedures

Trocar Placement

Cystoscopy is performed at the beginning of the operation to assess the location of the ureteral orifice and guide trocar placement. A ureteral catheter might be placed at this time to help laparoscopic dissection. Under direct view, two 5-mm balloon tip ports are inserted suprapubically into the completely distended bladder 1 fingerbreadth superior to the symphysis pubis with one each on either side of the midline. Attaching the two ports to continuous wall suction could potentially diminish fluid escape to extravesical space during the procedure. An additional trocar for telescope is described on the bladder dome in the original publishing of vesicoscopic cross-trigonal ureteroneocystostomy.

Techniques

Laparoscopic Extraperitoneal Trigonoplasty This technique is the first vesicoscopic procedure that was an adaptation of Gil Vernet trigonoplasty to laparoscopy introduced by Okamura et al. in 1995 [11]. This Japanese group further improved this technique, renaming it as trigonoplasty II in 1999. They proposed U-shaped incisions around the ureteral orifice to create a more significant flap of ureter and bladder muscle to avoid trigonal splitting and improve long-term success rates [14]. This group preferred to fill the bladder with carbon dioxide to improve visibility. As the narrow space seems to be the most important technical problem during these procedures, Simforoosh et al. [24] introduced pure extraperitoneal access and bladder splitting to enlarge working space in 2007. Standard trigonoplasty II as proposed by Okamura et al. consists of the following steps.

Creating Ureteral Flaps A ureteral catheter is placed and sutured to orifice for easier manipulation. The bladder mucosa just distal to ureteral orifice and detrusor muscle along each side of the ureter is incised using a resectoscope, and a 2–3-cm flap including the ureter is created. The mucosa distal to original ureteral orifice is resected to advance the ureter.

Creation of the Muscular Bed and Fixation of the Ureteral Flap Pneumobladder is created using carbon dioxide insufflation. The incised detrusor muscle and ureteral hiatus are reapproximated using 3-0 synthetic absorbable interrupted sutures to create muscular bed. Ureteral flap is laid on the muscular bed, advanced distally, and anchored using interrupted 3-0 synthetic absorbable sutures. Ureteral catheters are removed and abdominal trocar sides are closed primarily. A Foley catheter is left indwelling for 7 days and ultrasonographical follow-up for upper urinary tract dilatation is performed within 1–4 weeks.

Vesicoscopic Cross-trigonal Ureteroneocystostomy Gill and colleagues introduced this technique of laparoscopic transvesical cross-trigonal Cohen antireflux ureteroneocystostomy in 2001 [15].

Dissection of the Ureter and Creation of the Submucosal Bed Intramural ureter is circumferentially detached from the full-thickness bladder wall. The extravesical pelvic extraperitoneal fatty tissues are gently dissected bluntly off the ureter by the Collins knife, mobilizing 2–3 cm of extravesical ureter into the bladder. Using suprapubically inserted 5-mm laparoscopic grasping forceps and electrosurgical scissors, the bladder mucosa is elevated on either side of the previously scored marking to create a submucosal bed for the subsequent ureteral tunnel.

Anchoring of the Ureter Multiple 3-0 absorbable synthetic sutures are used to anchor the neoureteral orifice to the detrusor at the apex of the cross-trigonal submucosal bed. The posterior cystotomy at the original ureteral hiatus is narrowed with a stitch as necessary. The previously created mucosal flaps are then reapproximated over the ureter with 3–4 interrupted 4-0 or 5-0 synthetic absorbable sutures stitched to construct the submucosal tunnel [15]. Indwelling catheter is removed after 24–48 h and all patients are followed up with ultrasound and voiding cystogram at 3 months postoperatively.

Megaureter

Trocar Placement

For extracorporeal tailoring, the camera port is placed along the lower lip of the umbilicus in the midline, and further two trocars (5 and 10 mm) for working instruments are placed in the midclavicular lines on either side. Usually an additional trocar for traction is required during intracorporeal tailoring. This trocar is placed in anterior axillary line for right ureter and in midline midway between umbilicus and pubic symphysis for left side.

Extracorporeal Tailoring Technique

The colon is reflected medially to expose the retroperitoneal course of the ureter. The ureter is dissected circumferentially down to the bladder and divided close to the bladder. To obtain additional length, it is slightly dissected upward and subsequently the free ureteral end is taken out of the abdomen through the ipsilateral 5-mm port. The lower end is tailored over an 8-Fr catheter. After a 6-Fr double-J stent is placed, the entire assembly is placed back in the abdomen.

Intracorporeal Tailoring Technique

The ureter is left attached to the bladder during the dissection and a vessel loop encircling the ureter is used for traction. This approach allows the surgeon to work in a fix anatomic orientation and provides him a firm platform for additional excisional tailoring and resuturing. Excisional tailoring is performed using cold scissor and ureterotomy is closed using 4-0 synthetic absorbable sutures. After completing the tailoring, the ureterovesical junction is divided and 4.8-Fr double-J stent is placed through the laparoscopic ports.

Ureteral Reimplantation

Ureteral reimplantation is performed on the lateral wall of the bladder using suprahiatal extravesical method. Seromuscular cystotomy is performed on distended bladder followed by suburothelial undermining of detrusor to provide enough space for housing of the implanted ureter. Approximately 5-mm disk of urothelium is excised at the distal end of cystotomy. Subsequently, ureter is reimplanted using interrupted 4-0 synthetic absorbable sutures; distalmost suture traverse full thickness of the bladder wall. Detrusor is closed over the implanted ureter for a length of 4–5 cm using 3-0 synthetic absorbable sutures [25].

Urinary catheter and DJ catheter are removed during first and fourth week following surgery, respectively. Voiding cystogram and diuretic renogram are performed 4 weeks after removal of stent to look for residual VUR or ureteral obstruction [25].

Robotic-Assisted Ureteroneocystostomy

Patient Position

The patient is placed supine on the table, with the legs apart. The table is kept flat without flexion. Urinary catheter is placed and the bladder is distended with saline. Robotic-assisted correction of VUR can be performed extravesically as well as intravesically.

Port Placement for Extraperitoneal Intravesical Technique

Securing the ports to the bladder wall is critical to efficient performance. The initial midline port, located at the dome of the bladder, is for the camera using a 12-mm Versa Step sheath and cannula. Two additional 8-mm robotic cannulas are then placed halfway between the umbilicus and the pubis. Purse-string sutures are placed as with the first port and used to close the bladder punctures at completion. Once the robotic working ports are positioned in the bladder, the saline is evacuated by insufflating with CO_2 at a pressure of 8–10 mmHg. The robotic device is moved to the foot of the bed, and the arms are engaged.

Port Placement for Transperitoneal Extravesical Technique

Cystoscopy is performed prior to docking and colored ureteral catheters are placed to ease robotic-assisted dissection. An umbilical trocar is placed for robotic camera and two additional ports for working arms are placed each lateral to rectus muscle at the level of the anterosuperior iliac spine.

Surgical Technique

The surgical technique reported in the only two literatures available does not differ from laparoscopic technique.

Outcomes and Discussion

Extravesical Techniques

Initial attempts at laparoscopic correction of reflux were made in children using a modified Lich–Gregoir reimplant technique transperitoneally. In 1994, Ehrlich et al. [8] reported on two patients with successful outcomes after laparoscopic extravesical reimplantation. The following year, Janetschek et al. reported outcomes in six children, one of whom required postoperative ureteral stenting for 6 weeks. The authors felt that the procedure was complex and unwieldy and offered no significant advantage compared to open surgery [10]. Despite this, others have pursued the extravesical laparoscopic reimplantation in children. Lakshmanan and Fung published on their experience of 71 extravesical reimplants in 47 children (23 unilateral and 24 bilateral). They reported 100% success rate with mean follow-up of 34 months. They experienced three ureteral injuries which they relate to excessive ureteral handling. Although one case was managed conservatively by placing a DJ catheter, two further cases required open reimplantation [22]. In 2006, Riquelme et al. [26] reported series of 17 patients with 94.7% success rate and three children requiring catheterization for 3–4 days for mucosal perforation.

In 2004 Shu et al. published excellent outcomes (100%) in postpubertal female with mean operative time of 105 min. They documented minimal postoperative morbidity during a mean follow-up period of 11.4 months [23]. One of the patients experienced persistent abdominal pain without known reason. Another patient experienced symptoms suggesting an ureteral obstruction which responded to ureteral catheterization and resolved over the next 24 h.

There are limited reports of robotic ureteral reimplantations being performed in children [19]. Casale et al. [20] reported a series of 41 children with a mean age of 33 months treated with bilateral robotic extravesical reimplantation. All children voided well after catheter removal on the first day following operation. No patient had retention as documented by ultrasonic bladder scanning. Reflux was cured in 97% and no ureters were obstructed.

Intravesical Techniques

The first results on intravesical trigonoplasty were published by Okamura et al. in 1995. They reported outcomes in 12 adult patients with low- and moderate-grade vesicoureteral reflux with a 100% reflux correction rate and 178 min mean surgical time. No major complications were noted and the most common minor complication observed was trocar displacement and subsequent pneumoperitoneum [11].

On the other hand, preliminary results published by Cartwright et al. 1 year later on the same technique pointed to a reflux-resolving rate of 62.5%. Operative time ranged between 60 and 240 min and complications included a vesicovaginal fistula hyponatremia and perivesical fluid collection. They concluded that the technique needed to be further modified to achieve acceptable success rates [12].

In 1999, the Japanese group published their long-term follow-up on 36 patients (51 renal units), 15 of whom were children. Their resolution rates at 1–3 months were 96 and 70%, which had decreased to 74 and 59% at 12 months for adults and children, respectively. The problem seemed to be trigonal splitting [27].

Further modifications on their procedure, namely trigonoplasty II, improved reflux resolution rates to 86% at 1 year follow-up; however, Japanese group's conclusion was that their technique could not be recommended, as their success rate was lower than other laparoscopic techniques for the treatment of VUR [14]. However 1 year after this conclusion was made, Simforoosh et al. reported their results on this technique on 41 refluxing units with a mean follow-up of 8.2 moths. With a mean operative time of 147 min and blood loss of less than 50 ml, they achieved a success rate of 93% [24].

In 2001, Gill et al. first described laparoscopic cross-trigonal ureteral reimplantation using two working ports and cystoscopic guidance and published their initial experience on three patients. They reported operative time between 2.5 and 4.5 h with minimal blood loss. Reflux resolved in two patients, whereas it downgraded from grade IV to grade II in the other patients [15]. Yeung et al. reported their initial experience with pneumovesical approach in 16 children with 23 refluxing ureters in 2005. They reported a mean operative time of 136 min with a success rate of 96%. In three cases, they experienced dislocation of trocar, of which two could be managed laparoscopically, whereas the third case needed to be converted to open surgery. Both of the laparoscopically managed cases experienced scrotal and suprapubic emphysema that resolved spontaneously over the next 24 h. There were also two cases of persistent mild hematuria for more than 72 h which ceased spontaneously [3].

Thakre et al. reported their operative success rate of 97.5% for laparoscopic Cohen performed in 60 children. Similar to results reported by Yeung et al., this group also did not experience any major complication and the most common problem was trocar displacement [4].

Canon et al. reported on their series of 52 consecutive children undergoing vesicoscopic ureteral reimplantation. Postoperative VUR resolution rate was 91% with a mean operative time of 199 min. Average length of hospital stay was 2 days and less oral and intravenous analgesia was needed postoperatively compared to open surgery. The only major complication they experienced was a child who experienced acute renal failure due to bilateral ureteral obstruction. This case was primarily treated with bilateral nephrostomies and required an open reimplantation afterward [17].

Kutikov et al. reported on their experience with a total of 32 patients undergoing laparoscopic transvesical reimplantation. Five of the patients had primary obstructing megaureters and 27 had vesicoureteral reflux. Transvesical laparoscopic cross-trigonal ureteral reimplantation was performed in patients with reflux, and a Glenn–Anderson reimplantation was used in patients with a primary obstructing megaureter. The operative success rates were 92.6 and 80% for vesicoureteral reflux and primary obstructing megaureter cases, respectively. Complications included a postoperative urinary leak in four patients (12.5%) and ureteral stricture at the neoureterovesical anastomosis in two patients (6.3%). The authors experienced higher complication rate in patients 2 years or younger with bladder capacity less than 130 cm^3 [16].

In 2009, Kawauchi et al. compared their outcome and complications between adult and pediatric cases. The median operating time was 145 min in the unilateral cases and 230 min in the bilateral cases with a success rate of 96%. No intraoperative complications were observed. They encountered one persistent reflux and one ureterovesical stricture. The operation time was similar between pediatric and adult patients and one operative failure was observed in each group [28].

Peters et al. performed robotic-assisted transtrigonal reimplantation operation in six children aged 5–15 years old with no open conversions. The hospital stay ranged from 2 to 4 days. One girl had a urine leak postoperatively secondary to inadequate port-site closure. One patient had persisting low-grade reflux at the early period. There has been no evidence of obstruction [19].

Outcomes published in major English literature is summarized in Table 14.1.

Conclusion

Laparoscopic urologic reconstructive surgery in correction of vesicoureteral reflux has lagged behind as it is a technically very demanding surgery to be performed within a very small space. However, with advances in both technical and equipment aspects, laparoscopic reconstructive surgery is becoming more feasible and routinely performed in daily urological practice. However, standardization of these techniques is still needed to encourage standard urological surgeon performing these procedures more frequently. It is our opinion that robotic-assisted surgery will also have an increasingly important role in the treatment of pediatric population in the future.

Critical Operative Steps

Extravesical Reimplantation

1. The ureter can be identified by shearing the lateral peritoneal fold below the common iliac artery.
2. Care should be taken to avoid injury to the ovaries in women and vas in men when freeing the ureter.
3. Care should be taken to identify the pelvic plexus, avoiding injury while ureteral mobilization at the hiatus.

Table 14.1 Outcomes of laparoscopic ureteral reimplantation procedures published in major English literature

	Patients	Ureter	Mean age (years)	Grade	Mean operation time (min) (unilateral/bilateral)	Success (%)	Complication (*n*)	Technique
Kawauchi [28]	30	54	14.5	1–5	145/230	96	1: Ureterovesical stricture	Transtrigonal
Casale [20]	41	82	3.2	3–5	153	97.6	–	Extravesical (robotic)
Capolicchio [6]	20	31	7.3	2–4	120	75	3: Mucosal perforation 1: Distal ureteral necrosis 1: Contralateral reflux	Extravesical
Jayanthi and Patel [18]	103	181	13 months–18 years	1–4	–	94	1: Contralateral reflux 3: Ureterovesical fistula 2: Ureteral obstruction 1: Bladder stones	Transtrigonal
Simforoosh et al. [24]	27	41	8.2	1–4	147	93	4: Peritoneal perforation	Extravesical
Canon et al. [17]	52	87	5.7	1–4	199	91	1: Bladder stones 1: Urine leakage 1: Bilateral obstruction	Transtrigonal
Kutikov et al. [16]	27		5	3–5	168	92.6	4: Urine leakage 2: Ureteral stricture	Transtrigonal
Riquelme et al. [26]	15	19	–	2–3	94.7 (110/180)	94.7	3: Mucosal perforation	Extravesical
Peters and Woo [19]	6	12	5–15	2–3	210	100	1: Urine leakage	Transtrigonal (robotic)
Yeung et al. [3]	16	23	4.1	2–5	136 (80/230)	96	1: Scrotal emphysema 1: Persistent mild hematuria	Transtrigonal
Tsuji et al. [14]	8	14	21.5	1–4	245	86	1: Persisted reflux 1: Ureterovesical fistula	Trigonoplasty II
Shu et al. [23]	6	6	18.7	–	105	100	1: Hydronephrosis 1: Persistent abdominal pain	Extravesical
Gill et al. [15]	3	3	17.7	–	150–270	66		Transtrigonal
Lakshmanan and Fung [22]	47	71	–	1–5	–	100	3: Ureteral injury	Extravesical
Cartwright et al. [12]	22	32	14 months–18 years	2–5	60–240	62.5	1: Vesicovaginal fistula 1: Perivesical fluid collection 1: Hyponatremia	Trigonoplasty
Okamura et al. [11]	12	15	26.8	1–3	178	100	3: Trocar placement	Trigonoplasty

4. Detrusor tunnel should course slightly laterally to avoid kinking of the ureter. The tunnel should obtain a 5:1 ratio of length to width.
5. An optional traction suture placed just beyond the end of the detrusor tunnel would facilitate subsequent bladder manipulations.
6. No angulation or torsion on the ureter is mandatory.
7. The continuous detrusorrhaphy suture should avoid ureteral obstruction, and the wall of the ureter should tightly cling to the bladder so that there remains no gap or tension.

Intravesical Reimplantation

Transtrigonal

1. Optic trocar at the dome and working trocars at lateral walls of the bladder should be securely attached to the bladder wall.
2. Circumferential incision of the ureteral orifice and blunt dissection of the periureteral tissue.
3. Creation of submucosal tunnel.
4. Tension-free anastomosis of the ureter at the apex of submucosal tunnel.
5. Closure of the bladder trocar sites.

Trigonoplasty

1. Creating the U-shaped flap around the ureteral orifices.
2. Creation of the muscular bed and closure of the native ureteral orifice.
3. Advancing and anchoring of the U-shaped flap including ureter at the midline.

Critical Instruments and Supplies

Extravesical Technique

- Hasson trocar (5 mm)
- Working ports (3 mm, 1×)
- Working port (5 mm, 2×)
- Reducer seal (3–5 mm)
- 0° laparoscope (5 mm)
- Curved scissors (3 mm), insulated, with rotatable shaft
- Tapered curved jaw dissectors (3 mm, 2×)
- Babcock forceps (5 mm)
- Allis grasper (3 mm)
- Needle driver (3–5 mm)
- Bipolar and monopolar cable used with special endodissector

Intravesical Technique

- 5 mm in 30° laparoscope
- Instruments (3 mm): hook, grasper, dissector, needle holder
- Trocars (5 mm) for the laparoscope
- Balloon tip trocar (5 mm)
- Bipolar and monopolar cable used with special endodissector

Robotic Surgery

- da Vinci® Surgical System (Intuitive Surgical, Sunnyvale, CA)
- 0° telescope (12 mm; Intuitive Surgical)
- Hook cautery (Intuitive Surgical)
- DeBakey forceps (Intuitive Surgical)
- Round-tip scissors (Intuitive Surgical)
- Fine-point needle driver (Intuitive Surgical)
- VersaStep® (12 mm) radially expanding cannula (US Surgical, Norwalk, CT)
- InStep® (5–10 mm) radially expanding sheath (2×) (US Surgical)
- Laparoscopic grasper (5 mm)
- Micro forceps (Intuitive Surgical)

References

1. Atala A, Kavoussi LR, Goldstein DS, et al. Laparoscopic correction of vesicoureteral reflux. J Urol. 1993;150:748–51.

2. Kim C, Docimo SG. Use of laparoscopy in pediatric urology. Rev Urol. 2005;7(4):215–23.
3. Yeung CK, Sihoe JD, Borzi PA. Endoscopic cross-trigonal ureteral reimplantation under carbon dioxide bladder insufflation: a novel technique. J Endourol. 2005;19:295–9.
4. Thakre AA, Sreedhar B, Yeung CK. Laparoscopy in the management of pediatric vesicoureteral reflux. Indian J Urol. 2007;23(4):414–9.
5. Valla JS, Steyaert H, Griffin SJ, et al. Transvesicoscopic Cohen ureteric reimplantation for vesicoureteral reflux in children: a single-centre 5-year experience. J Pediatr Urol. 2009;5(6):466–71.
6. Capolicchio JP. Laparoscopic extravesical ureteral reimplantation: technique. Adv Urol. 2008;2008:5679–80.
7. Schimberg W, Wacksman J, Rudd R, et al. Laparoscopic correction of vesicoureteral reflux in the pig. J Urol. 1994;151:1664–7.
8. Ehrlich RM, Gershman A, Fuch G. Laparoscopic vesico-ureteroplasty in children: initial case reports. Urology. 1994;43:255–61.
9. Reddy PK, Evans RM. Laparoscopic ureteroneocystostomy. J Urol. 1994;152:2057–9.
10. Janetschek G, Radmayr C, Batsch G. Laparoscopic ureteral antireflux plasty reimplantation. First clinical experience. Ann Urol. 1995;29:101–5.
11. Okamura K, Ono Y, Yamada Y, Kato T, Tsuji Y, Miyake K. Endoscopic trigonoplasty for primary vesico-ureteric reflux. Br J Urol. 1995;75:390–4.
12. Cartwright PC, Snow BW, Mansfield JC, Hamilton BD. Percutaneous endoscopic trigonoplasty: a minimally invasive approach to correct vesico-ureteral reflux. J Urol. 1996;156:661–4.
13. Okamura K, Kato N, Takamura S, et al. Trigonal splitting is a major complication of endoscopic trigonoplasty at 1-year follow up. J Urol. 1997;157:1423–5.
14. Tsuji Y, Okamura K, Nishimura T, et al. A new endoscopic ureteral reimplantation for primary vesicoureteral reflux (endoscopic trigonoplasty II). J Urol. 2003;169(3):1020–2.
15. Gill IS, Ponsky LE, Desai M, Kay R, Ross JH. Laparoscopic cross-trigonal Cohen ureteroneocystostomy: novel technique. J Urol. 2001;166:1811–4.
16. Kutikov A, Guzzo TJ, Canter DJ, Casale P. Initial experience with laparoscopic transvesical ureteral reimplantation at the Children's Hospital of Philadelphia. J Urol. 2006;176:2222–6.
17. Canon SJ, Jayanthi VR, Patel AS. Vesicoscopic crosstrigonal ureteral reimplantation: a minimally invasive option for repair of vesicoureteral reflux. J Urol. 2007;178:269–73.
18. Jayanthi V, Patel A. Vesicoscopic ureteral reimplantation: a minimally invasive technique for the definitive repair of vesicoureteral reflux. Adv Urol. 2008;973616. Epub 5 Nov 2008.
19. Peters CA, Woo R. Intravesical robotically assisted bilateral ureteral reimplantation. J Endourol. 2005;19(6):618–21.
20. Casale P, Patel PR, Kolon TF. Nerve sparing robotic extravesical ureteral reimplantation. J Urol. 2008;179:1987–90.
21. Smaldone MC, Sweeney DD, Ost MC, Docimo SG. Laparoscopy in paediatric urology: present status. BJU Int. 2007;100(1):143–50.
22. Lakshmanan Y, Fung LC. Laparoscopic extravesicular ureteral reimplantation for vesicoureteral reflux: recent technical advances. J Endourol. 2000; 14:589–93.
23. Shu T, Cisek LJ Jr, Moore RG. Laparoscopic extravesical reimplantation for postpubertal vesicoureteral reflux. J Endourol. 2004;18(5):441–6.
24. Simforoosh N, Mohammad NS, Shahrokhi S. Extraperitoneal laparoscopic trigonoplasty for treatment of vesicoureteral reflux: novel technique duplicating its open counterpart. J Urol. 2007; 177:321–4.
25. Agarwal MM, Singh SK, Agarwal S, Mavuduru R, Mandal AK. A novel technique of intracorporeal excisional tailoring of megaureter before laparoscopic ureteral reimplantation. Urology. Jan 2010;75(1):96–9. Epub 2 Oct 2009.
26. Riquelme M, Aranda A, Rodriguez C. Laparoscopic extravesical transperitoneal approach for vesicoureteral reflux. J Laparoendosc Adv Surg Tech A. 2006;16:312–6.
27. Okamura K, Kato N, Tsuji Y, Ono Y, Ohshima S. A comparative study of endoscopic trigonoplasty for vesicoureteral reflux in children and in adults. Int J Urol. 1999;6(11):562–6.
28. Kawauchi A, Naitoh Y, Soh J, et al. Transvesical laparoscopic cross-trigonal ureteral reimplantation for correction of vesicoureteral reflux: initial experience and comparisons between adult and pediatric cases. J Endourol. 2009;23(11):1875–8.

Chapter 15

Robotic Ureteral Reimplant Surgery to Correct Reflux Disease

Craig A. Peters and Ryan P. Smith

This chapter contains a video segment which can be found at the URL: http://www.springerimages.com/ost

Introduction

Atala et al. initially described the laparoscopic approach for the correction of vesicoureteral reflux over a decade ago in animals [1]. The technique was subsequently modified by several other investigators in porcine models [2–4]. Ehrlich and colleagues were the first to introduce this technique in children [5]. Over time, various technical refinements have been described, thus establishing laparoscopic ureteral reimplantation as an alternative to open repair. Utilization of conventional laparoscopic reimplantation has been limited, however, due to the technical difficulty inherent in this approach. Parental preference for minimally invasive techniques has only burgeoned interest in the endoscopic, laparoscopic, and robotic correction of vesicoureteral reflux [6–8].

Robotic-assisted laparoscopic surgery in urology emerged after an initial report by Partin et al. in 1995 [9]. The robot has facilitated the acquisition of laparoscopic skills for the open surgeon. The goal of robotic assistance is to diminish the learning curve of traditional laparoscopy, while attaining the reconstructive precision of open surgery and the reduced pain and morbidity of laparoscopy [10]. Pediatric uses have been adopted slowly but seek to gain the advantages of laparoscopy including reduced incision size, morbidity, postoperative pain, and length of stay. The core advantages of the robotic system are high-resolution three-dimensional vision, tremor-filtered instrument control with movement scaling, and wrist-like articulation, all of which are limited in traditional laparoscopy [11]. Primary deterrents for the robotic approach have included increased cost, lack of tactile feedback and lack of pediatric sized ports and instruments [10, 12]. Some early applications in pediatric urology have included robotic-assisted dismembered pyeloplasty, appendicovesicostomy, extravesical and intravesical bilateral ureteral reimplantation and more recently, partial nephrectomy [13–19].

The demonstration of successful intravesical and extravesical laparoscopic ureteral reimplantation allowed for implementation of the robotic approach to ureteral reimplantation [11, 13, 16]. This chapter will focus on the general principles and techniques associated with the intravesical and extravesical approaches to pediatric robotic-assisted antireflux surgery. Results, complications, and potential advancements of this technique in the pediatric population will also be discussed.

C.A. Peters (✉)
Division of Pediatric Urology, University of Virginia Children's Hospital, Charlottesville, VA 22908, USA
e-mail: cap9b@virginia.edu

M.C. Ost (ed.), *Robotic and Laparoscopic Reconstructive Surgery in Children and Adults*,
Current Clinical Urology, DOI 10.1007/978-1-60327-914-7_15,

Background

Indications for Intervention

Indications for extravesical or intravesical robotic reimplantation are identical to the laparoscopic and open approaches including breakthrough infections, progressive renal scarring, and persistent reflux despite watchful waiting. Bilateral reflux has traditionally favored an intravesical approach as the potential for transient postoperative urinary retention is reportedly higher with bilateral extravesical reimplantation [20]. Lakshmanan and Fung [21], however, found a diminished risk with the laparoscopic approach. Despite these findings, several authors' experience suggests that the same risk remains and therefore an intravesical approach which uses the transtrigonal or Cohen technique has been explored [11, 13, 16, 22]. Extravesical reimplantation is primarily indicated when confronting unilateral reflux and maintains a role in bilateral reflux with the caveat that transient retention is a risk.

Patient Selection

Patient selection is identical to that of the laparoscopic approach with surgeon experience playing a significant role. Conditions which may impose significant technical difficulty for a robotic approach in children include obesity, extensive prior abdominal or pelvic surgery, and pelvic fibrosis [23]. These relative contraindications require careful risk–benefit analysis and discussion of operative risk with the patient and their family.

Anesthetic Risk and Pediatric Laparoscopy

Associated risks of anesthesia also play a role in patient selection for laparoscopic procedures. The risks associated with laparoscopy result from the physiologic effects created by pneumoperitoneum. Careful screening should be applied to those with restrictive airway disease and cardiac insufficiency [24]. Intraabdominal pressure is significantly elevated and the insufflation of carbon dioxide results in its absorption across the peritoneum. The reduced lung volumes created by pneumoperitoneum more significantly impact children, as compared to adults. This is inherent in a child's decreased pulmonary reserve and low functional reserve capacity. However, the hypercarbia resultant from carbon dioxide absorption is generally well tolerated in children [25, 26]. Cardiovascular function is similarly altered by pneumoperitoneum resulting in decreased venous return and cardiac output. This is generally without consequence in children with normal cardiac function [25, 27]. For most bladder procedures, steep Trendelenburg position is needed, putting increased pressure on the thorax. Increased abdominal pressure is also associated with reduced intraoperative urine output. This effect is transient and has not been shown to result in any permanent renal injury [28–30].

Patient Preparation and Setup

Bowel preparation is initiated 24 h prior to surgery and consists of a clear liquid diet and a glycerin suppository the evening before surgery. A rectal tube may additionally be placed after the induction of general anesthesia to aid in decompression of the rectosigmoid colon. The bladder catheter is introduced on the sterile field. The experience of the operative room team and their familiarity with the robotic equipment are paramount in ensuring safe positioning for robotic surgery. The anesthesia team should be aware of the constraints of positioning in robotic-assisted cases as the accessible space can be limited and the robotic arms require a large degree of clearance.

For both the transvesical and extravesical approaches, the patient is placed in the supine position with feet at the end of the bed (Fig. 15.1). The robot is brought in from the patient's feet.

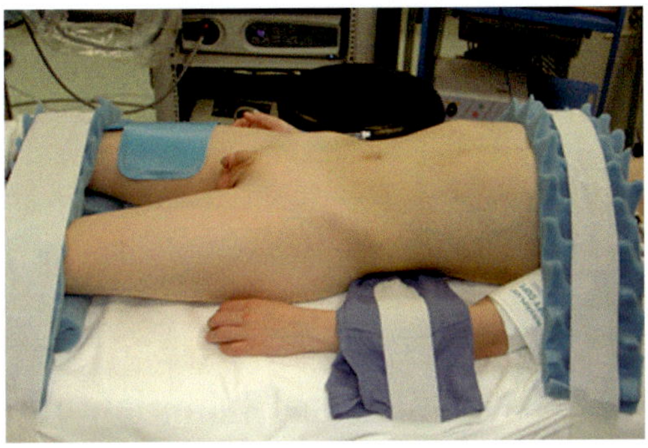

Fig. 15.1 For both reimplant approaches the patient is placed supine. All adjustments in positioning are made prior to docking of the robot

All aspects of the robotic system should be turned on and evaluated prior to initiation of surgery. The extravesical approach requires placing the patient in Trendelenburg's position. No flexion of the table is necessary. All table adjustments and patient positioning should be completed prior to engagement and docking of the robot [11, 13, 31].

Port Placement and Selection of Instruments

The basic principles of laparoscopic port placement apply to both the transvesical and extravesical approaches. Ports should be placed symmetrically in relationship to the operative site. If the arms are not symmetric, there will be limited range of movement or interference with the camera arm. Careful placement is essential in children where working space is limited. The authors prefer a box-stitch modification of the Hasson technique for trocar insertion [32]. This technique assures direct visual placement of the trocar, fastening of the trocar to the abdominal wall, and ease of closure. The central port is typically placed at the umbilicus and is reserved for the 30°, 12-mm camera. Care should be taken to ensure that the camera is aligned with the central axis of the robot. Insertion of the additional working ports is performed under direct visualization after insertion of the 12-mm camera port. The lateral, 5-mm working ports are placed equidistant along a line that is perpendicular to the central camera axis and at an appropriate distance to the operative site. This is at the level of the umbilicus in children over 3 years of age and slightly above the umbilicus in younger ages. In children, these working ports are either 5 or 8 mm.

The da Vinci Robot System (Intuitive Surgical, Sunnyvale, Ca) has both 8- and 5-mm working instruments. For bladder applications, the DeBakey forceps or the 5-mm Maryland dissector are all-purpose instruments for tissue manipulation, dissection, and control. The hook cautery is a versatile instrument, facilitating hemostasis and dissection. The 5-mm curved scissors are not electrified, while the 8-mm curved scissors are electrified. The 8-mm needle drivers are useful for suturing and come in two types: large and fine. The large needle driver can handle sutures of 4-0 and above. Neither needle driver is suitable for tissue manipulation. The 5-mm needle drivers are useful for sutures from 3-O to 6-O. These are more effective in tissue manipulation but require more room to move into a right angle, which may limit movement in the confined space of a pediatric abdomen [11, 31].

Specifics of the Robotic Approach

General Principles

Atala and colleagues' description of the laparoscopic correction of vesicoureteral reflux was a modification of the Lich–Gregoir technique in a porcine model [1]. Ehrlich and others, using this technique in humans, were able to demonstrate the safety and efficacy of this approach [5, 33, 34]. Early reports of laparoscopic repair of reflux focused on the extravesical approach with good results. A difficult learning curve was evident in several early series. Open extravesical ureteroneocystostomy has been associated with decreased incidence of postoperative hematuria and bladder spasm [35, 36]. The extravesical technique, however, has the potential disadvantage of postoperative voiding dysfunction as well as the inherent complications of a transperitoneal approach. The open Cohen, cross-trigonal reimplantation is well established and has been associated with reflux resolution rates above 97% [37]. Concerted efforts were subsequently applied to replicate this approach laparoscopically. In 2001, Gill and colleagues outlined a novel technique of laparoscopic cross-trigonal Cohen ureteroneocystostomy for reflux [38]. This approach offers the potential efficiency and durability of the open transtrigonal repair without the risk of urinary retention associated with bilateral extravesical repair.

Cartwright and Okamura [39, 40], independently in 1996, published reports of endoscopic trigonoplasty for the correction of vesicoureteral reflux. Okamura et al. in their initial report had resolution in all 11 refluxing units in a 3–12-month timeframe. Cartwright and Snow performed percutaneous endoscopic trigonoplasty with a success rate of 62.5%. Long-term outcomes with patients observed up to 37 months were published in 1999. Patients who underwent Gil-Vernet trigonoplasty had dropped to a resolution rate of 47%, while those who underwent a Cohen cross-trigonal technique exhibited reflux resolution of 83% with a trend toward longer operative times [41]. Simforoosh [42] et al. described an extraperitoneal laparoscopic trigonoplasty in 2007 with resolution rates approaching 93% over 4–19 months of follow-up. None of these laparoscopic techniques have been applied broadly due to the technical challenges of the procedure and the uncertainty of outcomes in light of the minimal morbidity and high reflux resolution rates of open repair.

The potential of robotic-assisted laparoscopic surgery lies in enhanced visualization and instrument control. These advantages over the traditional laparoscopic technique have the potential to permit broader application of the robotic-assisted transvesical and extravesical correction of reflux. Both techniques have been applied robotically, thus offering a more technically facile approach to surgeons without extensive laparoscopic training [11]. The initial report of robotic-assisted pneumovesical ureteral reimplantation was performed in a porcine model by Olsen in 2003 [16]. Robotic-assisted intravesical and extravesical reimplantation were described in the pediatric population shortly thereafter [11, 13].

Extravesical Ureteral Reimplantation

Positioning and Port Placement

The patient is placed supine and then moved into Trendelenburg's position. Access for the robotic-assisted extravesical approach is transperitoneal using a Lich–Gregoir technique [43]. Port placement is as shown in Fig. 15.2. Prior to trocar placement, fascial sutures are placed in a box-stitch fashion [32]. This assists in fascial closure following the procedure as well as securing the ports to the abdominal wall. The 12-mm camera port is positioned infraumbilically using the described Bailez technique [44].

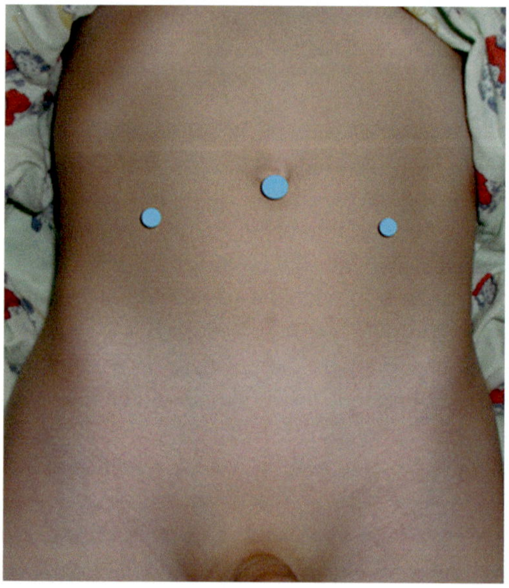

Fig. 15.2 Port-site placement for robotic extravesical ureteral reimplantation. The camera port is at the umbilicus with the working ports placed equidistant just below the level of the umbilicus

Pneumoperitoneum is established with carbon dioxide insufflation to a pressure of 12 mmHg. The additional 5- or 8-mm working ports are then placed laterally below the level of the umbilicus and under direct visualization. Fascial sutures are also used here. Once satisfactory access is gained, the robot is engaged and docked with the camera axis centrally aligned.

Description of Robotic-Assisted Extravesical Technique

The operation begins with identification of the obliterated umbilical artery, which is then followed into the pelvis. The ureter can be found passing inferiorly and medially to the obliterated umbilical artery. Incising the anterior peritoneum exposes the ureter. In boys, the vas deferens should be spared by sweeping it superiorly with the peritoneum. In girls, the peritoneal incision is made between the bladder and the uterus and the ureter is identified by blunt dissection along the posterior wall. Using careful dissection, the ureter is then mobilized for approximately 4–5 cm to the level of the ureterovesical junction (Fig. 15.3). While it has been reported that the bladder nerves presumed to be at risk of injury can be seen and avoided, this author has not been able to discern them. Staying as close to the ureter as possible is likely the best means to limit the risk of retention. Excessive mobilization should be avoided which risks devascularization. A hitch stitch using Vicryl suture may be placed to draw the bladder toward the contralateral side and enhance visualization. This may be passed through the abdominal wall and out again or in older children sutured within the pelvis. The posterior bladder wall is then cleared and the bladder is partially filled. A 2.5–3-cm detrusor incision is made down to the level of the mucosa. The detrusor muscle is then peeled away from the mucosa laterally to create the muscle flaps which will be used to wrap the ureter in its detrusor tunnel (Fig. 15.4).

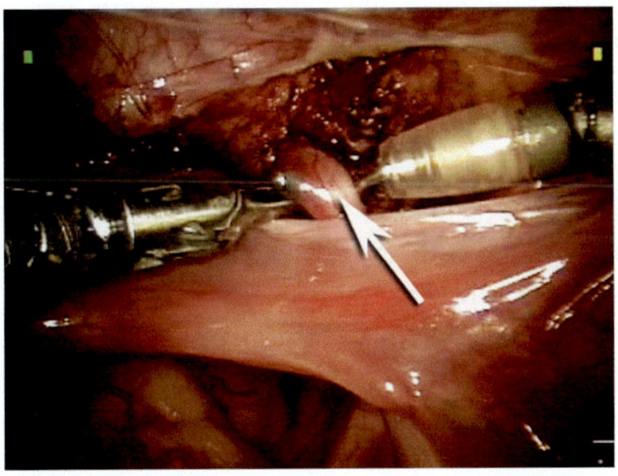

Fig. 15.3 Extravesical ureteral mobilization. The ureter is mobilized from 4 to 5 cm to the level of ureterovesical junction with care to stay as close as possible to the ureter (*marked with arrow*)

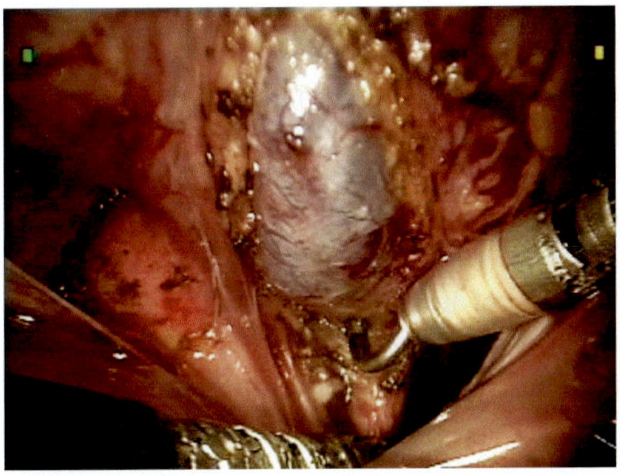

Fig. 15.4 Creation of the detrusor flaps following incision of the muscularis of the bladder. The mucosa and detrusor edges are visible with the ureteral hiatus at the base of the tunnel

A Y-shaped mobilization is then carried out at the level of the ureteral hiatus. Dissection should be adjacent to the ureter and noncircumferential with care to avoid extending the dissection dorsomedially [45]. The detrusor flaps are then wrapped along the mobilized ureter and reapproximated using interrupted 4-O Polydioxanone or Vicryl suture. By closing distal to proximal, one has clearer visualization of all structures; however, needle passage is subureteric for each suture (Fig. 15.5). Closing from top down or proximal to distal approximates the detrusor edges, but the first suture must be tied under tension. Following creation of the tunnel, the peritoneum is closed with a loose running stitch.

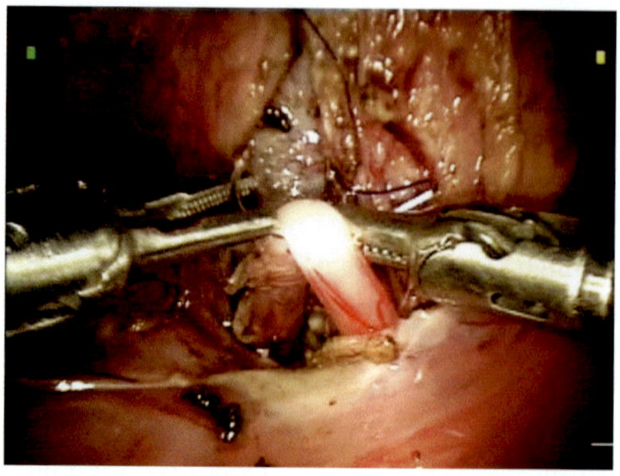

Fig. 15.5 Closure of the detrusor tunnel with interrupted, absorbable sutures. Note subureteric passage of the suture

The working ports are removed and the previously placed box-stitch fascial sutures are closed under direct visualization. The camera port is closed in similar fashion. The subcutaneous layer is reapproximated with a 4-O Vicryl and the skin is closed with a 5-O Monocryl in a subcuticular fashion. In bilateral cases, a bladder catheter is left postoperatively, but in unilateral repairs, a catheter is not routinely left in place [11, 13, 31].

Results

The author's initial results with robotic-assisted extravesical reimplantation for reflux were reported in 2004. Twenty-four children underwent extravesical reimplantation with ages ranging from 4.6 to 140 months. Mean age was 6.5 years. Nineteen patients were female and five were male with a range of reflux grades II–IV. Twenty-one patients had a unilateral reimplant, while the three remaining children had bilateral reimplants. Four of these cases were associated with contralateral nephrectomy. Operative times for unilateral implantation approached 2 h with an additional 1.5 h for bilateral procedures. At the time of initial publication, patients had been followed for a mean of 5.7 months in the unilateral group and 8.7 months in the bilateral group.

Reflux was persistent in three patients; however, reflux was reduced to grade I or II in two of these patients and the third patient had unchanged grade II reflux. Complications included voiding dysfunction in two patients, one of whom had a bilateral reimplantation. Two children, including one patient with postoperative voiding dysfunction, had a bladder leak which responded to prolonged drainage. One child who underwent contralateral nephrectomy at the time of extravesical reimplantation developed postoperative hydronephrosis and a rising creatinine necessitating ureteral stent placement. One month after stent removal, the patient had a normal creatinine with no residual reflux or hydronephrosis. The author has since recommended ureteral stent placement in patients with solitary kidneys undergoing unilateral laparoscopic reimplantation procedures [11, 31].

The author's reflux cessation rate based on this series was 87%. This falls below the success rates quoted in the literature for open extravesical reimplantation. When further age-matched analysis was performed comparing the author's open and robotic extravesical reflux cessation rates, there was no statistically significant difference noted. Further series will be required to see if the quoted success rate is low due to the learning curve associated with adopting new technology. Larger series will be required to continue to compare success rates in both open and robotic extravesical reimplantation [31]. As in open series, obtaining adequate tunnel length, muscular backing, and tissue quality are paramount for performance.

Casale and colleagues published a series of 41 patients who underwent robotic extravesical reimplantation for bilateral vesicoureteral reflux in 2008. Reflux was grade III in eight patients and five patients each had grade IV and grade V reflux, respectively. Twenty-three patients had mixed grade (III–V) with or without duplication anomalies. The outcomes were reviewed retrospectively in attempt to determine whether the extravesical approach diminished the incidence of postoperative voiding dysfunction. The hypothesis being that the enhanced visualization afforded by robotic assistance provides better visualization and sparing of the pelvic plexus. Postoperative VCUG was performed in all patients with a reflux resolution rate of 97.6%, which approaches that of open extravesical reimplantation (92.5–98%) [46]. The patient who failed robotic reimplantation in this series underwent dextranomer/hyaluronic acid injection with subsequent resolution of reflux demonstrated 3 months later on VCUG [47].

Mean operative time was 2.33 h including cystoscopy and placement of ureteral catheters. The ureteral catheters were secured to the urethral catheter. By the author's report, operative time decreased significantly after the first five cases. Average length of stay was 26.1 h. All patients had their urethral and ureteral catheters removed on postoperative day 1 followed by a post-void residual. All 41 patients voided spontaneously with a mean residual of 13 ml. No episodes of retention were noted and postoperative uroflow assessments were unchanged from preoperative results. The authors reported that they no longer routinely perform postoperative VCUG and patients are followed clinically. VCUG is used only if pyelonephritis were to develop which mirrors the approach after open ureteroneocystostomy. All patients underwent 3- and 6-month ultrasounds which were reportedly normal in all cases [47]. Lendvay additionally described an initial series of 16 patients who underwent extravesical robotic reimplantation. They reported three VCUG-documented failures of reflux resolution or only downgrading of reflux and one case of de novo contralateral reflux. All complications arose in patients with preexisting voiding dysfunction [48].

Evaluation of the robotic approach to extravesical reimplantation continues. As with any new technology, its use must hold up to the gold standard, in this case, open cross-trigonal reimplantation. As operative times decrease and familiarity with the technology improves, further comparative studies will be required to assure that adequate tunnel length and resolution of reflux can be achieved with the robotic extravesical approach. The success rates and operative times published by the authors above are an early indication of the promise of this new technology; however, larger robotic-assisted series are required to more soundly evaluate this promise and assess its impact as a minimally invasive technique. At this early phase of exploration, a postoperative VCUG should continue to be routine. In an era where open extravesical reimplantation can be performed as an outpatient procedure, we must assess whether this new technology has the potential to advance current practice [49].

Intravesical Ureteral Reimplantation

Positioning and Port Placement

The robotic-assisted intravesical reimplant is performed using a transvesical approach with a cross-trigonal Cohen technique. The patient is placed supine on the table with the legs apart and the feet at the end of the bed. Prior to trocar insertion, a urethral catheter is inserted and the bladder is filled with saline. The catheter may also be used to evacuate blood and urine which may disrupt visualization during the procedure. Suction may be intermittently applied to the catheter to facilitate drainage.

Bladder distention also aids in the placement of the working ports which are placed equidistant at the palpable, lateral bladder edge (Fig. 15.6). A 12-mm vertical incision is made overlying the palpable bladder dome and blunt dissection is carried down to the space of Retzius. A 3-O Vicryl suture is placed in box-stitch fashion which lifts the bladder dome into the incision. A small cystotomy is made and the trocar is then placed through the box stitch, entering the bladder. This stitch again aids in elevation of the bladder wall throughout the procedure and in closure of the cystotomy. Securing the ports to the bladder wall is paramount in ensuring efficient performance. One should avoid making too large a cystotomy which may result in leakage of insufflated carbon dioxide and fluid during the procedure. The camera is subsequently introduced and the bladder inspected [13, 31].

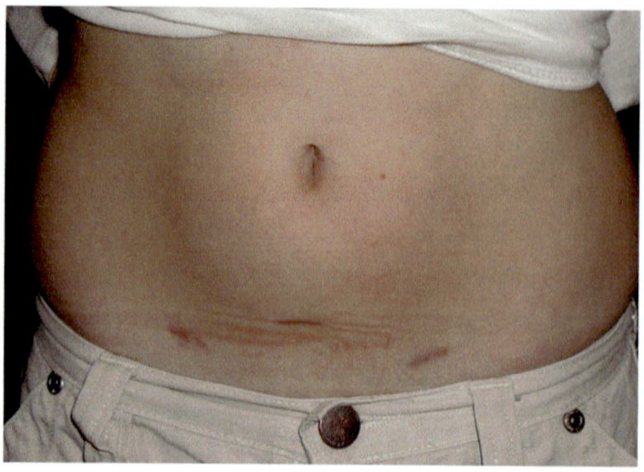

Fig. 15.6 Port-site placement for robotic intravesical ureteral reimplantation as seen 3 months following the procedure. The camera port is below the umbilicus at the dome of the bladder as detected on palpation. The working ports are placed at the palpable bladder edge after saline distension

The working ports are subsequently placed symmetrically halfway between the umbilicus and the pubis along the lateral, palpable bladder edge. A box stitch is again used to facilitate closure of the bladder punctures at completion. Obtaining an adequate seal around each port site avoids leakage and retroperitoneal insufflation. Yeung et al. [50] described a technique of passing sutures via two angiocatheters, one of which contains a loop snare, thus enabling a purse-string suture in patients with a large volume of subcutaneous fat. Following trocar placement, insufflation of carbon dioxide is initiated to a pressure of 8–10 mmHg to displace the saline. The author has found that withholding insufflation until all port sites have been placed is more effective than placing the working ports after insufflation. The intravesical pressure is higher with saline present, thus preventing bladder collapse when external pressure is applied during port placement. During instrument changes, pneumovesical pressure may fall and cause the field to contract. The traction sutures placed in the bladder wall at the skin level will minimize this complication. The retroperitoneum may also become insufflated during periureteral dissection and compress the operative field. Following insufflation, the ports are then secured and the robot is docked at the foot of the bed.

Description of Robotic-Assisted Intravesical Technique

After docking the robot and engaging the arms, a 6-cm segment of a 5-Fr feeding tube and an 8 cm length of 4-O Vicryl suture are passed into the bladder using the 5-mm laparoscopic grasper. The Maryland dissector and fine needle holders are used to manipulate the feeding tube into each ureteral meatus. The tube is then secured with a 4-O Vicryl suture. This facilitates dissection in enabling the operator to place traction on the ureter. Mobilization of the ureters follows that of the traditional transtrigonal, open technique; however, assessment of adequate mobilization relies heavily on visual inspection as opposed to tactile feedback (Fig. 15.7). The mucosa is incised circumferentially leaving a cuff of mucosa, which is reapproximated with the vesicular mucosa after tunnel creation.

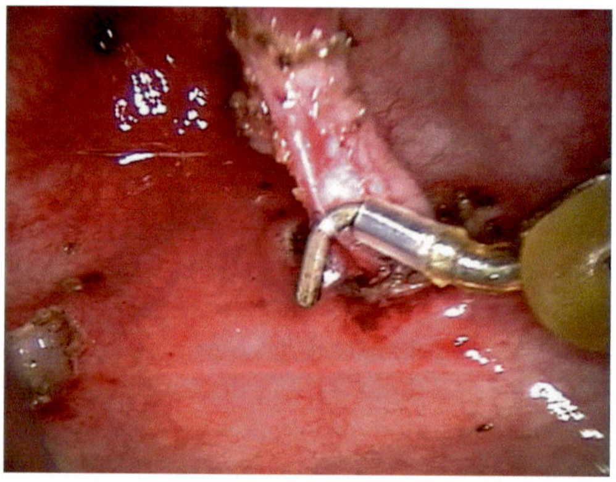

Fig. 15.7 Intravesical ureteral mobilization. Mobilization follows that of the open Cohen technique. Adequate mobilization relies heavily on visual inspection

Mobilization of both ureteral orifices should occur prior to submucosal tunnel creation.

Each ureteral hiatus is reduced using 4-O Vicryl suture. The submucosal tunnels are then created via sharp dissection with the scissors. The dissection is carried from the original hiatus to the contralateral portion of the trigone. The right angle articulation of the robotic instrument greatly facilitates this maneuver (Fig. 15.8).

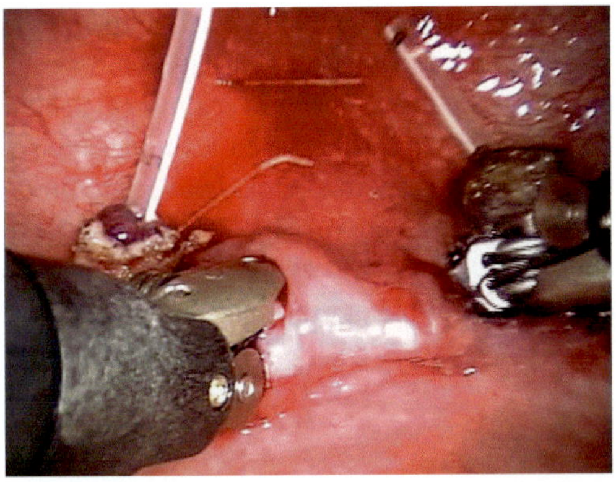

Fig. 15.8 Creation of submucosal ureteral tunnels. Dissection is carried out from the original ureteral hiatus to the contralateral portion of the trigone. Note the feeding tube within the ureteral orifice to aid in manipulation of the ureter

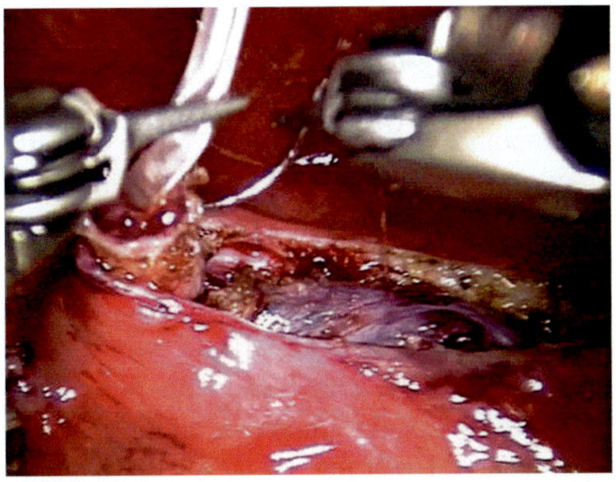

Fig. 15.9 Anastomosis of the ureter to the newly created hiatus. Three anchoring 4-O Monocryl sutures secure the ureter to the mucosa and underlying detrusor. The remainder of the cuff and mucosal defect are sutured with 5-O Monocryl

A small incision is then made in the vesical mucosa, thus creating a new mucosal opening. The lower ureter may exit the submucosal tunnel at the original ureteral hiatus of the contralateral ureter. The ureters are brought through the newly created tunnels using the 5-Fr feeding tube previously sewn in place. The feeding tubes are then removed as each ureter is secured to the previously created vesicular mucosal cuff. Three anchoring, 4-O Monocryl sutures re-approximate each ureter to the underlying detrusor and mucosa. The remainder of the ureteral cuff is closed with 5-O Monocryl (Fig. 15.9). Ureteral patency is tested by insertion of a 5-Fr feeding tube into the lumen. The remaining mucosal defects at the ureteral hiatus are closed with 5-O Monocryl.

The bladder is then irrigated and hemostasis is assessed. The balloon of the bladder catheter is inflated and left in position. The working ports are removed, thus evacuating the pneumovesicum. The pre-placed box-stitch sutures are then tied down under direct visualization to ensure closure of the bladder wall. The suture ends should not be cut until satisfactory closure of the port sites is assured. This permits the port site to be lifted into the incision and if necessary, a second suture may be placed in a figure-of-eight fashion for more secure closure. The camera port is closed in a similar fashion. Each fascial defect is then closed in the standard fashion. The subcutaneous layer is reapproximated with a 4-O Vicryl and the skin is closed with a 5-O Monocryl in subcuticular fashion. The urethral catheter is left in place for 24 h [13, 31].

Results

The traditional laparoscopic approach to intravesical reimplantation has been described as one of the most difficult laparoscopic operations in pediatric urology. Yeung et al. reported a novel technique of endoscopic cross-trigonal ureteral reimplantation using carbon dioxide pneumovesicum in 2005. Ten boys and six girls with primary reflux ranging in age from 10 months to 13 years underwent endoscopic, cross-trigonal ureteroneocystostomy. Preoperatively, there were eight grade V, ten grade IV, four grade III, and one grade II refluxing ureters. Grade III or milder refluxing ureters were reimplanted only when concomitant grade IV or grade V reflux was present on the contralateral side. Complete resolution of reflux was documented in 96% of children. The patient who failed to resolve was downgraded from grade V to grade I reflux. Reported complications included extravesical port displacement in three patients requiring open conversion in two and transient scrotal and suprapubic emphysema in two patients. Mean operatives times approached 136 min with a steep learning curve. Hospital stays ranged from 1 to 4 days with no narcotic use reported postoperatively [50].

Kutikov and colleagues reported an initial experience of 27 patients with varying degrees of reflux who underwent pure laparoscopic transvesical reimplantation in 2006. They reported a success rate of 92.6% with patients aged from 14 months to 11 years. Complications included two urinary leaks from the camera port sites, two patients with persistent reflux, and one ureteral stricture in a tapered ureter. These complications primarily arose in patients with small bladder capacities. In their conclusion, they comment on the potential benefit of using robotic actuators to assist in tissue manipulation and suturing in these tight spaces [51]. Valla and Cannon have independently had similar success rates of 92 and 91%, respectively, in children undergoing laparoscopic intravesical ureteral reimplantation [52, 53]. Both authors, however, comment on the technical demands and steep learning curve in this approach.

Peters and Woo reported an initial series of six children who underwent intravesical, cross-trigonal ureteral reimplantation with robotic assistance in 2005. These cases were performed without the need for open conversion. Patient's ages ranged from 5 to 15 years old. Length of stay ranged from 2 to 4 days. One girl developed a urine leak postoperative secondary to inadequate port-site closure. This resolved with catheterization for 1 week. Of the patients who underwent postoperative VCUG testing, only one boy had persistent low-grade reflux. At 6 months, his VCUG showed reflux downgraded from grade III to grade II. No evidence of obstruction was found postoperatively [13].

As originally alluded to by Kutikov and colleagues, the robotic approach to intravesical reimplantation affords a more facile development of the submucosal tunnel due to the articulation capabilities of the robot. In addition, it has the potential to create longer tunnel length and muscular backing, which approach that of the open technique. The intravesical technique may also be expanded to other realms of pediatric urology. The author has used a similar approach to perform a ureterocele excision and common sheath reimplantation. The intravesical robotic approach continues to evolve and has the potential for wide applicability.

Summary

The correction of vesicoureteral reflux in children by the open, Cohen, cross-trigonal technique remains the gold standard. The high reflux resolution rates, low postoperative pain, short length of stay, and cosmetic closure make the advantages of minimally invasive approaches difficult to establish [54–56]. The popularity of minimally invasive approaches to antireflux surgery, however, is reinforced by parental preference. The appeal of technology to the public and medical community, combined with the advantages of enhanced visualization and instrument control for surgeons, will continue to increase the demand for practitioners to acquire these techniques. Early series show promising reflux resolution rates approaching those of the open technique and a diminished learning curve from traditional laparoscopy. Further prospective series comparing open and robotic antireflux surgeries will be required to elucidate the potential benefits of smaller incisions, minimal blood loss, diminished postoperative pain, shorter hospital stays, and rapid recovery afforded to the robotic approach. With this evolving technology, we can expect smaller working instruments and improved tools for delicate tissue handling. As robotic usage becomes more widespread, we should also see the cost-prohibitive nature of this new technology improve. Robotic assistance also brings the possibility of remote surgery, thus providing patients with equal access to an experienced surgeon [57, 58]. In summary, the initial results of robotic antireflux surgery are promising and warrant further investigation.

Critical Instruments and Supplies: Robotic Intravesical and Extravesical Reimplantation

- da Vinci® Surgical System (Intuitive Surgical, Sunnyvale, CA) [13]
- A 12-mm 0° telescope (Intuitive Surgical)
- Hook cautery 5 or 8 mm (Intuitive Surgical)
- Maryland 5 or 8 mm (bipolar) (Intuitive Surgical)
- Curved scissors 5 or 8 mm (monopolar) (Intuitive Surgical)
- Needle driver (5 mm; Intuitive Surgical)
- Ethicon 12 mm × 100 mm XCEL trocar (Ethicon)
- da Vinci trocar (5 mm) (2) (Intuitive Surgical)
- Laparoscopic grasper for needle transfer (5 mm)
- Urethral catheter

Critical Operative Steps: Extravesical Reimplantation

- Camera port insertion with Bailez technique (12 mm) [11]
- Working port insertion (5 mm)
- Docking of robot
- Mobilization of ureter
- Bladder hitch-stitch placement for improved visualization (optional)
- Bladder filling and incision of detrusor
- Creation of detrusor muscle flaps
- Y-shaped mobilization of ureteral hiatus
- Wrapping of detrusor flaps
- Reapproximation of detrusor flaps

Critical Operative Steps: Intravesical Reimplantation

- Urethral catheter placement with saline installation [13]
- Vertical cystotomy (12 mm) with placement of camera port
- Working port (5 mm) placement (2)
- Docking of robot with saline evacuation and insufflation
- Intubation of both ureters with 6-cm 5-Fr feeding tubes
- Mobilization of ureters
- Tunneling of ureteral hiatus
- Creation of transtrigonal tunnels
- Anastomosis of ureteral meatus
- Port-site closure

References

1. Atala A, Kavoussi LR, Goldstein DS, et al. Laparoscopic correction of vesicoureteral reflux in the pig. J Urol. 1993;150:748.
2. Schimberg W, Wacksman J, Rudd R, et al. Laparoscopic correction of vesicoureteral reflux in the pig. J Urol. 1994;151:1664.
3. McDougall EM, Urban DA, Kerbl K, et al. Laparoscopic repair of vesicoureteral reflux utilizing the Lich–Gregoir technique in the pig model. J Urol. 1995;153:497.
4. Janssen T, Bassi S, Cussenot O, et al. Laparoscopic treatment of vesico-ureteral reflux in the pig. Preliminary report. Prog Urol. 1994;4:70.
5. Ehrlich RM, Gershman A, Fuchs G. Laparoscopic vesicoureteroplasty in children: initial case reports. Urology. 1994;43:255.
6. Ogan K, Pohl HG, Carlson D, et al. Parental preferences in the management of vesicoureteral reflux. J Urol. 2001;166:240.
7. Capozza N, Lais A, Matarazzo E, et al. Treatment of vesico-ureteric reflux: a new algorithm based on parental preference. BJU Int. 2003;92:285.
8. Callaghan K, Gray E, Caldamone A, et al. Factors involved in parental decision making for surgical correction of vesicoureteral reflux. J Urol. 2008;180:701.
9. Partin AW, Adams JB, Moore RG, et al. Complete robot-assisted laparoscopic urologic surgery: a preliminary report. J Am Coll Surg. 1995;181:552.
10. Hayn MH, Smaldone MC, Ost MC, et al. Minimally invasive treatment of vesicoureteral reflux. Urol Clin North Am. 2008;35:477.
11. Peters CA. Robotically assisted surgery in pediatric urology. Urol Clin North Am. 2004;31:743.
12. Smaldone MC, Sweeney DD, Ost MC, et al. Laparoscopy in paediatric urology: present status. BJU Int. 2007;100:143.
13. Peters CA, Woo R. Intravesical robotically assisted bilateral ureteral reimplantation. J Endourol. 2005;19:618.

14. Lee RS, Retik AB, Borer JG, et al. Pediatric robot assisted laparoscopic dismembered pyeloplasty: comparison with a cohort of open surgery. J Urol. 2006;175:683.
15. Olsen LH, Jorgensen TM. Computer assisted pyeloplasty in children: the retroperitoneal approach. J Urol. 2004;171:2629.
16. Olsen LH, Deding D, Yeung CK, et al. Computer assisted laparoscopic pneumovesical ureter reimplantation a.m. Cohen: initial experience in a pig model. APMIS Suppl. 2003;109:23–5.
17. Yee DS, Shanberg AM, Duel BP, et al. Initial comparison of robotic-assisted laparoscopic versus open pyeloplasty in children. Urology. 2006;67:599.
18. Lee RS, Sethi AS, Passerotti CC, et al. Robot assisted laparoscopic partial nephrectomy: a viable and safe option in children. J Urol. 2009;181:823.
19. Pedraza R, Weiser A, Franco I. Laparoscopic appendicovesicostomy (Mitrofanoff procedure) in a child using the da Vinci robotic system. J Urol. 2004;171:1652.
20. Lipski BA, Mitchell ME, Burns MW. Voiding dysfunction after bilateral extravesical ureteral reimplantation. J Urol. 1998;159:1019.
21. Lakshmanan Y, Fung LC. Laparoscopic extravesicular ureteral reimplantation for vesicoureteral reflux: recent technical advances. J Endourol. 2000;14:589.
22. Cohen SJ. Uretero cystoneostomie: eine neue antireflux technik. Aktuelle Urologie. 1975;6:1–6.
23. Eichel L, McDougall EM, Clayman RV. Basics of laparoscopic urologic surgery. In: Campbell MF, Wein AJ, Kavoussi LR, editors. Campbell–Walsh urology. editor-in-chief, Alan J. Wein; editors, Louis R. Kavoussi ... [et al.]. 9th ed. Philadelphia, PA: W.B. Saunders; 2007. pp. 4 v (xlii, 3945, cxv p.).
24. Lorenzo AJ, Karsli C, Halachmi S, et al. Hemodynamic and respiratory effects of pediatric urological retroperitoneal laparoscopic surgery: a prospective study. J Urol. 2006;175:1461.
25. Docimo S, Peters C. Pediatric endourology and laparoscopy. In: Campbell MF, Wein AJ, Kavoussi LR, editors. Campbell–Walsh urology. editor-in-chief, Alan J. Wein; editors, Louis R. Kavoussi ... [et al.]. 9th ed. Philadelphia, PA: W.B. Saunders; 2007. pp. 4 v. (xlii, 3945, cxv p.).
26. Tobias JD. Anesthetic considerations for laparoscopy in children. Semin Laparosc Surg. 1998;5:60.
27. Gentili A, Iannettone CM, Pigna A, et al. Cardiocirculatory changes during videolaparoscopy in children: an echocardiographic study. Paediatr Anaesth. 2000;10:399.
28. Chang DT, Kirsch AJ, Sawczuk IS. Oliguria during laparoscopic surgery. J Endourol. 1994;8:349.
29. Chiu AW, Chang LS, Birkett DH, et al. The impact of pneumoperitoneum, pneumoretroperitoneum, and gasless laparoscopy on the systemic and renal hemodynamics. J Am Coll Surg. 1995;181:397.
30. Cisek LJ, Gobet RM, Peters CA. Pneumoperitoneum produces reversible renal dysfunction in animals with normal and chronically reduced renal function. J Endourol. 1998;12:95.
31. Copp H, Peters C. Pediatric robotic-assisted antireflux surgery. In: Smith AD, editor. Smith's textbook of endourology. 2nd ed. Hamilton, ON: BC Decker Inc; 2007. pp. 951–5.
32. Poppas DP, Bleustein CB, Peters CA. Box stitch modification of Hasson technique for pediatric laparoscopy. J Endourol. 1999;13:447.
33. Sakamoto W, Nakatani T, Sakakura T, et al. Extraperitoneal laparoscopic Lich–Gregoir antireflux plasty for primary vesicoureteral reflux. Int J Urol. 2003;10:94.
34. Kawauchi A, Fujito A, Soh J, et al. Laparoscopic correction of vesicoureteral reflux using the Lich–Gregoir technique: initial experience and technical aspects. Int J Urol. 2003;10:90.
35. Houle AM, McLorie GA, Heritz DM, et al. Extravesical nondismembered ureteroplasty with detrusorrhaphy: a renewed technique to correct vesicoureteral reflux in children. J Urol. 1992;148:704.
36. Wacksman J, Gilbert A, Sheldon CA. Results of the renewed extravesical reimplant for surgical correction of vesicoureteral reflux. J Urol. 1992;148:359.
37. Elder JS, Peters CA, Arant BS Jr, et al. Pediatric Vesicoureteral Reflux Guidelines Panel summary report on the management of primary vesicoureteral reflux in children. J Urol. 1997;157:1846.
38. Gill IS, Ponsky LE, Desai M, et al. Laparoscopic cross-trigonal Cohen ureteroneocystostomy: novel technique. J Urol. 2001;166:1811.
39. Cartwright PC, Snow BW, Mansfield JC, et al. Percutaneous endoscopic trigonoplasty: a minimally invasive approach to correct vesicoureteral reflux. J Urol. 1996;156:661.
40. Okamura K, Yamada Y, Tsuji Y, et al. Endoscopic trigonoplasty in pediatric patients with primary vesicoureteral reflux: preliminary report. J Urol. 1996;156:198.
41. Gatti JM, Cartwright PC, Hamilton BD, et al. Percutaneous endoscopic trigonoplasty in children: long-term outcomes and modifications in technique. J Endourol. 1999;13:581.
42. Simforoosh N, Nadjafi-Semnani M, Shahrokhi S. Extraperitoneal laparoscopic trigonoplasty for treatment of vesicoureteral reflux: novel technique duplicating its open counterpart. J Urol. 2007;177:321.
43. Gregoir W. Lich–Gregoir operation. In: Surgical pediatric urology. Philadelphia, PA: W.B. Saunders; 1977. pp. 265–8.
44. Franc-Guimond J, Kryger J, Gonzalez R. Experience with the Bailez technique for laparoscopic access in children. J Urol. 2003;170:936.
45. Leissner J, Allhoff EP, Wolff W, et al. The pelvic plexus and antireflux surgery: topographical findings and clinical consequences. J Urol. 2001;165:1652.

46. Heidenreich A, Ozgur E, Becker T, et al. Surgical management of vesicoureteral reflux in pediatric patients. World J Urol. 2004;22:96.
47. Casale P, Patel RP, Kolon TF. Nerve sparing robotic extravesical ureteral reimplantation. J Urol. 2008;179:1987.
48. Lendvay T. Robotic-assisted laparoscopic management of vesicoureteral reflux. Adv Urol. 2008:732942.
49. Palmer JS. Extravesical ureteral reimplantation: an outpatient procedure. J Urol. 2008;180:1828.
50. Yeung CK, Sihoe JD, Borzi PA. Endoscopic cross-trigonal ureteral reimplantation under carbon dioxide bladder insufflation: a novel technique. J Endourol. 2005;19:295.
51. Kutikov A, Guzzo TJ, Canter DJ, et al. Initial experience with laparoscopic transvesical ureteral reimplantation at the Children's Hospital of Philadelphia. J Urol. 2006;176:2222.
52. Valla JS, Steyaert H, Griffin SJ, et al. Transvesicoscopic Cohen ureteric reimplantation for vesicoureteral reflux in children: a single-centre 5-year experience. J Pediatr Urol. 2009;5:466–71.
53. Canon SJ, Jayanthi VR, Patel AS. Vesicoscopic cross-trigonal ureteral reimplantation: a minimally invasive option for repair of vesicoureteral reflux. J Urol. 2007;178:269.
54. McCool AC, Joseph DB. Postoperative hospitalization of children undergoing cross-trigonal ureteroneocystostomy. J Urol. 1995;154:794.
55. Chen HW, Yuan SS, Lin CJ. Ureteral reimplantation for vesicoureteral reflux: comparison of minimally invasive extravesical with transvesical and conventional extravesical techniques. Urology. 2004;63:364.
56. Duong DT, Parekh DJ, Pope JCT, et al. Ureteroneocystostomy without urethral catheterization shortens hospital stay without compromising postoperative success. J Urol. 2003;170:1570.
57. Challacombe B, Patriciu A, Glass J, et al. A randomized controlled trial of human versus robotic and telerobotic access to the kidney as the first step in percutaneous nephrolithotomy. Comput Aided Surg. 2005;10:165.
58. Challacombe BJ, Kavoussi LR, Dasgupta P. Transoceanic telerobotic surgery. BJU Int. 2003;92:678.

Part VI
Laparoscopic Orchiopexy in Children

Chapter 16

Laparoscopic and Robotic Orchiopexy for the Impalpable Undescended Testicle

Ahmad Z. Mohamed, Regina Norris, and Francis X. Schneck

This chapter contains a video segment which can be found at the URL: http://www.springerimages.com/ost

Laparoscopic Orchiopexy

Introduction

Approximately 1% of males are diagnosed with cryptorchidism [1]. In the majority of cases the undescended testicle is palpable. However, as many as 20% of cryptorchid patients will have a non-palpable testis [2]. In these cases, the testis might be absent, intra-abdominal, or within the inguinal canal (canalicular). Prior to the advent of laparoscopic exploration for the non-palpable testicle in 1976, management of the undescended testicle consisted of an inguinal exploration with extension into the peritoneum [3]. The testicle was either absent (vanishing), removed, positioned scrotally, or in the worst case scenario, not located by the surgeon.

Preoperative Assessment

At the initial evaluation of the patient, a history of palpable gonads, hypospadias, and previous genital surgery including inguinal herniorrhaphy should be elicited. A careful physical exam (non-threatening in a warm environment with warm lubricant on the groin) is crucial to identify a subtle, but palpable, testicle. Contralateral testicular size should be documented to assess for compensatory hypertrophy [4]. Bilateral non-palpable testicles represent a distinct subgroup that is discussed later.

Diagnostic Workup

Any diagnostic test for the non-palpable testicle must reliably determine the presence or the absence of gonadal tissue and localize it if present. Radiologic testing, including inguinal/abdominal ultrasound, MRI/MRA, herniography, venography, and arteriography, has been shown to have limited value in detection or localization of non-palpable testicles [5–7]. Radiographic imaging studies may be useful in certain clinical circumstances, especially in the obese child. Examination under anesthesia at the time of exploration is generally more cost effective and sensitive [8]. Hormonal therapy to promote testicular descent is rarely therapeutic and not cost effective [9, 10]. This therapy has not been shown to compliment either open or laparoscopic orchiopexy. While the value of this therapy may be increasing the number and maturation of germ cells, evidence supporting preservation

A.Z. Mohamed (✉)
Department of Urology, Children's Hospital of Pittsburgh of UPMC, Pittsburgh, PA, USA
e-mail: ahmad.mohamed@chp.edu

M.C. Ost (ed.), *Robotic and Laparoscopic Reconstructive Surgery in Children and Adults*, Current Clinical Urology, DOI 10.1007/978-1-60327-914-7_16, © Springer Science+Business Media, LLC 2011

of fertility is lacking [11, 12]. Surgery, open or laparoscopic, has been the only modality proven to accurately diagnose, localize, and concurrently treat the non-palpable testicle [8, 13, 14].

Timing of Surgery

At birth, the undescended testicle has been shown to have normal histology. Although this may continue into the first year of life, delayed germ cell development has been described by 6–8 months of age. These histologic changes are progressive with both light and electron microscopies, and consistent with deterioration of the germ cell population detectable by 18 months [15]. Histology correlates with testicular position, with worse features seen in higher testicles. Spontaneous testicular descent has been noted as late as 4–6 months of age. Therefore, in order to allow adequate time for a testis to descend spontaneously while minimizing the risk for irreversible developmental damage, the generally accepted recommendation is to perform orchiopexy at 6–12 months of age. Early orchiopexy has been shown to have a positive impact on testicular growth [16] and adult Leydig function [17] supporting these recommendations. Decisions regarding orchiopexy after 2 years of age are based on the risks/benefits of the testicle to the individual. In prepubertal children, the usefulness of androgen production must be considered especially in cases of a solitary testicle. In postpubertal males with a persistently undescended testis, sperms are rarely noted [18] and the testes are at risk for malignant change, leading some authors to recommend orchiectomy in all healthy, postpubertal cryptorchid males [19].

Open Surgical Management of the Non-palpable Testicle

The principles of abdominal exploration and orchiopexy including identification of testicular tissue, mobilization of the spermatic cord, repair of the associated hernia, and adequate scrotal fixation without tension have essentially remained the same since originally described by Bevan in 1899 [20]. Predominantly employed techniques for the intra-abdominal testis prior to the advent of diagnostic laparoscopy included the transabdominal approach, extended inguinal orchiopexy (Jones technique) [21], Fowler–Stephens orchiopexy, staged Fowler–Stephens orchiopexy [22, 23], and testicular autotransplantation [24]. Successful orchiopexy is related to the preoperative testicular position and loosely defined as satisfactory scrotal position with lack of atrophy. The need for impeccable technique to protect the vasculature to the testicle while obtaining sufficient cord length is indisputable. The early assumption that orchiopexy is a largely successful operation and failures are few and far between was likely due to the more common practice of inguinal orchiopexy for the distal undescended testicle. In a meta-analysis of open orchiopexy techniques, Docimo [25] reported success rates by type of procedure (inguinal 89%; Fowler–Stephens 67%; staged Fowler–Stephens 77%; transabdominal 81%; two-stage 73%; microvascular 84%) and concluded that the high failure rates left significant room for improvement.

Laparoscopic Management of the Non-palpable Testicle

Diagnostic Laparoscopy

The principle goal of diagnostic laparoscopy is to determine the presence of a non-palpable testicle. Intraoperatively, the position and mobility of the testicle, its paratesticular structures including the epididymis and vas deferens, and its vascular supply are assessed to determine if the testicle is amenable to orchiopexy or best served by removal. The indications/goals of diagnostic and therapeutic laparoscopy are identical to the goals of open surgical management, i.e., to preserve potential fertility, identify and relocate the testicle to the scrotum for easier examination, and ablate the associated inguinal hernia. Historically, laparotomy was performed to localize an intra-abdominal testis or diagnose blind-ending vessels if cord vessels were not observed on initial inguinal exploration. This was most often accomplished with a high inguinal (i.e., Jones incision) or Pfannenstiel incision. It is now standard practice at most centers to proceed with diagnostic laparoscopy when the testicle is non-palpable.

Initially described by Cortesi et al. [26] in 1976, diagnostic laparoscopy has become the gold standard for the evaluation of the non-palpable testicle. In six early series [27–32], laparoscopy identified 42 testicles in 86 patients after prior negative open exploration. Recent studies report that blind-ending cord structures or an intra-abdominal testis is found during laparoscopic evaluation of non-palpable testis between 31 and 83% of the time [30, 33–38]. Barqawi et al. [30] reviewed 27 patients who had undergone previous inguinal exploration and identified a viable canalicular or intra-abdominal testicle in 67%. Cisek et al. [8] reported that laparoscopic findings precluded unnecessary abdominal exploration in 13% of cases and that the typical surgical incision for inguinal exploration would have left the surgeon compromised in 66% of the cases compared to the approach optimized as a result of laparoscopic testicular localization. In many of these patients, diagnostic laparoscopy can eliminate the need for further open exploration or facilitate open or laparoscopic orchiopexy.

Alternative strategies in the evaluation of the non-palpable testicle have been described. To reduce the number of unnecessary intra-abdominal laparoscopic procedures, Kanemoto et al. [39] suggested initial inguinal exploration followed by trans-inguinal laparoscopy. In 22 patients with a hypertrophied unilateral palpable testicle, Belman et al. [40] reported that scrotal exploration prior to laparoscopic evaluation identified an atrophic testicular remnant in 91% of patients. Schleef et al. [41] described a technique in which they proceeded first with laparoscopic evaluation of the inguinal canal to avoid unnecessary open exploration. The decision to proceed with an inguinal or a laparoscopic abdominal exploration first depends on the surgeon's certainty on physical exam and is still currently a source for debate. However, the evidence clearly suggests that if an initial open inguinal exploration is inconclusive, laparoscopic exploration should be the next step in the diagnosis and treatment of the non-palpable testicle. Our current protocol is to perform examination under anesthesia. If any tissue suggestive of a scrotal nubbin is felt, then open scrotal exploration is performed. If this exam is negative or inconclusive, only then do we perform laparoscopic exploration.

Laparoscopic Orchiopexy

Laparoscopic techniques have been applied to the therapy of intra-abdominal testes as an extension of diagnosis. The impetus for development of these techniques has been the difficulty of achieving successful open orchiopexy for the high undescended testicle [25]. There have been many technical descriptions of laparoscopic orchiopexy with success rates reported ranging from 63 to 97% [31, 42]. Initial laparoscopic orchiopexy series, although viewed as promising, were criticized for originating from high-volume centers with increased laparoscopic experience and low patient numbers [43–50]. To address this issue, in a large multi-institutional analysis, Baker et al. [31] reported excellent success rates superior to those of historical open orchiopexy and no significant difference in success or complication rates between low- and high-volume centers.

Parents or guardians are made aware of the approximate 8–25% risk of testicular atrophy associated with performing an orchiopexy regardless of operative technique [25]. Orchiopexy on the intra-abdominal testicle may carry the highest risk for failure (25%). Recent long-term data, however, suggest that atrophy rates following laparoscopic orchiopexy can be as low as 7% at 6 years follow-up irrespective of whether or not a staged Fowler–Stephens approach is utilized (Table 16.1) [31, 36, 51, 52]. The goal of laparoscopic orchiopexy is to adequately mobilize the testicular vessels and vas deferens to

Table 16.1 Laparoscopic orchiopexy

Study	*N*	Mean operative time (min)	Testicular atrophy (%)	Unsatisfactory scrotal position
Baker et al. [31]	310	124	2[a] 22[b] 10[c]	1[a] 7[b] 2[c]
Radmayr et al. [36]	57	49[a] 38/53[c] (by stage)	0[a] 7[c]	n/a
Samadi et al. [51]	197	n/a	0[a] 7[c]	9[a] 0[c]
El-Anany et al. [52]	93	n/a	0[a] 4[c]	3[a] 3.5[c]

[a]Primary laparoscopic
[b]One-stage Fowler–Stephens
[c]Two-stage Fowler–Stephens

enable relocation of the testicle to the orthotopic scrotal position. Ultimate "success" of laparoscopic orchiopexy will therefore be measured by maintenance of the testicle in proper scrotal position without evidence of atrophy. Equally important is avoiding the associated complications inherent to this laparoscopic procedure. In light of this, it is critical to know the different steps that will maximize successful outcomes.

In the open inguinal approach, the canal from the internal ring to the scrotal inlet is first explored. If a testicular remnant is found (hemosiderin deposit or atrophic testicle), it is removed and the procedure is terminated [53]. If the inguinal exploration is negative, the incision is extended, the peritoneum is entered, and exploration for an intra-abdominal testis is carried out. Open exploration is still a viable option in managing the non-palpable testis, especially among urologic surgeons without laparoscopic experience. One recent single-surgeon open orchiopexy series reported success rates of 98–100% for staged Fowler–Stephens and open primary orchiopexy , respectively [54], although these success rates are higher than generally reported. It can be argued that a laparoscopic approach to the non-palpable testicle can be used to perform a Fowler–Stephens orchiopexy [55] with the advantage of less morbidity [56]. Cost, formerly higher for laparoscopic approaches, can no longer be used as a bias against initial laparoscopic exploration when planning to manage the non-palpable testicle [57].

The decision to perform a single-stage procedure leaving the vessels intact or to perform a staged or non-staged Fowler–Stephens procedure is challenging and no specific set of criteria has been determined. Baker et al. [31] reported the incidence of testicular atrophy after laparoscopic orchiopexy (2.2%), non-staged Fowler–Stephens (22%), and staged Fowler–Stephens (10%). Some centers advocate universal staged procedures, whereas others are more selective. Intraoperatively measuring the distance between the testis and the internal ring, observation of the cord anatomy, or the ability of the intra-abdominal testicle to reach the opposite inguinal ring can be helpful [58]. Laparoscopy has also been used as an adjunct to microvascular testicular autotransplantation [59]. Compared to open orchiopexy, the early data show that laparoscopic orchiopexy is a successful approach with low risk in the management of the non-palpable undescended testicle.

Laparoscopic Technique for the Non-palpable Testicle

Immediate considerations prior to commencing with the procedure include re-examination, patient positioning, and starting an ongoing dialogue with the anesthesia team. A difficult intra-office exam may have yielded a false exam.

Indeed, in approximately 18% of boys, a previously non-palpable testis will be palpable when the child is examined under anesthesia [8]. In this regard, the child should be completely relaxed anesthetically. In the instance of a unilateral non-palpable testicle, assessment of the contralateral testicle may be helpful in determining if indeed the intrabdominal testicle is present. For example, a contralateral palpable testicle length exceeding 2 cm and an average volume of >2 cm^3 have been cited as being predictive of monorchia in over 90% of cases [40, 60], although not reliable enough to forego exploration. These findings may also support the concept of primary scrotal exploration in the child who has an empty hemiscrotum and a hypertrophied descended testicle. If a remnant is not found on scrotal exploration, laparoscopic exploration should follow.

Anesthesia maintenance with N_2O should be avoided to decrease bowel distention and maximize visualization within the abdomen. When starting with a laparoscopic approach, the arms are tucked and the legs are slightly spread as one would for an inguinal orchiopexy. Four-inch tape can be used to secure the child to the table, placing it without tension over the chest and legs. Securing the child to the table permits placement in the Trendelenburg or rolled position. Draping to allow access to the entire abdomen is used. In the sterile field, an appropriately sized Foley catheter is placed. Figure 16.1 demonstrates our preferred setup and trocar placement for performing a laparoscopic orchiopexy.

Blind access for pneumoperitoneum with a Veress needle or a trocar is not commonly used in the pediatric population as an overly compliant abdomen may increase the risk of injury to intra-abdominal structures. It is our preference to use the Bailez technique for open access [61], modified to employ the use of a radially dilating trocar [62]. In our current technique a 2-0 Vicryl suture is first placed in the umbilicus to provide continual anterior traction. A 3-mm hidden infraumbilical incision is made in the skin and a scissor is then used at an approximate 15–20° angle to cut through the umbilical fascia into the underlying adherent peritoneum. Alternatively, the rectus fascia and underlying peritoneum may be entered sharply at 90° under direct vision.

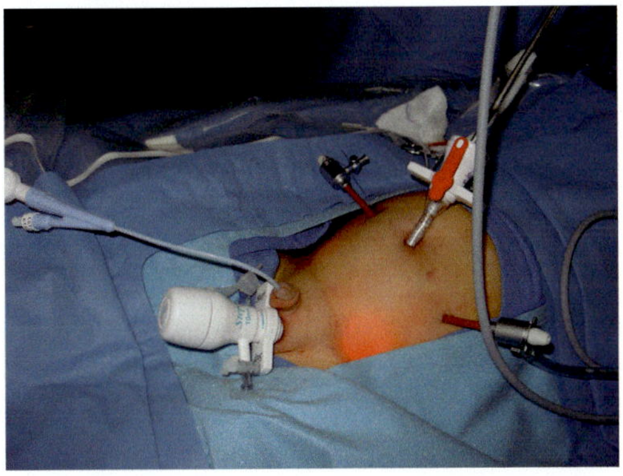

Fig. 16.1 Preferred setup for a *left single*-stage laparoscopic orchiopexy. A 5-mm radial dilating trocar is placed at the umbilicus. Two 3-mm working ports are placed lateral to the rectus muscles just inferior to the umbilicus. Care is taken to avoid injury to the epigastric vessels. In the event that either a single-stage or staged Fowler–Stephens procedure is performed, a 5-mm trocar would be used on the contralateral side to accommodate a 5-mm clip applier to ligate the testicular vessels. A 10-mm scrotal port is placed in the final stage of the case when the mobilized intra-abdominal testicle is delivered into the scrotum

For the umbilical camera port, we utilize a 5-mm radially dilating trocar to accommodate a 5-mm camera with a 0° lens [63]. The child is placed in Trendelenburg position and the abdomen is insufflated at 1–2 l/min to a pressure of 10–12 cmH_2O. After inspecting the underlying bowel for injury, the pelvis is examined. If an instrument is needed to aid in the inspection, only then is a 3-mm port placed on the ipsilateral side lateral to the rectus and just caudal to the umbilicus. An atraumatic 3-mm instrument may then be used to sweep bowel cephalad. Placement of a 5-mm trocar on the contralateral side (lateral to the rectus and just caudal to the umbilicus) is reserved for use of a 5-mm clip applier. Clinical circumstances in which this would be necessary are if an atrophic nubbin is to be excised and if a viable testicle is found far from the internal ring and a staged Fowler–Stephens orchiopexy is to be performed.

In the case of a unilateral undescended testicle, the internal ring of the descended testicle is examined first to gain an appreciation of the anatomy. Possible findings on inspecting the affected side of the "non-palpable" testicle may include the following.

Blind-Ending Testicular Vessels

The finding of blind-ending gonadal vessels is evident of a "vanishing" testicle. Intra-abdominal blind-ending vessels were found in approximately 10% of boys with non-palpable testes in one series [8]. This is considered to be a result of in utero testicular torsion, which is most likely a scrotal event rather than an abdominal or inguinal event. Vessels will have a "horse tail" appearance that diverge, do not exit the internal ring, and do not supply obvious testicular tissue (Fig. 16.2). If found during exploration, no further investigation is needed and the procedure is terminated. It has been argued however that fixation of the contralateral testicle might be considered at this point to safeguard against testicular torsion of the solitary testicle. Bellinger [64], for example, described the presence of a bell-clapper deformity in 83% of children with a vanishing testis whose contralateral scrotum was explored. Clinical torsion of the solitary testis is such a rarely reported event, however, that the risk of exposure and fixation of an otherwise healthy testis may be as significant as the risk of eventual torsion. There is no consensus on the need for contralateral fixation in this situation.

The sole finding of a blind-ending vas during laparoscopy is insufficient to conclude the absence of testicular tissue; it is assumed that gonadal disunion has occurred. Further cephalad inspection toward the aortic origin of the gonadal vessels is then necessary.

Cord Structures Entering the Internal Ring

Laparoscopically, cord structures may be visualized entering a closed internal ring or a patent processus vaginalis (open ring) (Fig. 16.3). In either scenario, further exploration may be warranted to determine what lies distally along the line of testicular descent [65]. In the instance of a closed internal ring, a groin or a scrotal exploration may be performed (Fig. 16.4). If a patent processus vaginalis is present, then the laparoscope may be used to inspect the inguinal canal antegrade. Alternatively, gentle manual retrograde pressure can be applied over the inguinal canal in an attempt to manipulate the contents (viable testicle) intra-abdominally. A single-stage laparoscopic or open orchiopexy may be carried out when a viable testicle is encountered (described below). In the instance of a nubbin or a testicular remnant, laparoscopic orchiectomy is performed. This is accomplished by either clipping and dividing the cord structures

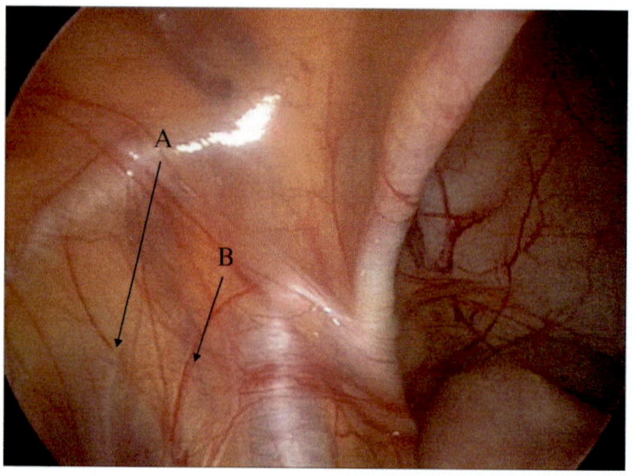

Fig. 16.2 Finding blind-ending and divergent testicular vessels (**a**) is evidence of a vanishing testicle. The sole finding of a blind-ending vas (**b**) is insufficient evidence to conclude that there is absence of ipsilateral testicular tissue

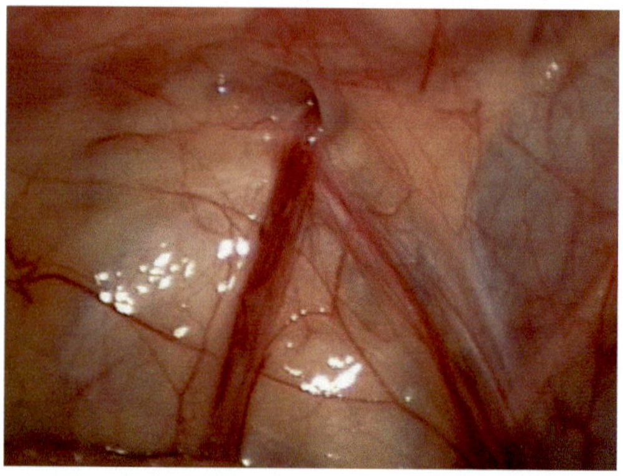

Fig. 16.3 Laparoscopic view of a *left* patent processus vaginalis (hernia) with normal cord structures exiting the internal rings. *Left* groin exploration revealed a high viable intracanalicular testicle. Inguinal orchiopexy with hernia sac ligation was performed

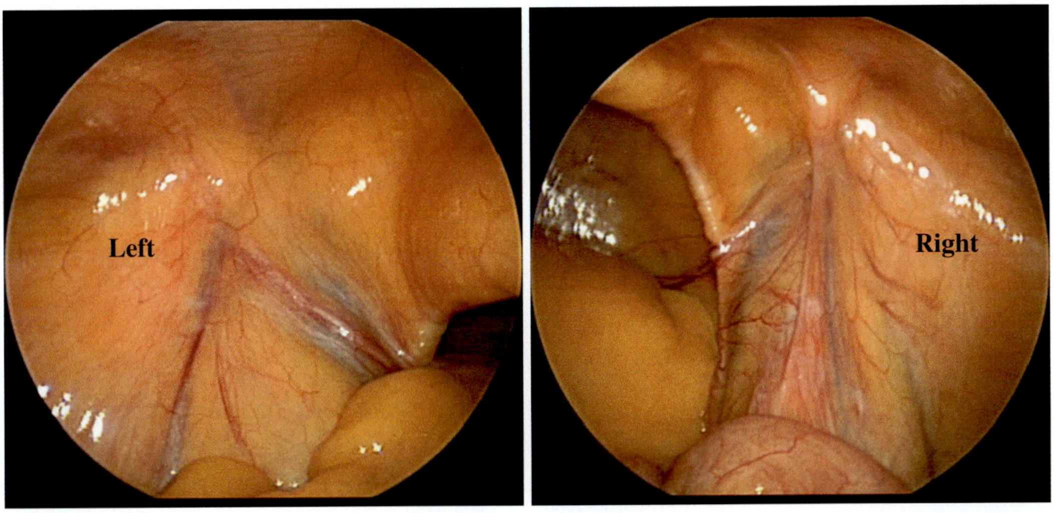

Fig. 16.4 Bilateral closed processus vaginalis with normal cord structures exiting the internal rings. This morbidly obese 8-year-old boy underwent exploratory laparoscopy for a "non-palpable" *left* testicle. The findings on diagnostic laparoscopy of cord structures exiting the *left* internal ring proceeded to a left groin exploration. A high viable intracanalicular testicle was found and open orchiopexy was performed

or using a 5-mm instrument designed to seal and divide smaller vessels (i.e., Ligasure or Harmonic Scalpel). The specimen is grasped and removed from the contralateral 5-mm port.

Intra-abdominal Testis

There are three minimally invasive reconstructive options to address when encountering a viable intra-abdominal testicle: (1) primary laparoscopic orchiopexy, (2) laparoscopic Fowler–Stephens orchiopexy, and (3) staged laparoscopic Fowler–Stephens orchiopexy. In a multi-institutional analysis, success rates for these procedures have been quoted as 97.2, 74.1, and 87.9%, respectively [31]. Interestingly, these results show an advantage over the open approach when outcomes from an earlier study are compared. For example, meta-analysis by Docimo reported success rates of 81.3, 66.7, and 76.8% for open primary orchiopexy, Fowler–Stephens orchidopexy, and staged Fowler–Stephens orchidopexy, respectively [25].

Laparoscopic orchiectomy is reserved for a non-viable intra-abdominal testicle (atrophic nubbin) or a testicle that cannot be brought into the scrotum based on a very long distance from the scrotum (i.e., pararenal) or an extreme ectopic location, limiting blood supply length. Older children found to have an intra-abdominal testis are better served with a laparoscopic orchiectomy, provided the contralateral testicle is normal and intrascrotal. Although an intra-abdominal testicle may remain hormonally active indefinitely, spermatogenic potential tends to decline after 18 months.

The initial measured distance of the testicle from the internal ring will determine which laparoscopic approach should be utilized and is therefore a predictor of success rates. "Peeping testes" or those located in close proximity to the internal ring (<2 cm) can usually be mobilized into the scrotum in a single stage without dividing the testicular vessels (Fig. 16.5). It is important to counsel parents that although an overall 7% atrophy rate is expected, intra-abdominal ectopic testicles and those testicles located >2 cm from the internal ring are at increased risk for surgical failure. In light of this, if an intra-abdominal testicle is found at a significant distance from the internal ring and is thought to be amenable to a staged Fowler–Stephens orchiopexy, the testicular vessels are doubly clipped (Fig. 16.6).

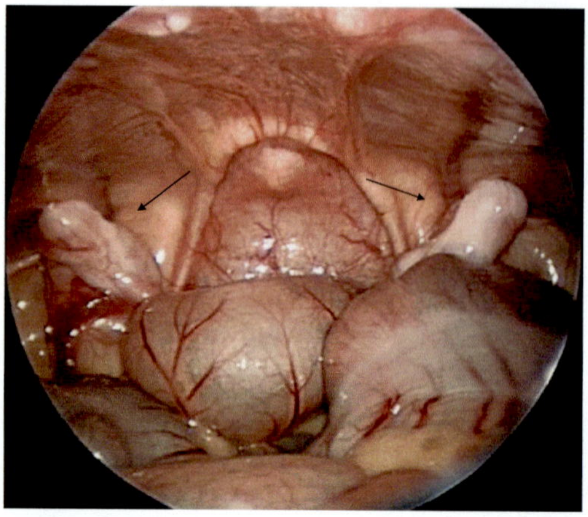

Fig. 16.5 Bilateral intra-abdominal "peeping" testicles at the internal rings in a 6-month old with non-palpable gonads. Bilateral single-stage laparoscopic orchiopexies were performed

A laparoscopic second-stage Fowler–Stephens orchiopexy should be performed approximately 6 months later when collateral blood flow from the deferential artery has matured.

In 1991, Bloom [49] reported using laparoscopy to ligate the testicular vessels in the first stage of a Fowler–Stephens approach. Jordan [48] further advanced the role of laparoscopy as a therapeutic modality when he reported the first laparoscopic orchiopexy in 1992. There have been many subtle variations described for performing this procedure. Herein our preferred laparoscopic technique is described. Figure 16.1 should be referred to as our preferred operative setup when either a primary laparoscopic orchiopexy or a second-stage Fowler–Stephens laparoscopic orchiopexy is performed. Keep in mind that a 5-mm trocar must be used at the port site lateral to the rectus (contralateral to operative site) if a stapler or a vascular sealing device is going to be used.

Primary Laparoscopic Orchiopexy

Establishing a Peritoneal Pedicle Flap

Following abdominal access, insufflation, and additional trocar placement as described previously, attention is focused on the intra-abdominal testicle and internal ring. Figure 16.7 demonstrates the surgical "map" needed to mobilize a triangular flap of peritoneum demarcated by the testicular vessels laterally and vas deferens medially. The preliminary goal is to create two continuous peritoneotomies parallel to the testicular vessels and vas in order to mobilize the testicle on a well-vascularized peritoneal pedicle.

The first survey requires evaluation of the testicle, epididymis, and extent of vasal course distally into the inguinal canal. It is critical from

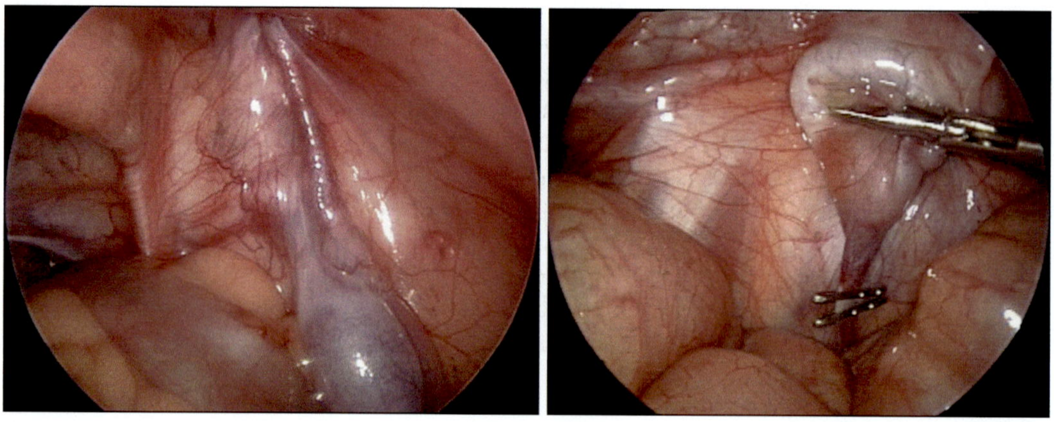

Fig. 16.6 A right intra-abdominal testicle in a 9-month-old boy was found >2 cm from the internal ring. The testicular vessels were clipped in the first stage of a staged Fowler–Stephens reconstruction. Note that clips are applied without dissecting the peritoneal attachments free from the vessels

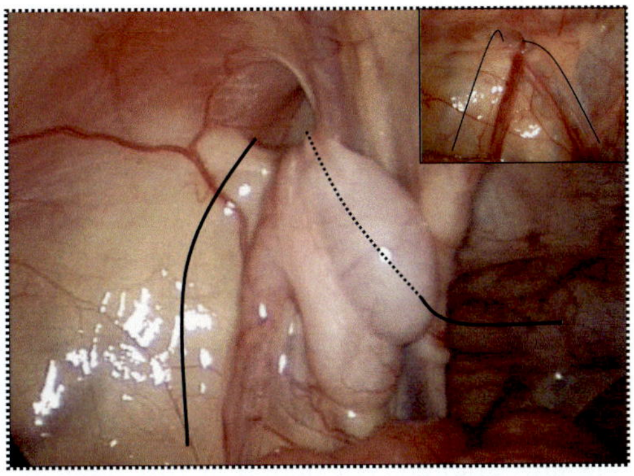

Fig. 16.7 A left intra-abdominal testicle in an 8-month-old boy at the internal ring. The *dark lines* represent where peritoneotomies are made parallel to the testicular vessels (lateral) and vas deferens (medial) in order to mobilize the testicle on a vascularized peritoneal pedicle flap. The *inset* shows the same landmarks when a non-palpable intra-canalicular testicle is milked into the abdomen and then mobilized via laparoscopic orchiopexy

the onset to define the distal attachments and identify a long-looping vas, if present. A scissors is used in the preliminary dissection. Care must be taken not to activate cautery in too close proximity to the vessels and vas. The first peritoneotomy is made lateral to the testicular vessels at the most proximal position. The incision is directed toward the internal ring. Often after the first incision, pneumoperitoneum will diffuse into the plane between the peritoneum and the pelvic side wall. In this regard, CO_2 can aid in isolating the peritoneum to be dissected.

The second line of dissection will begin at the level of the internal ring distally but will parallel the vas medially. Care is taken not to injure the iliac vessels and ureter that lie beneath the vas. It is also critical that dissection is not performed within the distal triangular area enclosed by the gonadal vessels and vas (Fig. 16.8). Critical collateral microvasculature within this flap will flow from the vasal artery to the testicle and should be maintained if possible. This is especially relevant when Fowler–Stephens orchiopexy is performed; dividing the testicular vessels and interrupting collateral blood flow will invariably lead to testicular atrophy [66]. Widely mobilizing the peritoneal flap laterally and medially leaves only the distal gubernacular attachments. A window is created distally allowing the distal attachments to be divided while visualizing the course of the vas deferens. An indication that dissection has maximized the flap length is that the testicle can

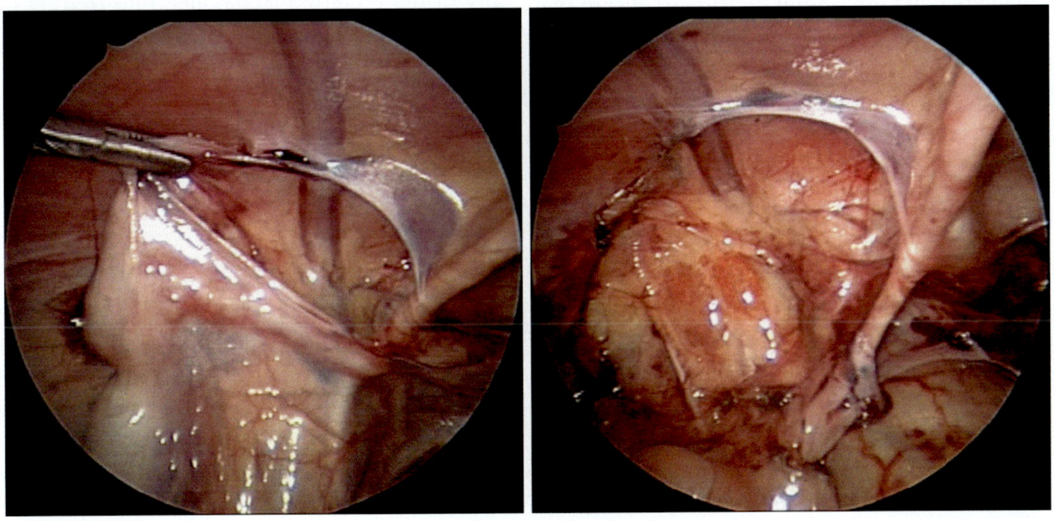

Fig. 16.8 After lateral mobilization, medial dissection follows the course of the vas deferens (*left*). Collateral para-vasal blood supply to the testicle is visualized. Cephalad traction following release of the distal gubernacular attachments (*right*) demonstrated the extent of the peritoneal flap and clarifies the boundaries where the neo-inguinal hiatus is to be created between the inferior epigastric vessels and the medial umbilical ligament

reach the contralateral internal ring without tension. The ipsilateral ring is not closed since there is no increased risk for a clinically significant hernia to develop. The patent processus is ablated by the peritoneal incisions, the division of the distal attachments, and, if necessary, the incision of the anterior peritoneum. Subsequently, the peritoneum obliterates the previously patent tract.

Creating a Neo-inguinal Hiatus and Testicular Delivery into the Scrotum

Various methods to deliver the testicle into the scrotum have been described. It is our belief that the testis may be most safely and effectively delivered to the scrotum using 2- or 3-mm instruments and a radially dilating trocar system [67]. A 1-cm ipsilateral scrotal incision is first made and a sub-dartos pouch is created. A 2-mm laparoscopic grasper is placed through the ipsilateral 3-mm lateral trocar directed toward the scrotal incision. Care is taken to place the instrument over the pubis and between the medial umbilical ligament and the inferior epigastric vessels. The surgeon's free hand should palpate the pubic area and the scrotal incision to ensure that the instrument is being guided over the pubis and through the scrotal incision. After the instrument is passed through the scrotum, the Foley catheter is checked for hematuria. A bladder injury, which is very rare, would most likely occur during this step of the procedure. Proper placement of the instrument in the position described above should minimize this complication from occurring (Fig. 16.9). The step sheath is then passed onto the end of the 2- or 3-mm instrument ex vivo and brought through the scrotum. The 5- or 10-mm trocar obturator, depending on the size of the testicle, is then inserted creating the neo-inguinal hiatus. A locking grasper is introduced into the abdomen through the scrotal trocar, the testicle is grasped at the distal attachments, and then delivered into the scrotum (Fig. 16.10). It is imperative for the surgeon to personally monitor the tension on the cord during scrotal delivery so that the vessels are not avulsed.

Gaining Additional Cord Length and Securing the Testicle

Delivering the testicle into the scrotum provides the traction and assistance of what we have termed "a third arm." If there is tension and/or if additional length is needed, further dissection can be carried out laterally and cranially toward the kidney. In most instances, the cord length will still be inadequate and additional maneuvers are required. An option at this point is to divide the peritoneum overlying the testicular vessels to provide extra cord length and release any remaining tension (Fig. 16.11). If incising the peritoneum has not helped, consideration can be given to dividing the testicular vessels, therefore performing a non-staged Fowler–Stephens orchiopexy. The contralateral 3-mm port must be upsized to a 5-mm port in order to accommodate a clip applier. Consideration must be given to the higher risk of testicular atrophy prior to performing a non-staged Fowler–Stephens maneuver.

When the testicle lays tension free in the scrotum, the orchiopexy can be completed (Fig. 16.12). The testicle is harnessed in the dartos pouch and the scrotal skin is closed by any of the preferred technique(s) utilized by the surgeon.

Closure and Exiting the Abdomen

The abdomen is surveyed a final time and the pneumoperitoneum pressure is lowered. Any occult bleeding should be identified and addressed. While maintaining pneumoperitoneum, the two lateral ports are removed sequentially and inspected for bleeding. The fascial layers of these trocar sites are closed with 2-0 Vicryl sutures through the fascia. The laparoscopic view is maintained on the port sites during closure to ensure that it is airtight and free of any intra-abdominal contents (i.e., bowel or omentum). Through the umbilical port the pneumoperitoneum is evacuated. Larger tidal volumes given by the anesthesiologist and mild

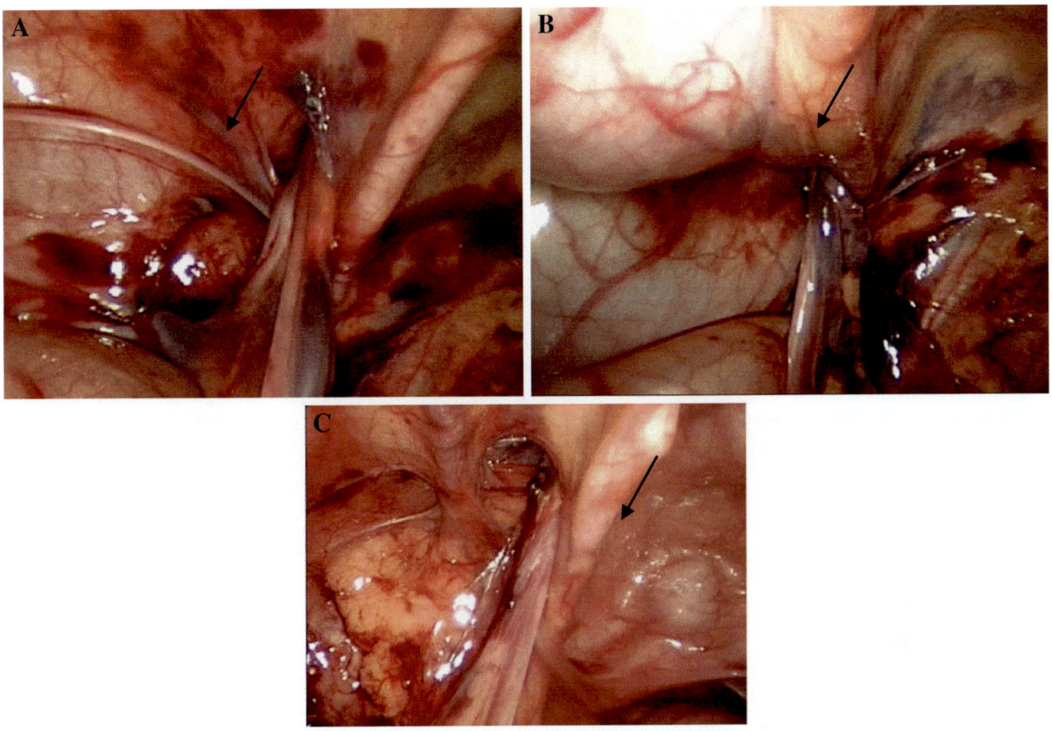

Fig. 16.9 During delivery of the testicle into the scrotum, the bladder edge (*arrows*) is at increased risk for perforation. The risk is increased if the neo-inguinal hiatus is not created anterior to the pubis and lateral to the medial umbilical ligament. Following delivery of the testicle medial to the ligament in a *right* laparoscopic orchiopexy, there was concern that the bladder was perforated (**a**). Filling the bladder demonstrated no evidence of a leak (**b**). After delivery of the testicle through a 12-mm scrotal trocar in the final stage of a *left* laparoscopic orchiopexy, there is little concern of a bladder injury. The neo-hiatus was created in a plane lateral to the medial umbilical ligament and medial to the epigastric vessels (**c**)

abdominal pressure help with the expulsion of CO_2. The umbilical trocar and camera are removed while inspecting for bleeding. Final fascial stitches are placed in the umbilical port, the skin is closed, and dressings are applied.

Second-Stage Fowler–Stephens

As a general rule, the further the intra-abdominal testicle lies from the internal ring (i.e., > 2 cm), the higher the likelihood that a staged procedure is necessary. Staging the procedure will enable delivery of the testicle into the scrotum without tension at a decreased risk for atrophy. This may be accomplished laparoscopically by using a 5-mm stapler through the contralateral port. After 6 months, the second stage is performed exactly as described above with the addition of dividing the previously clipped testicular vessels and maintaining a "tongue" of peritoneum overlying the vas deferens and its associated vessels.

Bilateral Non-palpable Testicles and Laparoscopic Orchiopexy

Bilateral non-palpable testicles in a newborn should raise the suspicion of an intersex condition, especially with coincidental genital ambiguity (i.e., proximal hypospadias). Other

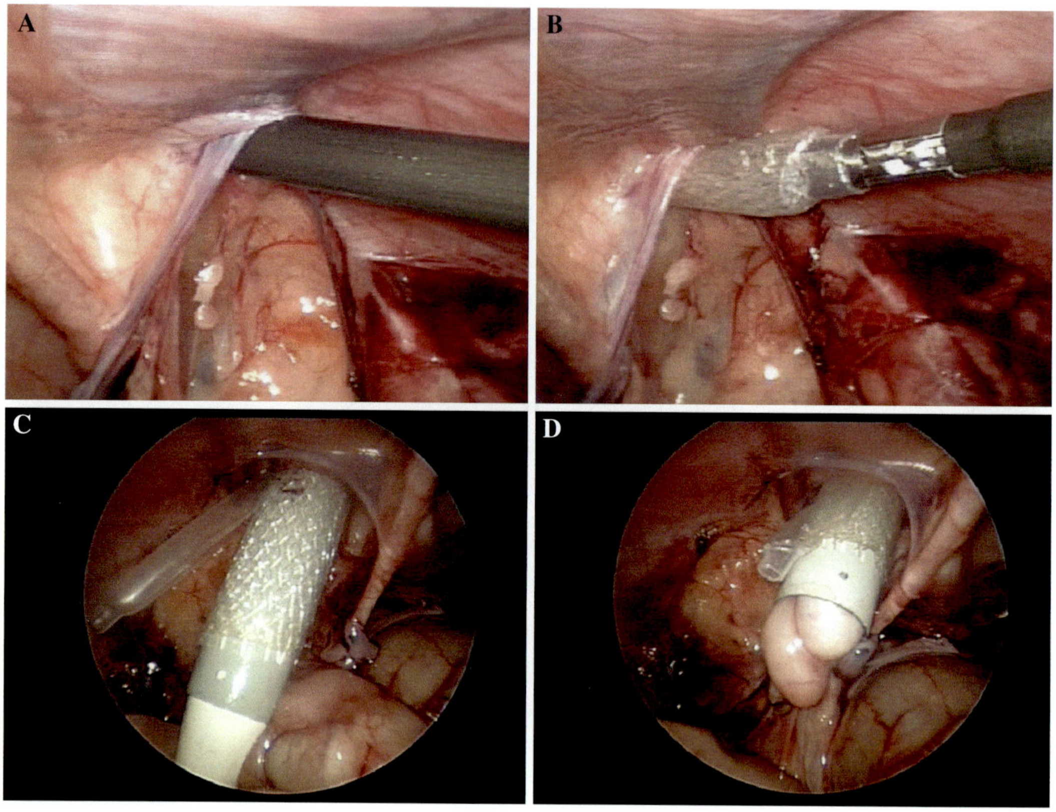

Fig. 16.10 Delivering the testicle into the scrotum requires developing a neo-hiatus (**a–c**) to facilitate passage of the testicle, epididymis, and cord structures into the scrotum without resistance. This technique minimizes the risk of an avulsion injury (**d**)

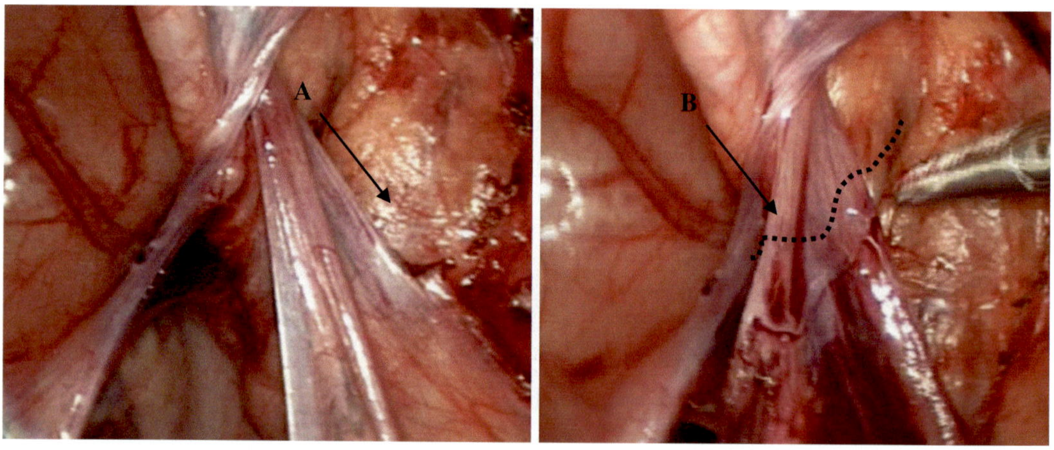

Fig. 16.11 Delivering the testicle into the scrotum provides the traction and assistance of "a third arm." If there is tension and/or additional length is needed, further dissection can be carried out laterally and cephalad. The peritoneum overlying the testicular vessels (**a**) may also be divided (**b**) to release tension and provide extra cord length

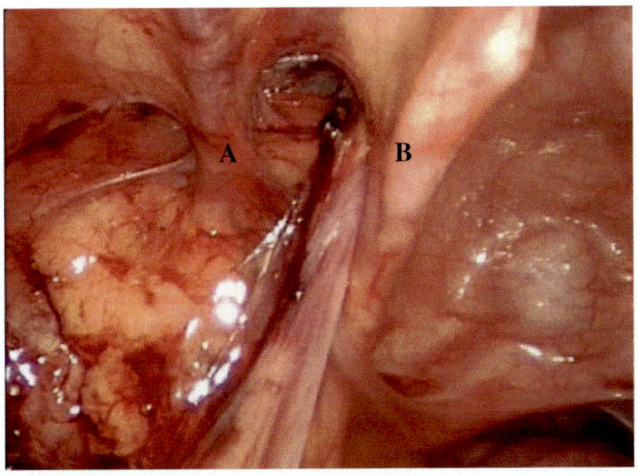

Fig. 16.12 Antegrade view of a *left* neo-inguinal hiatus created between the inferior epigastric vessels (**a**) and the medial umbilical ligament (**b**). The testicle is fixed to the scrotum after maximal length on the cord has been reached without residual tension

possibilities include bilateral anorchia or bilateral intra-abdominal testicles. It is urgent to institute a workup to rule out life-threatening intersex conditions such as congenital adrenal hyperplasia (CAH). Once an intersex disorder has been excluded, endocrine studies including a human chorionic gonadotropin (hCG) stimulation test and/or serum Müllerian inhibitory substance (MIS) if available will be useful in differentiating anorchia from bilateral cryptorchidism [68]. Regardless of such laboratory findings, however, exploratory laparoscopy will be needed for either a gonadal biopsy, a gonadectomy, or a orchiopexy (Fig. 16.13).

Laparoscopy in the Management of High-Palpable Undescended Testicle

In addition to the value of laparoscopy in the management of non-palpable testicle, several researchers suggested the use of laparoscopy in the treatment of the high-palpable testis. This includes patients diagnosed in the office as well as those in whom a testicle is only felt when performing examination under anesthesia. Results were similar to open inguinal orchiopexy with a complications rate ranging from 0 to 13, 3% [47, 68, 69].

Complications

The number of complications associated with laparoscopic orchiopexy compares quite favorably to that of an open approach. In a large

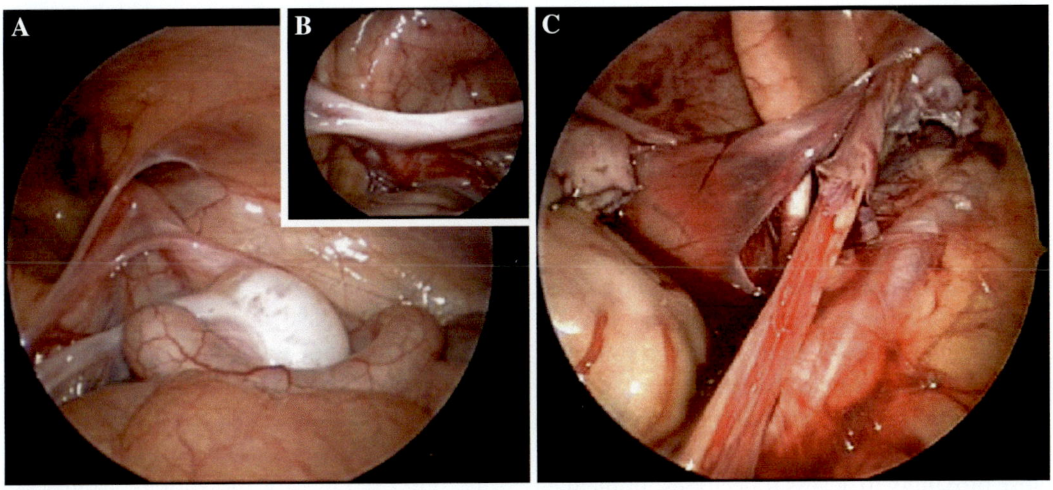

Fig. 16.13 An 8-month-old XY phenotypic male with bilateral undescended testicles and Müllerian inhibiting substance (MIS) deficiency. MIS hormone level was 0.1 ng/ml (normal 48–83). Diagnostic laparoscopy revealed bilateral intra-abdominal testicles (**a**) with Müllerian (uterus) and Wolffian (vas) structures intimately associated (**b**). *Left* laparoscopic orchiopexy was performed, aided by releasing the contralateral round ligament (**c**)

multi-institutional review, Baker reported a major complication rate of 3.0% and a minor complication rate of 2.0% [31]. Major complications that have been reported include acute testicular atrophy, bowel perforation [50], cecal volvulus, vascular injury [69], bladder perforation [70], ileus, laceration of the vas [34], testicular vessel avulsion [71], and wound dehiscence/infection. In addition, there are the potential complications that are inherent to any laparoscopic procedure that are important to recognize (i.e., pneumothorax and trocar site hernia) [72].

The prevention of complications associated with laparoscopy starts with proper positioning and padding to reduce the risk of neuromuscular injuries. Although injuries are less likely to occur with pelvic laparoscopy, extremes in table positioning are often necessary. Close attention to placement of straps and/or tape and adequate padding should limit positioning-related injuries.

Complications related to access are a common concern. Indeed, the most frequent identifiable cause of complications within pediatric laparoscopy has been the method employed for abdominal access. The pediatric abdomen is highly compliant and limited in space. For this reason, open peritoneal access has been associated with fewer complications than when a Veress needle approach is used [69]. As previously mentioned, we prefer to gain access using an open Bailez technique. Regardless of the access technique used, preperitoneal insufflation may still occur. This complication can readily be identified when there is characteristically high opening pressure at low volumes. Additional sharp dissection and entry into the peritoneal cavity followed by repositioning of the trocar is necessary if this occurs. Prior to placing additional working ports, areas vulnerable to trocar injuries must be mapped and noted with the laparoscope. Due to great abdominal wall compliance, the epigastric vessels, iliac vessels, and bowel all come into close proximity to access trajectories. Immediate inspection of these loci before and after port placement is mandatory.

Surgical planning and an appreciation for the anatomical landmarks within the pelvis will aid in

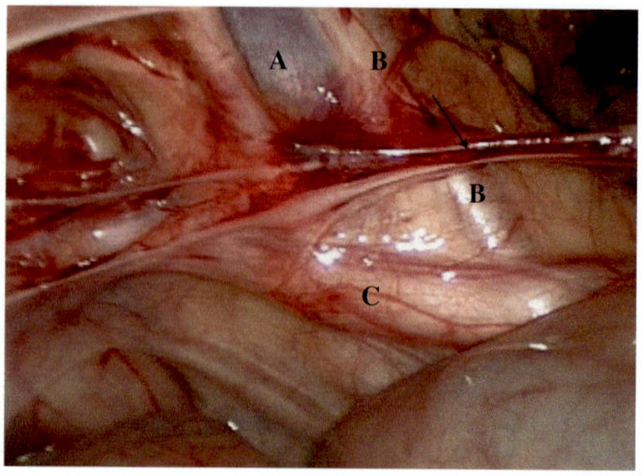

Fig. 16.14 Pelvic view during a right laparoscopic orchiopexy. During medial mobilization of the vas deferens, the cord structures (*arrow*) are held cranially and laterally. Care must be taken not to injure the iliac vein (**a**), iliac artery (**b**), and or ureter (**c**) that lie immediately posterior to the mobilized peritoneal flap

avoiding complications. During testicular mobilization, care must be taken to avoid injury to the vas, testicular, femoral and iliac vessels and the ureter. When mobilizing the vas on the medial aspect of the peritoneal flap, these structures lie directly posterior and medial (Fig. 16.14). In general, complications can be limited by careful intra-abdominal mobilization, using cautery in short bursts, and execution of meticulous technique. The laparoscopic approach helps to facilitate this by allowing extensive and high retroperitoneal mobilization of the testicular vessels in an atraumatic manner.

Conclusions

Laparoscopy has evolved from a diagnostic procedure to a surgical treatment of choice when managing the intra-abdominal testicle. The type of procedure used is reflective of the intra-abdominal anatomy of the testicle, the viability of the testicle, and its distance from the internal ring. Success rates for the various laparoscopic techniques are comparable to or exceed those reported in open series. Maintaining a mobilized testicle on a wide peritoneal flap free from tension is the key to minimizing the risk of testicular atrophy. Although there is a learning curve associated with this minimally invasive technique, it is surmountable. Laparoscopy has become the gold standard technique for diagnosis and reconstruction of the intra-abdominal testis.

References

1. John Radcliffe Hospital Cryptorchidism Study Group. Cryptorchidism: a prospective study of 7500 consecutive male births, 1984–8. Arch Dis Child. 1992;67:892–9.
2. Cendron M, Huff DS, Keating MA, Snyder HM 3rd, Duckett JW. Anatomical, morphological and volumetric analysis: a review of 759 cases of testicular maldescent. J Urol. 1993;149:570–3.
3. Abeyaratne MR, Aherne WA, Scott JE. The vanishing testis. Lancet. 1969;2:822–4.
4. Koff SA. Does compensatory testicular enlargement predict monorchism? J Urol. 1991;146:632–3.
5. Elder JS. Ultrasonography is unnecessary in evaluating boys with a nonpalpable testis. Pediatrics. 2002;110:748–51.
6. Hrebinko RL, Bellinger MF. The limited role of imaging techniques in managing children with undescended testes. J Urol. 1993;150:458–60.
7. Kanemoto K, Hayashi Y, Kojima Y, Maruyama T, Ito M, Kohri K. Accuracy of ultrasonography and magnetic resonance imaging in the diagnosis of nonpalpable testis. Int J Urol. 2005;12:668–72.
8. Cisek LJ, Peters CA, Atala A, Bauer SB, Diamond DA, Retik AB. Current findings in diagnostic laparoscopic evaluation of the nonpalpable testis. J Urol. 1998;160:1145–9; discussion 50.
9. Polascik TJ, Chan-Tack KM, Jeffs RD, Gearhart JP. Reappraisal of the role of human chorionic gonadotropin in the diagnosis and treatment of the nonpalpable testis: a 10-year experience. J Urol. 1996;156:804–6.
10. Docimo SG. Re: Is human chorionic gonadotropin useful for identifying and treating nonpalpable testis? J Urol. 2001;166:1010–1.
11. Henna MR, Del Nero RG, Sampaio CZ, Atallah AN, Schettini ST, Castro AA, Soares BG. Hormonal cryptorchidism therapy: systematic review with meta-analysis of randomized clinical trials. Pediatr Surg Int. May 2004;20(5):357–9.
12. Hadziselimovic F. Successful treatment of unilateral cryptorchid boys risking infertility with LH–RH analogue. Int Braz J Urol. May–Jun 2008;34(3):319–26; discussion 27–8.
13. Moore RG, Peters CA, Bauer SB, Mandell J, Retik AB. Laparoscopic evaluation of the nonpalpable tests: a prospective assessment of accuracy. J Urol. 1994;151:728–31.
14. Tennenbaum SY, Lerner SE, McAleer IM, Packer MG, Scherz HC, Kaplan GW. Preoperative laparoscopic localization of the nonpalpable testis: a critical analysis of a 10-year experience. J Urol. 1994;151:732–4.
15. Huff DS, Hadziselimovic F, Snyder HM 3rd, Blythe B, Ducket JW. Histologic maldevelopment of unilaterally cryptorchid testes and their descended partners. Eur J Pediatr. 1993;152(Suppl 2):S11–4.
16. Nagar H, Haddad R. Impact of early orchidopexy on testicular growth. Br J Urol. 1997;80:334–5.
17. Lee PA, Coughlin MT. Leydig cell function after cryptorchidism: evidence of the beneficial result of early surgery. J Urol. 2002;167:1824–7.
18. Rogers E, Teahan S, Gallagher H, et al. The role of orchiectomy in the management of postpubertal cryptorchidism. J Urol. 1998;159:851–4.
19. Oh J, Landman J, Evers A, Yan Y, Kibel AS. Management of the postpubertal patient with cryptorchidism: an updated analysis. J Urol. 2002;167:1329–33.
20. Howards SS. Surgery of the scrotum and testis in childhood. In: Walsh PC, Retik AB, Stamey T, Vaughn ED, editors. Campbell's Urology. 6th ed. Philadelphia, PA: WB Saunders; 1992.
21. Jones PF, Bagley FH. An abdominal extraperitoneal approach for the difficult orchidopexy. Br J Surg. 1979;66:14–8.
22. Corkery JJ. Staged orchiopexy – a new technique. J Pediatr Surg. 1975;10:515–8.
23. Ransley PC, Vordermark JS, Caldamone AA, Bellinger MF. Preliminary ligation of the gonadal vessels prior to orchiopexy for the intra-abdominal testicle: a staged Fowler–Stephens procedure. World J Urol. 1984;2:266.
24. Silber SJ, Kelly J. Successful autotransplantation of an intra-abdominal testis to the scrotum by microvascular technique. J Urol. 1976;115:452–4.
25. Docimo SG. The results of surgical therapy for cryptorchidism: a literature review and analysis. J Urol. 1995;154:1148–52.
26. Cortesi N, Ferrari P, Zambarda E, Manenti A, Baldini A, Morano FP. Diagnosis of bilateral abdominal cryptorchidism by laparoscopy. Endoscopy. 1976;8:33–4.
27. Boddy SA, Corkery JJ, Gornall P. The place of laparoscopy in the management of the impalpable testis. Br J Surg. 1985;72:918–9.
28. Perovic S, Janic N. Laparoscopy in the diagnosis of non-palpable testes. Br J Urol. 1994;73:310–3.
29. Lakhoo K, Thomas DF, Najmaldin AS. Is inguinal exploration for the impalpable testis an outdated operation? Br J Urol. 1996;77:452–4.
30. Barqawi AZ, Blyth B, Jordan GH, Ehrlich RM, Koyle MA. Role of laparoscopy in patients with previous negative exploration for impalpable testis. Urology. 2003;61:1234–7; discussion 7.
31. Baker LA, Docimo SG, Surer I, et al. A multi-institutional analysis of laparoscopic orchidopexy. BJU Int. 2001;87:484–9.

32. Koyle MA, Rajfer J, Ehrlich RM. The undescended testis. Pediatr Ann. 1988;17(39):42–6.
33. Galvin DJ, Bredin H. The role of laparoscopy in the management of the impalpable testicle. Ir J Med Sci. 2002;171:73–5.
34. Esposito C, Damiano R, Gonzalez Sabin MA, et al. Laparoscopy-assisted orchidopexy: an ideal treatment for children with intra-abdominal testes. J Endourol. 2002;16:659–62.
35. Alam S, Radhakrishnan J. Laparoscopy for nonpalpable testes. J Pediatr Surg. 2003;38:1534–6.
36. Radmayr C, Oswald J, Schwentner C, Neururer R, Peschel R, Bartsch G. Long-term outcome of laparoscopically managed nonpalpable testes. J Urol. 2003;170:2409–11.
37. Rodriguez A, Freire U, Orpez R, Lorenzo G. Diagnostic and therapeutic laparoscopy for nonpalpable testis. Surg Endosc. 2003;17:1756–8.
38. Castilho LN, Ferreira U. Laparoscopy in adults and children with nonpalpable testes. Andrologia. 1987;19:539–43.
39. Kanemoto K, Hayashi Y, Kojima Y, Tozawa K, Mogami T, Kohri K. The management of nonpalpable testis with combined groin exploration and subsequent transinguinal laparoscopy. J Urol. 2002;167:674–6.
40. Belman AB, Rushton HG. Is an empty left hemiscrotum and hypertrophied right descended testis predictive of perinatal torsion? J Urol. 2003;170:1674–5; discussion 5–6.
41. Schleef J, von Bismarck S, Burmucic K, Gutmann A, Mayr J. Groin exploration for nonpalpable testes: laparoscopic approach. J Pediatr Surg. 2002;37:1552–5.
42. Stec AA, Tanaka ST, Adams MC, Pope JC 4th, Thomas JC, Brock JW 3rd. Orchiopexy for intra-abdominal testes: factors predicting success. J Urol. Oct 2009;182(4 Suppl):1917–20.
43. Lindgren BW, Darby EC, Faiella L, et al. Laparoscopic orchiopexy: procedure of choice for the nonpalpable testis? J Urol. 1998;159:2132–5.
44. Gill IS, Ross JH, Sung GT, Kay R. Needlescopic surgery for cryptorchidism: the initial series. J Pediatr Surg. 2000;35:1426–30.
45. Merguerian PA, Mevorach RA, Shortliffe LD, Cendron M. Laparoscopy for the evaluation and management of the nonpalpable testicle. Urology. 1998;51:3–6.
46. Lindgren BW, Franco I, Blick S, et al. Laparoscopic Fowler–Stephens orchiopexy for the high abdominal testis. J Urol. 1999;162:990–3; discussion 4.
47. Docimo SG, Moore RG, Adams J, Kavoussi LR. Laparoscopic orchiopexy for the high palpable undescended testis: preliminary experience. J Urol. 1995;154:1513–5.
48. Jordan GH, Winslow BH. Laparoscopic single stage and staged orchiopexy. J Urol. 1994;152:1249–52.
49. Bloom DA. Two-step orchiopexy with pelviscopic clip ligation of the spermatic vessels. J Urol. 1991;145:1030–3.
50. Caldamone AA, Amaral JF. Laparoscopic stage 2 Fowler–Stephens orchiopexy. J Urol. 1994;152:1253–6.
51. Samadi AA, Palmer LS, Franco I. Laparoscopic orchiopexy: report of 203 cases with review of diagnosis, operative technique, and lessons learned. J Endourol. 2003;17:365–8.
52. El-Anany F, Gad El-Moula M, Abdel Moneim A, et al. Laparoscopy for impalpable testis: classification-based management. Surg Endosc. Mar 2007;21(3):449–54.
53. Kirsch AJ, Escala J, Duckett JW, et al. Surgical management of the nonpalpable testis: the Children's Hospital of Philadelphia experience. J Urol. 1998;159:1340–3.
54. Dhanani NN, Cornelius D, Gunes A, Ritchey ML. Successful outpatient management of the nonpalpable intra-abdominal testis with staged Fowler–Stephens orchiopexy. J Urol. 2004;172:2399–401.
55. Ferro F, Spagnoli A, Zaccara A, De Vico A, La Sala E. Is preoperative laparoscopy useful for impalpable testis? J Urol. 1999;162:995–6; discussion 7.
56. Abolyosr A. Laparoscopic versus open orchiopexy in the management of abdominal testis: a descriptive study. Int J Urol. 2006;13:1421–4.
57. Lorenzo AJ, Samuelson ML, Docimo SG, Baker LA, Lotan Y. Cost analysis of laparoscopic versus open orchiopexy in the management of unilateral nonpalpable testicles. J Urol. 2004;172:712–6.
58. Banieghbal B, Davies M. Laparoscopic evaluation of testicular mobility as a guide to management of intra-abdominal testes. World J Urol. 2003;20:343–5.
59. Tackett LD, Wacksman J, Billmire D, Sheldon CA, Minevich E. The high intra-abdominal testis: technique and long-term success of laparoscopic testicular autotransplantation. J Endourol. 2002;16:359–61.
60. Hurwitz RS, Kaptein JS. How well does contralateral testis hypertrophy predict the absence of the nonpalpable testis? J Urol. 2001;165:588–92.
61. Docimo SG. Re: experience with the Bailez technique for laparoscopic access in children. J Urol. 2004;171:806.
62. Cuellar DC, Kavoussi PK, Baker LA, Docimo SG. Open laparoscopic access using a radially dilating trocar: experience and indications in 50 consecutive cases. J Endourol. 2000;14:755–6.
63. Schulam PG, Hedican SP, Docimo SG. Radially dilating trocar system for open laparoscopic access. Urology. 1999;54:727–9.
64. Bellinger MF. The blind-ending vas: the fate of the contralateral testis. J Urol. 1985;133:644–5.
65. Elder JS. Laparoscopy for impalpable testes: significance of the patent processus vaginalis. J Urol. 1994;152:776–8.
66. King LR. Orchiopexy for impalpable testis: high spermatic vessel division is a safe maneuver. J Urol. 1998;160:2457–60.
67. Ferrer FA, Cadeddu JA, Schulam P, Mathews R, Docimo SG. Orchiopexy using 2 mm laparoscopic

instruments: 2 techniques for delivering the testis into the scrotum. J Urol. 2000;164:160–1.
68. Jarow JP, Berkovitz GD, Migeon CJ, Gearhart JP, Walsh PC. Elevation of serum gonadotropins establishes the diagnosis of anorchism in prepubertal boys with bilateral cryptorchidism. J Urol. 1986;136: 277–9.
69. Peters CA. Complications in pediatric urological laparoscopy: results of a survey. J Urol. 1996;155:1070–3.
70. Jordan GH. Laparoscopic management of the undescended testicle. Urol Clin North Am. 2001;28: 23–9.
71. Esposito C, Lima M, Mattioli G, et al. Complications of pediatric urological laparoscopy: mistakes and risks. J Urol. 2003;169:1490–2; discussion 1492.
72. Yee DS, Duel BP. Omental herniation through a 3-mm umbilical trocar site. J Endourol. 2006;20: 133–4.

Part VII
Laparoscopic and Robotic Anastomoses for Radical Prostatectomy

Chapter 17

Laparoscopic Anastomoses and Bladder Neck Reconstruction Following Radical Prostatectomy

Ender Özden, Özcan Kılıç, Ali Serdar Gözen, Dogu Teber, and Jens Rassweiler

This chapter contains a video segment which can be found at the URL: http://www.springerimages.com/ost

Introduction

Laparoscopic radical prostatectomy (LRP) and robotic-assisted laparoscopic radical prostatectomy have gained increasing importance in the urologic oncology field and have become an established treatment for localized prostate cancer [1–3]. The goals in both open and laparoscopic radical prostatectomy are lifelong oncologic control of localized prostate carcinoma while maintaining continence and potency functions with minimization of operative morbidity that contribute to a global quality of life. Vesicourethral anastomosis is a critical step during laparoscopic prostatectomy with major implications for anastomotic leak and ultimately continence.

However, LRP requires prolonged learning curves even for experienced laparoscopic surgeons. One of the most difficult and time-consuming steps is the vesicourethral anastomosis [4]. Initial nine cases of transperitoneal radical prostatectomy were reported by Schuessler and he defined vesicourethral anastomosis part of the procedure as requiring the greatest time, taking twice as long as the removal of the prostate [5].

J. Rassweiler (✉)
Department of Urology, SLK-Klinikum Heilbronn, University of Heidelberg, Heilbronn, Germany
e-mail: jens.rassweiler@slk-kliken.de

One of the major advantages of LRP is its potential for performance of all sutures under total visual control. However, knotting of the sutures is time consuming and contributes to the prolonged operating time. This critical component presents as a barrier to widespread introduction of LRP. However, this technique needs to be standardized at the very beginning of the laparoscopic experience in order to improve its ergonomics and accuracy.

It is obvious to say that anastomosis comes at the end of the radical prostatectomy and quality of sutures is affected by surgeon's fatigue and anatomy of the patients.

Position of the Patient and the Surgeon

The patient is put in a deflected supine position with his arms by his sides and the adducted legs. Additionally, a 30° Trendelenburg decline is made, which displaces the bowel cephalad by gravity. During vesicourethral anastomosis, usually there is no need to give a special position rather than rest of the procedure. A rectal balloon catheter should be deflated before anastomosis if it is used.

A right-handed surgeon stands on the left side of the patients to perform surgery. An assistant who works with suction device stands on the right

M.C. Ost (ed.), *Robotic and Laparoscopic Reconstructive Surgery in Children and Adults*, Current Clinical Urology, DOI 10.1007/978-1-60327-914-7_17, © Springer Science+Business Media, LLC 2011

side. The vesicourethral anastomosis is generally carried out with preferably two needle holders, eventually with one needle holder in the dominant surgeon's hand, assisted by a straight or Maryland forceps. The choice of the trocars defines the spatial relationship between the needle holders and hence also has a direct impact on the suturing technique.

Preparations for the Anastomosis

The optimum preparation of the bladder neck and the urethral stump is of paramount importance for cancer control, continence, and eventually for achieving an adequate vesicourethral anastomosis. Complete removal of the prostate inevitably reduces the significant part of the urethra, depending on the prostate size. So, optimal preparation of urethral stump and bladder neck is crucial for the quality of the vesicourethral anastomosis.

As the dorsal vein complex and striated sphincter are very closely associated, control of bleeding from dorsal vein complex affects the precise division of the urethra and sphincter and helps in the anastomosis. After the cutting of dorsal venous complex, urethra is exposed and usually cut under tension. Therefore sometimes, urethral stump retracts and cannot be seen clearly to perform anastomosis. Transurethral insertion of catheter or metal bougie can be used to expose urethral stump.

Identification of the exact dissection area between bladder neck and prostate requires different perceptions because of the lack of manual palpation. The bladder is covered with prevesical fat tissue, in contrast to the prostate, which is covered by endopelvic fascia laterally. The bladder neck and prostate are also distinguished from each other with the help of tactile sensation of balloon and tissues. Care must be taken while dividing the bladder neck from prostate to maintain clear detrusor margin which helps during vesicourethral anastomosis. In general, laparoscopic prostatectomy does not incorporate with bladder neck mucosal eversion.

Preparation of bladder neck in patients with history of TURP can be more difficult because perforation of the prostatic capsule during TURP with extravasation of blood and irrigation fluid can result in periprostatic fibrosis and distortion of the surgical planes. In a study of our group, the dissection was described as more difficult in the TURP group and resulted in a significantly longer operating time. In particular, the identification of the anterior bladder neck remains a difficult step after TURP owing to fibrosis and distortion of the position of the ureteral orifices [6].

A larger median lobe during laparoscopic radical prostatectomy presents several challenges for the surgeon. To remove the median lobe completely, wide excision of the trigone results in a larger bladder defect. Therefore there is a risk of ureteral injury during bladder neck dissection and risk of ureteral obstruction during anastomosis since the ureteral orifices can be so close to bladder neck. This would need special precautions during the reconstruction since the ureteral orifices are closer to the edge of the bladder neck.

On the contrary, bladder neck mucosal everting sutures may cause additional tension on anastomosis and may lead to increased tissue ischemia and fibrosis [7].

Reconstruction of the bladder neck before the anastomosis is rarely required. If bladder neck preservation was not possible or not performed because of surgeon's preference, the bladder neck may then be reconstructed with a racquet-handle technique. Posterior reconstruction may be required when ureteric orifices are very close to bladder mucosa. Posterior reconstruction can be carried out either by interrupted or running sutures. Bladder neck is reconstructed anteriorly rather than posteriorly in LRP. If necessary, after completing anastomosis, the remaining open bladder neck can be repaired either by interrupted or running sutures. The final appearance is like a reverse "racquet."

After preparation of urethral stump and bladder neck, before anastomosis, Rocco and coworkers propose to reconstruct the musculofascial plate by approximating dorsal wall of the rhabdosphincter to the residuum of the Denonvilliers' fascia and to suspend it to the posterior wall of the bladder, 1–2 cm cranially and dorsally to the new bladder neck. By this technique, anatomical and functional length of the rhabdosphincter is restored and firm support for its posterior aspect is provided by fixing the whole structure in its natural position [8].

The anastomosis becomes more difficult when performed under tension, with a higher risk of tearing the urethra. To reduce the tension, some maneuver and instruments can be used. To approximate bladder neck to urethral stump, a sponge stick can be employed to place the perineal pressure. This maneuver also helps to expose the urethral stump more clearly. Garrett and colleagues [9] described the use of Lowsley tractor to reduce the tension on urethra while performing vesicourethral anastomosis. Lowsley tractor is passed through the urethral stump and a single traction stitch is placed in posterior bladder neck. Traction stitch is then grasped with the wings of Lowsley and retracted into the urethra during first three anastomotic sutures.

Modified Vest suture for reduction of tension can also be used. A straight needle with nylon thread is inserted into the pubic cavity from the perineal region, anchored in the bladder neck, and an exit is made from the perineal region again. The bladder neck was towed by the nylon thread extracorporeally, bringing the bladder neck close to the urethra [10].

Two main techniques and the modifications of them were defined in the literature to perform vesicourethral anastomosis: the interrupted sutures defined by Montsouris group [11] and running sutures defined by Creteil group [12].

Interrupted Suture Technique

This technique was described by Guillonneau and Vallancien [11] after a continuous cohort of 260 patients operated in 23 months. Authors stated that it is not necessary to evert the bladder mucosa or to narrow the bladder neck. Knots may be formed inside or outside of the anastomotic lumen. The surgeon works with two needle holders all along this step. Anastomosis is performed with interrupted 3-0 resorbable 4/8 or 5/8 sutures on a No. 26 needle. For internally tied interrupted sutures, a 6-in. length is sufficient.

The metal Benique catheter with a depressed tip allows the needle into the urethra and the metal bougie can also help by allowing the needle to slide along the catheter.

The first suture is placed at the 5 o'clock position, running inside out on the urethra (right hand, forehand) and outside in on the bladder neck (right hand, forehand). The second suture is placed at the 7 o'clock position, running inside out on the urethra (right hand, forehand) and outside in on the bladder neck (right hand, forehand). The two sutures are tied inside the urethral lumen. Then four sutures are symmetrically placed at the 2, 4, 8, and 10 o'clock positions and tied outside the lumen. For a right-handed surgeon, the right-sided sutures run outside in on the bladder (right hand, forehand) and inside out on the urethra (left hand, backhand), and the left-sided stitches run outside in on the urethra (right hand, forehand) and inside out on the bladder neck (right hand, forehand).

The final two sutures are placed at the 11 o'clock position, running outside in on the urethra (right hand, forehand) and inside out on the bladder neck (right hand, forehand), and at the 1 o'clock position, running outside in on the urethra (right hand, forehand) and inside out on the bladder neck (left hand, forehand). The Foley catheter is inserted and position in the bladder is checked, and then the sutures can be tied safely. These two sutures are tied after the Foley catheter insertion. The balloon is blocked and the bladder is filled with saline to figure out for watertightness of the anastomosis. The choreographed sequence of all sutures is described in Table 17.1.

Similarly our group [13] described a modified interrupted technique with an initially placed 6 o'clock suture before catheterization. Anastomosis is performed with 15–17-cm polyglactin 3-0 interrupted endoscopic sutures using an RB-1 needle (Ethicon) after transurethral insertion of a metal bougie for exposure of the urethral stump. We start with a suture at the 6 o'clock position, taking the posterior urethra together with the rectourethral muscle. There are two further stitches subsequently made at the

Table 17.1 Choreographed sequence of successive stitches in interrupted vesicourethral anastomosis

Stitch	Location	Start	Hand	End	Hand	Knot
1	5 o'clock	Inside out on the urethra	Right hand, forehand	Outside in on the bladder neck	Right hand, forehand	Inside
2	7 o'clock	Inside out on the urethra	Left hand, forehand	Outside in on the bladder neck	Left hand, forehand	Inside
3	8 o'clock	Outside in on the bladder neck	Left hand, forehand	Inside out on the urethra	Left hand, forehand	Outside
4	4 o'clock	Outside in on the bladder neck	Right hand, forehand	Inside out on the urethra	Left hand, backhand	Outside
5	9–10 o'clock	Outside in on the bladder neck	Left hand, forehand	Inside out on the urethra	Right hand, backhand	Outside
6	2–3 o'clock	Outside in on the bladder neck	Right hand, forehand	Inside out on the urethra	Left hand, backhand	Outside
7	11–12 o'clock	Outside in on the urethra	Left hand, forehand	Inside out on the bladder neck	Right hand, forehand	Outside
8	12–01 o'clock	Outside in on the urethra	Left hand, forehand	Inside out on the bladder neck	Left hand, forehand	Outside

Source: From [11, 13]

5 and 3 o'clock positions followed by two at 7 and 9 o'clock positions. The latter stitches require a second needle driver in the left hand to start with the stitch at the bladder neck. The bougie is then withdrawn, and a 20-Fr Foley catheter is inserted into the bladder followed by anterior reconstruction, that is, tennis racket, of the bladder neck with 15-cm polyglactin 3-0 interrupted sutures using an SH needle (Ethicon, Norderstedt, Germany). Subsequently, the anterior part of the anastomosis is closed over the indwelling catheter.

Running Suture Technique

Hoznek and colleagues [12] described a novel technique using two hemicircumferential running sutures for anastomosis. In their technique, the patient is positioned in dorsal decubitus, with the legs slightly spread to allow intraoperative rectal examination. Five trocars are used.

The vesicourethral anastomosis consists of a posterior and an anterior hemicircumferential running suture. Two needle holders are used simultaneously.

The right needle holder is inserted through the 12-mm disposable trocar situated at the right margin of the rectus sheath. This trocar also allows the passage of the suturing material: a 3-0 Vicryl suture with a 26-mm needle, where the optimal length of the suture is about 20 cm. The left needle holder is passed through the 5-mm port near the left anterior superior iliac spine. One will notice here again that this implies an angle of at least 60° between the needle holder axes. The surgeon manipulates these two needle holders. The first assistant holds the 0° lens which is passed through the 12-mm trocar at the umbilicus. On the other hand, he holds the suction–irrigation device, passed through the left 12-mm trocar. The suction–irrigation device allows exposing the bladder neck and removing the accumulated urine from the operating field. A second assistant or the instrumentalist uses a narrow forceps to hold the long tail of the running suture. On the urethral side, the long tail is maintained under traction in the direction of the symphysis, while on the bladder side, it is pulled cephalad. A starter knot is done at the 3 o'clock position. The suture is placed from outside in on the bladder and then from inside of the urethra to the outside. The suture is then tightened with intracorporeal technique. Next, the needle is passed from outside to inside of the bladder, below the starter knot, at the lower margin of the bladder neck in the 4 o'clock position. This is done with the right needle holder. One or two sutures are then placed near the 6 o'clock position of the bladder and the urethra.

For the terminal knot of the posterior hemicircumferential suture, a closed loop is prepared at the 9 o'clock position. The needle is passed from inside to outside on the bladder, then from outside to inside on the urethra, thus forming a loop, and again from inside to outside on the bladder side. All the sutures are done with the right needle holder with a forehand position. The suture line is thus finished extramurally by a triple-knot. The Foley catheter is pushed without any difficulty into the bladder.

Then, a second running suture is realized on the anterior margin of the bladder and the urethra, beginning at the 2 o'clock position on the bladder side, then in the urethra with the help of the right needle holder. Two or three needle passages are sufficient to entirely close the anterior aspect of the anastomosis. A loop is again formed at the 10 o'clock position and the knot is tied. These different sutures are performed with deliberate structured and error-free choreography, which has evolved progressively during the developmental phase of laparoscopic radical prostatectomies. The choreographed sequence of all sutures is described in Table 17.2.

Single-Knot Method

After defining running suture technique, some modifications of this technique have evolved. Van Velthoven and colleagues described a simple running suture technique that requires just one intracorporeal knot [14]. This technique has gained popularities among laparoscopists.

After laparoscopic removal of the prostate has been accomplished, the bladder neck is identified. The running suture is prepared by tying together the ends of two 6–in. sutures of 3-0 or 2-0 monolayer polyglycolic acid or polydioxanone; when available one thread is dyed and the other is not dyed, for easy identification purposes. The running stitch is initiated by placing both needles (RB-1 or CV-23) outside in through the bladder neck and inside out on the urethra, one at 5:30 position and the other needle at 6:30. The sutures are run from the 6:30 and 5:30 positions to the 9 o'clock and 3 o'clock positions, respectively, approximating the bladder and the urethra at each pass. The posterior lip of the bladder neck is left apart from the posterior urethra as long as the two first runs on the urethra and the three first runs on the bladder are not completed. When this is achieved, a gentle traction is exerted on each thread simultaneously or alternatively, and the system of loops acts as a "winch" to bring the bladder in contact with the urethra without any excessive traction on the latter. For that purpose, the presence of the knot at 6 o'clock position allows keeping two equal suture branches when pulling and forces the bladder to move as the fixed point of the winch. At this point, the 16-Fr silastic catheter used during the whole procedure is placed into the bladder. Proceeding in this manner, both knots might reside on the bladder side of the anastomosis; this is avoided between sutures 7 and 8 to end on the urethral side with the right thread and on the bladder side with the left one. Carrying the suturing up to the 12 o'clock position on both sides, going outside in on the urethra and inside out on the bladder completes the remaining closure (Table 17.4). At 12 o'clock position, the ends of the running sutures are tied to one another on the outside of the bladder. The choreographed sequence of all sutures is described in Table 17.3. This table also illustrates the reduced need to sew with the left or non-dominant hand, although ambidextrous skills remain useful to some extent.

If some discrepancy persists between the diameters of the urethra and of the bladder neck, some residual anterior opening of the bladder is closed at that moment in two layers with the same sutures; in that case, both lengths of threads are increased accordingly to about 20 cm. The balloon on the 20-Fr silastic catheter is filled with 10 cm^3 of water; the bladder is irrigated until clear with approximately 60 cm^3 of sterile water. A drain is placed and is usually removed on the first postoperative day. The catheter is normally left in place for 5–6 days and removed after a retrograde cystogram.

Additionally, Menon and colleagues published a modification of this technique for robotic LRP [15]. A single anastomotic suture is prepared by extracorporeally tying the tails of two 3-0 monofilament sutures (one dyed

Table 17.2 Choreographed sequence of successive stitches in running vesicourethral anastomosis

Stitch	Location	Start	Hand	End	Hand
1	3 o'clock	Outside in on the bladder neck	Right hand, forehand	Inside out on the urethra	Right hand, forehand
2[a]	4 o'clock	Outside in on the bladder neck	Right hand, forehand	Inside out on the urethra	Right hand, forehand
3	5–6 o'clock	Outside in on the bladder neck	Left hand, forehand	Inside out on the urethra	Right hand, forehand
4	7 o'clock	Outside in on the bladder neck	Left hand, forehand	Inside out on the urethra	Right hand, backhand
5	8 o'clock	Outside in on the bladder neck	Left hand, forehand	Inside out on the urethra	Right hand, backhand
6[b]	9 o'clock	Outside in on the bladder neck	Left hand, forehand	Inside out on the urethra	Right hand, backhand
7	2 o'clock	Outside in on the urethra	Left hand, forehand	Inside out on the bladder neck	Left hand, forehand
8	1 o'clock	Outside in on the urethra	Left hand, forehand	Inside out on the bladder neck	Left hand, forehand
9	11–12 o'clock	Outside in on the urethra	Left hand, forehand	Inside out on the bladder neck	Left hand, forehand
10[b]	10 o'clock	Outside in on the urethra	Left hand, forehand	Inside out on the bladder neck	Left hand, forehand

[a]Needle is passed from outside to the inside of the bladder
[b]A closed loop is prepared and knotted
Source: From [12]

Table 17.3 Choreographed sequence of successive stitches in running "single-knot" vesicourethral anastomosis

Stitch	Location (o'clock)	Start	Hand	End	Hand
1	5–6	Outside in on the bladder neck	Right hand, forehand	Inside out on the urethra	Right hand, forehand
2	6–7	Outside in on the bladder neck	Right hand, forehand	Inside out on the urethra	Right hand, forehand
3	4	Outside in on the bladder neck	Right hand, forehand	Inside out on the urethra	Right hand, forehand
4	3	Outside in on the bladder neck	Right hand, forehand	Inside out on the urethra	Left hand, backhand
5	8	Outside in on the bladder neck	Left hand, forehand	Inside out on the urethra	Left hand, forehand
6	9	Outside in on the bladder neck	Left hand, forehand	Inside out on the urethra	Right hand, backhand
7	10	Outside in on the urethra	Right hand, forehand	Inside out on the bladder neck	Right hand, forehand
8	11	Outside in on the urethra	Right hand, forehand	Inside out on the bladder neck	Right hand, forehand
9	2	Outside in on the bladder neck	Right hand, forehand	Inside out on the urethra	Left hand, backhand
10	1	Outside in on the bladder neck	Right hand, forehand	Inside out on the urethra	Left hand, backhand
11	12	Outside in on the bladder neck	Right hand, forehand	Inside out on the urethra	Right hand, backhand

Source: From [14]

Table 17.4 Steps in single-knot running vesicourethral anastomosis

Surgeon	First assistant	Second assistant	Scrub nurse	Image
Insertion of bougie	Holds the camera and suction/irrigation			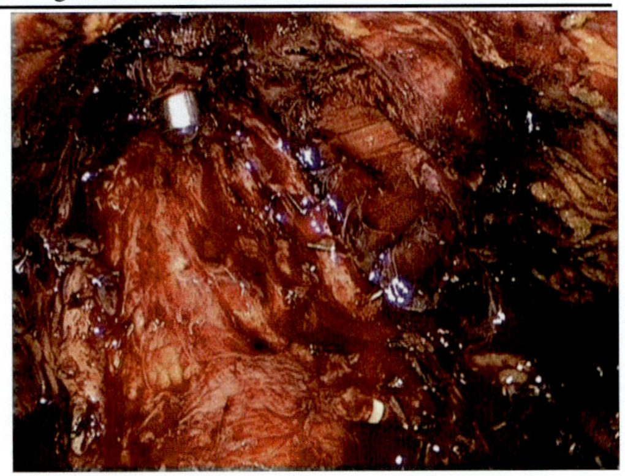
Places the needle holders in the left lateral and right medial trocars. Rocco suture for approximation of bladder and reconstruction of musculofascial plate	Sucks the blood and urine very gently in the bladder neck	Holds the bougie and compresses over the perineum for better visualization of urethral stump		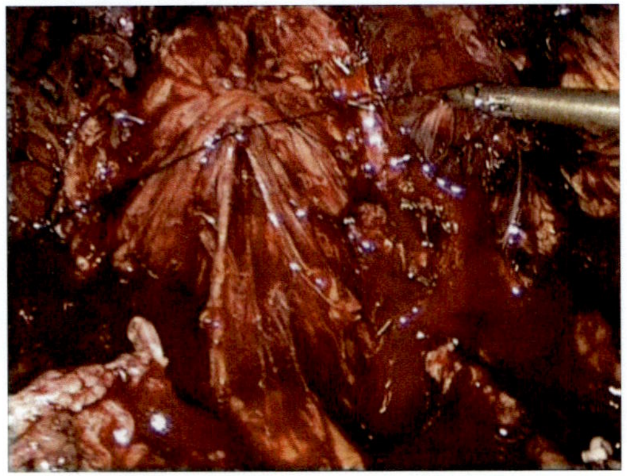

Table 17.4 (continued)

Surgeon	First assistant	Second assistant	Scrub nurse	Image
Reconstruction of the bladder neck in "racket" with running suture if needed	Gently pushes the bladder posteriorly, distal to the bladder neck for good visualization of the bladder neck	Keeps holding the bougie upward	Prepares the sutures for urethrovesical anastomosis	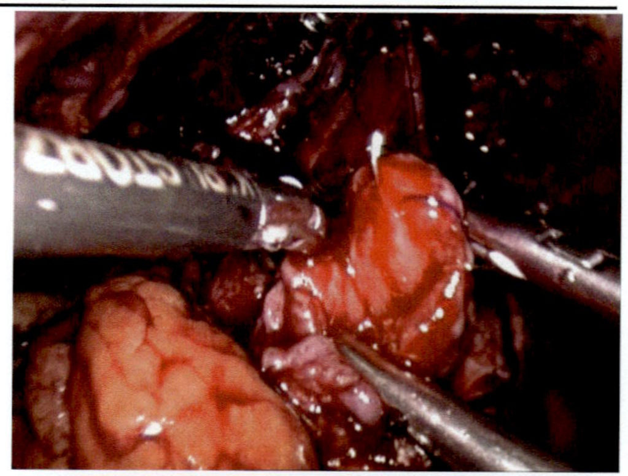
Urethrovesical anastomosis with single-knot running suture	Keeps on pushing gently the bladder. Sucks the blood and urine very gently in the bladder neck	Keeps bougie during posterior part of anastomosis, removes bougie, insert Foley at the end of posterior part of anastomosis	Tests the urinary catheter balloon twice for leakage Gives Foley catheter after removal of bougie	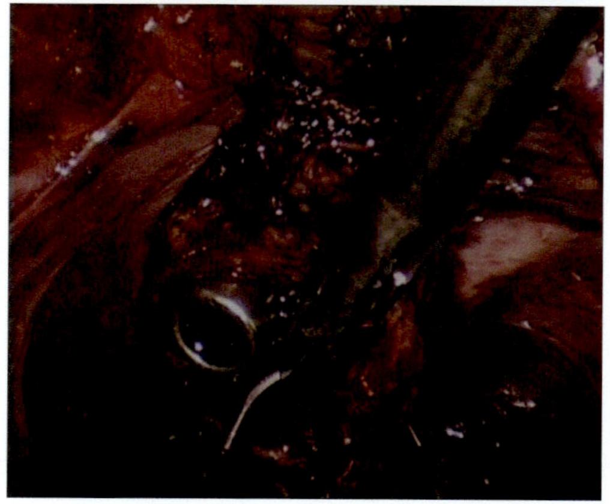

Table 17.4 (continued)

Surgeon	First assistant	Second assistant	Scrub nurse	Image
Makes the knot Cuts the suture		Blocks the Foley	Takes back the needle holders and needle. Prepares a syringe with 15 ml of sterile water	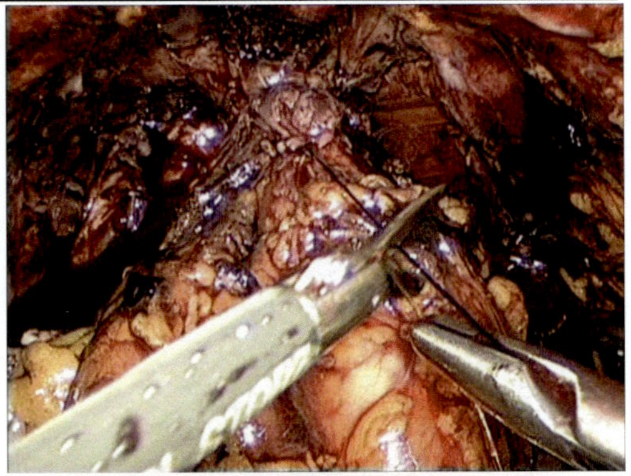
Looks for bladder or anastomosis leakage during injection of saline		Fills up the balloon with 100 ml to test for anastomosis leakage or bladder damage	Gives the syringe of 100 ml of saline	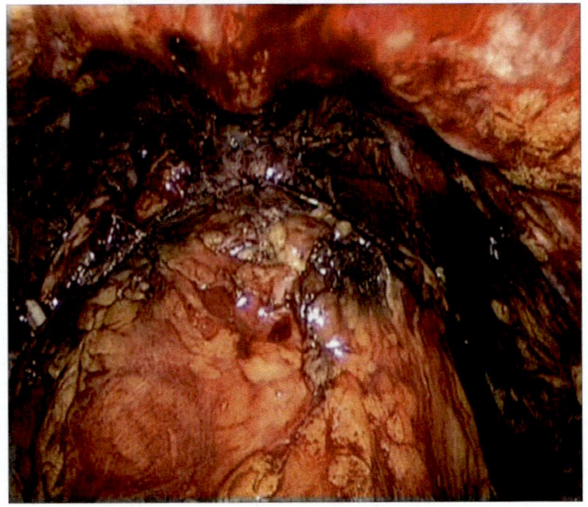

and one undyed). Anastomosis starts hemicircumferentially toward the left side, using the needle of the dyed end, by passing the needle outside in at the 4 or 5 o'clock position on the bladder neck and inside out on the urethra. After two or three throws on the urethra and three to four throws on the bladder to create an adequate posterior base, the bladder is cinched down against the knot of the sutures lying on the posterior surface of the bladder. The anastomosis is continued clockwise to the 9 o'clock position on the bladder. The suture is then turned into the bladder in such a way that it runs inside out on the bladder and outside in on the urethra to continue further up to the 11 or 12 o'clock position. Then the suture (dyed) is pulled cranially toward the left lateral side of the pelvis and maintained under traction by an assistant. Subsequently, the anastomosis is started on the right side of the urethra with the undyed end, passing it outside in on the urethra and then inside out on the bladder from the point where the anastomosis was started and continuing anticlockwise to the point where the other suture is met. The needle of the dyed end is cut off, and the free dyed end and undyed ends are tied together with several knots.

The "Bordeaux" technique, popularized by Richard Gaston and Thierry Piechaud, is a simple, single-running suture that starts at the 3 o'clock position. After the first throw at the bladder neck and at the urethra, the suture is tied immediately at the 3 o'clock position. The running suture is then continued clockwise and tied again at the 3 o'clock position [16].

Emiliozzi and colleagues [17] defined an anastomosis technique with a single-suture, single-knot, running procedure. In this technique, a single 24- to 26-cm 3-0 monofilament suture is used. A multiple (eight single knots) knot is prepared 4 cm from the end tail. The running suture is started outside in on the bladder neck at the 4 o'clock position. The bladder neck and the urethra stay apart, so it is easy to prolong the suture with a second passage at the bladder neck and the urethra at 5:30 o'clock and a third passage at the bladder neck at 6:30 o'clock (Table 17.4). At this point the suture is pulled, and the bladder neck and the urethra are approximated on the posterior plate. The running suture is continued clockwise while the assistant maintains the tension of the suture in the intervals between the passages. After a few throws (usually between seven and eight overall for completing the anastomosis), the needle end is tied to the 4-cm tail. A single-knot, watertight suture is obtained with this approach.

Besides these modifications, many different approaches have been proposed to improve vesicourethral anastomosis, including running anastomosis with posterior fixation [18], the use of absorbable clips [19], the use of a Lowsley tractor [9], extracorporeal bladder neck traction with nylon thread [10], and the use of a specifically designed urethral Benique sound [20].

Discussion

Laparoscopic radical prostatectomy was first performed by Schuessler and colleagues and presented in 1991. However, the technical difficulties did not allow widespread application of this procedure. An initial series with nine patients was published in 1997 by the same authors and they stated that the anastomosis required twice as long as the removal of the prostate and was one of the major reasons to convert to an open procedure. But they concluded that the procedure was not feasible due to the excessive operation time and multiple technical difficulties [5]. However, with the pioneering efforts of European surgeons, the technique of laparoscopic RP re-emerged in Europe, the UK, and the USA [13, 21–24].

Laparoscopic radical prostatectomy is now widespread among urologists. Probably one of the most difficult steps of the operation is still the anastomosis between the bladder neck and the urethral stump because laparoscopic suturing represents a demanding operative technique substantially differing from the open procedure. Laparoscopic instruments are usually limited to four degrees of freedom including pitch, jaw, rotation, extraction/insertion plus the actuation of the instruments. Translational movement is restricted by a pivot point, the trocar position which results in the fulcrum effect. Moreover, the posture of the surgeon can be unergonomic due to placement requirements of the trocars. Suturing in the pelvis requires the surgeon to cross the assistant's arm holding the camera. In addition to these factors, anastomosis takes place at the end of the surgery and all these factors require a higher muscle effort compared to the open surgical procedures [25].

One of the major advantages of laparoscopic radical prostatectomy is its potential to perform all the sutures under total visual control. However, knotting of the sutures is time consuming and contributes to prolonged operating time. The problems associated with laparoscopic suturing and knotting techniques are caused by spatial limitation and fixed trocar positions and, therefore, restricted movement and handling of instruments, which represents the principal limiting factor for the widespread use of laparoscopy. However, more important is the geometry such as angles and distances between instruments or angle to the horizontal line as well as camera or needle position. Frede and colleagues [26] described that acute angles between instruments of 25° and 45° and an angle of <55° between the instruments and the horizontal line maximize the efficiency of suturing and knotting.

The optimal anastomotic closure involves creating a watertight, tension-free anastomosis with mucosal apposition and correct alignment of urethra. Guillonneau and colleagues [27] reported about 57 cases out of 567 (10%) with early urine leakage resulting in aspiration of urine by the suction drain. Anastomotic leakage was defined as persistent urine in the suction drain for more than 6 days, justifying the maintenance of bladder drainage. They documented 46 cases of anastomotic leakage. In 43 cases the fistula healed spontaneously by continuing suction drainage until cure and by prolonging bladder drainage. Only one patient underwent reoperation via the laparoscopic approach due to a persistent urinary fistula, enabling creation of a watertight anastomosis. Percutaneous aspiration of uroperitoneum was necessary in two cases. In 11 cases, secondary anastomotic urine leakage was diagnosed after catheter removal in a context of acute pain, acute urinary retention, and the peritoneal irritation syndrome, requiring continued bladder catheterization for another week. Acute urinary retention developed as a function of the duration of catheterization in 26 cases (4.6%).

The difficulties in running vesicourethral anastomosis during laparoscopic prostatectomy reported by the group of Creteil [28], hemicircumferential running sutures for the anastomosis instead of interrupted sutures. The authors observed four cases of intraperitoneal urine extravasation in the beginning of their experience; three patients requested open and one requested laparoscopic repair. No reoperation was necessary for the second half of the experience in Creteil, although about 15% of patients have some degree of anastomotic leakage on postoperative cystography, performed at postoperative days 4–5.

To achieve a watertight anastomosis, Turk and colleagues emphasize the importance of an atraumatic and precise dissection of the bladder neck. They observed 13.6% anastomotic leakage in their series of 125 patients, almost all of them gathered during the learning curve; overzealous use of diathermy around the bladder neck was estimated responsible for these relatively poor results [29].

Van Velthoven and colleagues [14] described the single-knot method, which offers further simplification of the running suture technique. The first knot is prepared extracorporeally by joining the two ends of the threads together. With single-knot technique, Van Velthoven and colleagues performed 130 radical prostatectomies and they reported no cases of clinically evident postoperative urinary leakage or bladder neck contracture. In a multicenter study, 1,928 laparoscopic and 2,630 robotic-assisted cases of vesicourethral anastomosis after LRP and robotic-assisted laparoscopic prostatectomy, respectively, were analyzed. The mean anastomosis time was 16 min for experts, 23 min for second-generation surgeons, and 30 min for trainees. Early leakage, acute retention following catheter removal, and urethral stricture requiring internal urethrotomy were seen in 2.1, 0.5, and 0.8%, respectively [30].

Bladder neck contracture has been reported to occur in 0–3% of men following laparoscopic RP [13, 31, 32]. A watertight, well-vascularized bladder neck-to-urethra apposition is essential to successful healing and urinary function. There is no clear definitive known cause of BNC; however, multiple factors, as noted in Section "Introduction," have been correlated with its occurrence. The low rate of BNC in our study is perhaps attributable to the technique of reconstructing the bladder neck using a running anastomosis. Less tissue manipulation, finer surgical tools, and less use of cautery during bladder neck dissection may also play a role [32].

Comparison of different anastomosis techniques in a single center was performed by Teber and colleagues [33]. They evaluated the intra- and postoperative outcomes of three types of anastomotic techniques performed at Heilbronn Clinic. They retrospectively compared intracorporeal single-knot running (Van Velthoven) technique, classical interrupted (Montsouris) technique, and interrupted technique with placement of a 6 o'clock suture before division of the posterior wall of the urethra (Heilbronn).

Extravasation was assessed by cystourethrogram (at 5–7 days post-op). The presence of extravasation of contrast material and the location of leakage (dorsal, right, or left lateral) were evaluated. The presence of leakage was categorized depending on the site of leak as grade I (lateral leakage—left or right) and grade II (dorsal leakage—hemicircumferential). They also analyzed the incidence of urinary retention and anastomotic strictures after catheter removal.

They found no correlation between an initial extravasation in the cystogram and the formation of a stricture in the three groups. There was also no correlation between the initial grade of extravasation and subsequent formation of a stricture. The cystogram was useful in predicting duration of leakage. A comparison of the three anastomotic methods showed no difference in the incidence of strictures. To conclude, for the vesicourethral anastomosis, a modified circumferential running suture including only a single knot decreased anastomotic and overall operative time. Although the rate of severe dorsal leakage was reduced compared to interrupted techniques, the postoperative continence and stricture rates were not influenced by the method of anastomosis [33].

Although laparoscopic radical prostatectomy has gained great interest in the last few years, it has not obtained yet a widespread like the robot in the US. In Europe is still confined to 20–30% of the centers. This is due to the difficulty of the technique. To date, no single technique for vesicourethral anastomosis has prevailed, which means that probably the best procedure is not yet available.

The learning curve for LRP is characterized by a long operating time especially for vesicourethral anastomosis. To obtain optimal results, spending long hours in the operating field or in intensive training sessions is mandatory. When training with boxes and animals are used appropriately, they are extremely useful to avoid the negative impact of the learning curve. The effectiveness and the validity of these training programs are scientifically approved [34]. After adequate training, new generations of surgeons can perform LRP within the standard operating time.

Critical Operative Steps

Preparation of Anastomosis

- Optimum preparation of the bladder neck and the urethral stump is of paramount importance for cancer control, continence, and vesicourethral anastomosis.
- Control of bleeding from dorsal vein complex.
- Transurethral insertion of catheter or metal bougie can be used to expose urethral stump.
- Identification of the exact dissection area between bladder neck and prostate.
- No need for bladder neck eversion.
- Posterior reconstruction may be required when ureteric orifices are very close to bladder mucosa.
- Bladder neck is reconstructed anteriorly rather than posteriorly.

Interrupted Suture

- The metal Benique catheter is inserted through urethra.
- The first suture is placed at the 5 and second suture at 7 o'clock position inside out, outside in on the bladder neck.

- These two sutures are tied inside the urethral lumen.
- Then four sutures are symmetrically placed at the 2, 4, 8, and 10 o'clock positions and tied outside the lumen.
- The final two sutures are placed at the 11 and 1 o'clock position, running outside in on the urethra and inside out on the bladder neck (right hand, forehand at 11 o'clock position, left hand, forehand at the 1 o'clock position).
- These two sutures are tied after the Foley catheter insertion.
- Similarly in Heilbronn modified interrupted technique, an initially 6 o'clock suture is placed before catheterization.

Running Suture

- A starter knot is done at the 3 o'clock position outside in on the bladder, then inside out on the urethra.
- The suture is then tightened with intracorporeal technique.
- Running suture is passed from outside in on the bladder and inside out on urethra.
- n the terminal knot of the posterior hemicircumferential suture, a closed loop is prepared at the 9 o'clock position.
- The Foley catheter is pushed into the bladder.
- A second running suture is passed outside in on the bladder and the urethra and inside out on the urethra at the 2 o'clock position.
- A loop is formed at the 10 o'clock position and the knot is tied.

Van Velthoven Suture

- Both sutures are placed outside in through the bladder neck and inside out on the urethra, one at 5:30 o'clock position and the other needle at 6:30 o'clock position.
- The sutures are run to the 9 and 3 o'clock positions, respectively.
- A gentle traction is exerted on each thread simultaneously or alternatively to bring the bladder in contact with the urethra.
- The Foley catheter is inserted.

Both sutures are carried out up to the 12 o'clock position on both sides and are knotted together.

Critical Instruments and Supplies

- Optic (telescope) 10 mm, 30° (Storz)
- Bipolar cable used with special endodissector (Aesculap)
- A 10-mm 120° endodissect (Aesculap)
- Bipolar dissector (Aesculap)
- Two 5-mm needle holders
- A 10-mm endo-right angle (Storz)
- Endoscissors: 5 mm (Storz)
- Metal bougie

References

1. Laguna MP, Schreuders LC, Rassweiler JJ, Abbou CC, van Velthoven R, Janetschek G, Breda G, de la Rosette JJ. European Society of Uro-Technology. Development of laparoscopic surgery and training facilities in Europe: results of a survey of the European Society of Uro-Technology (ESUT). Eur Urol. 2005;47:346–51.
2. Rassweiler J, Stolzenburg J, Sulser T, Deger S, Zumbe J, Hofmockel G, John H, Janetschek G, Fehr JL, Hatzinger M, Probst M, Rothenberger KH, Poulakis V, Truss M, Popken G, Westphal J, Alles U, Fornara P. Laparoscopic radical prostatectomy – the experience of the German Laparoscopic Working Group. Eur Urol. 2006;49:113–9.
3. Menon M, Tewari A, Peabody JO, Shrivastava A, Kaul S, Bhandari A, Hemal AK. Vattikuti Institute prostatectomy, a technique of robotic radical prostatectomy for management of localized carcinoma of the prostate: experience of over 1100 cases. Urol Clin North Am. 2004;31:701–17.
4. Frede T, Erdogru T, Zukosky D, Gulkesen H, Teber D, Rassweiler J. Comparison of training modalities for performing laparoscopic radical prostatectomy: experience with 1,000 patients. J Urol. 2005;174:673–8; discussion 678.
5. Schuessler WW, Schulam PG, Clayman RV, Kavoussi LR. Laparoscopic radical prostatectomy: initial short-term experience. Urology. 1997;50:854–7.
6. Teber D, Cresswell J, Ates M, Erdogru T, Hruza M, Gozen AS, Rassweiler J. Laparoscopic radical prostatectomy in clinical T1a and T1b prostate cancer: oncologic and functional outcomes-a matched-pair analysis. Urology. 2009;73:577–81.
7. Srougi M, Paranhos M, Leite KM, Dall'Oglio M, Nesrallah L. The influence of bladder neck mucosal eversion and early urinary extravasation on patient

outcome after radical retropubic prostatectomy: a prospective controlled trial. BJU Int. 2005;95: 757–60.
8. Rocco F, Carmignani L, Acquati P, Gadda F, Dell'Orto P, Rocco B, Bozzini G, Gazzano G, Morabito A. Restoration of posterior aspect of rhabdosphincter shortens continence time after radical retropubic prostatectomy. J Urol. 2006;175:2201–6.
9. Garrett JE, LaGrange CA, Chenven E, Strup SE. Use of Lowsley tractor during laparoscopic prostatectomy to reduce urethrovesical anastomotic tension. J Endourol. 2006;20:220–2.
10. Kondo Y, Matsuzawa I, Watanabe J, Hamasaki T, Yoshida K, Nishimura T. Utility of extracorporeal traction with nylon thread for easier vesicourethral anastomosis in laparoscopic prostatectomy. Int J Urol. 2005;12:1082–4.
11. Guillonneau B, Vallancien G. Laparoscopic radical prostatectomy: the Montsouris technique. J Urol. 2000;163:1643–9.
12. Hoznek A, Salomon L, Rabii R, Ben Slama MR, Cicco A, Antiphon P, Abbou CC. Vesicourethral anastomosis during laparoscopic radical prostatectomy: the running suture method. J Endourol. 2000;14:749–53.
13. Rassweiler J, Sentker L, Seemann O, Hatzinger M, Rumpelt HJ. Laparoscopic radical prostatectomy with the Heilbronn technique: an analysis of the first 180 cases. J Urol. 2001;166:2101–8.
14. Van Velthoven RF, Ahlering TE, Peltier A, Skarecky DW, Clayman RV. Technique for laparoscopic running urethrovesical anastomosis: the single knot method. Urology. 2003;61:699–702.
15. Menon M, Hemal AK, Tewari A, Shrivastava A, Bhandari A. The technique of apical dissection of the prostate and urethrovesical anastomosis in robotic radical prostatectomy. BJU Int. 2004;93:715–9.
16. Curto F, Benijts J, Pansadoro A, Barmoshe S, Hoepffner JL, Mugnier C, Piechaud T, Gaston R. Nerve sparing laparoscopic radical prostatectomy: our technique. Eur Urol. 2006;49:344–52.
17. Emiliozzi P, Martini M, d'Elia G, Scarpone P, Pansadoro A, Pansadoro V. A new technique for laparoscopic vesicourethral anastomosis: preliminary report. Urology. 2008;72:1341–3.
18. Branco AW, Kondo W, de Camargo AH, Branco Filho AJ, de George MA, Stunitz LC. Laparoscopic running urethrovesical anastomosis with posterior fixation. Urology. 2007;70:799–802.
19. Shichiri Y, Kanno T, Oida T, Kanamaru H. Facilitating the technique of laparoscopic running urethrovesical anastomosis using Lapra-Ty absorbable suture clips. Int J Urol. 2006;13:192–4.
20. Ramani AP, Braasch M, Monga M, Ryndin I, Botnaru A. Novel device to assist urethrovesical anastomosis during laparoscopic radical prostatectomy. Urology. 2005;66:1099–100.
21. Hoznek A, Salomon L, Olsson LE, Antiphon P, Saint F, Cicco A, Chopin D, Abbou CC. Laparoscopic radical prostatectomy. The Creteil experience. Eur Urol. 2001;40:38–45.
22. Guillonneau B, Cathelineau X, Doublet JD, Vallancien G. Laparoscopic radical prostatectomy: the lessons learned. J Endourol. 2001;15:441–5; discussion 447–8.
23. Eden CG, Cahill D, Vass JA, Adams TH, Dauleh MI. Laparoscopic radical prostatectomy: the initial UK series. BJU Int. 2002;90:876–82.
24. Gill IS, Zippe CD. Laparoscopic radical prostatectomy: technique. Urol Clin North Am. 2001;28: 423–36.
25. Kenngott HG, Müller-Stich BP, Reiter MA, Rassweiler JJ, Gutt CN. Robotic suturing: technique and benefit in advanced laparoscopic surgery. Minim Invasive Ther. 2008;17:160–7.
26. Frede T, Stock C, Rassweiler JJ, Alken P. Retroperitoneoscopic and laparoscopic suturing: tips and strategies for improving efficiency. J Endourol. 2000;14:905–13; discussion 913–4.
27. Guillonneau B, Rozet F, Cathelineau X, Lay F, Barret E, Doublet JD, Baumert H, Vallancien G:. Perioperative complications of laparoscopic radical prostatectomy: the Montsouris 3-year experience. J Urol. 2002;167:51–6.
28. Nadu A, Salomon L, Hoznek A, Olsson LE, Saint F, de La Taille A, Cicco A, Chopin D, Abbou CC. Early removal of the catheter after laparoscopic radical prostatectomy. J Urol. 2001;166:1662–4.
29. Turk I, Deger S, Winkelmann B, Schonberger B, Loening SA. Laparoscopic radical prostatectomy. Technical aspects and experience with 125 cases. Eur Urol. 2001;40:46–52; discussion 53.
30. van Velthoven RF, Mottrie AM, Abbou CC, Erdoğru T, Teber D, Rassweiler JJ, Menon M, Gill IS, Ahlering TE. International multicentric survey about 4558 vesicourethral anastomosis after laparoscopic radical prostatectomy. J Endourol. 2006;20(Suppl 1):MP29–18.
31. Gonzalgo ML, Pavlovich CP, Trock BJ, Link RE, Sullivan W, Su LM. Classification and trends of perioperative morbidities following laparoscopic radical prostatectomy. J Urol. 2005;174:135–9; discussion 139.
32. Msezane LP, Reynolds WS, Gofrit ON, Shalhav AL, Zagaja GP, Zorn KC. Bladder neck contracture after robot-assisted laparoscopic radical prostatectomy: evaluation of incidence and risk factors and impact on urinary function. J Endourol. 2008;22: 377–83.
33. Teber D, Erdogru T, Cresswell J, Gozen AS, Frede T, Rassweiler JJ. Analysis of three different vesicourethral anastomotic techniques in laparoscopic radical prostatectomy. World J Urol. 2008;26: 617–22.
34. Sugiono M, Teber D, Anghel G, Gozen AS, Stock C, Hruza M, Frede T, Klein J, Rassweiler JJ. Assessing the predictive validity and efficacy of a multimodal training programme for laparoscopic radical prostatectomy (LRP). Eur Urol. 2007;51:1332–9; discussion 1340.

Chapter 18

Robotic Anastomoses and Bladder Neck Reconstruction Following Radical Prostatectomy

Marc C. Smaldone, Tina K. Schuster, and Stephen V. Jackman

This chapter contains a video segment which can be found at the URL: http://www.springerimages.com/ost

Introduction

Prostate cancer surgery has dramatically evolved since the radical perineal prostatectomy was introduced by Hugh Hampton Young over 100 years ago [1]. In 1947, Terrence Millin introduced the radical retropubic approach [2] but this did not gain acceptance until the 1970s due to significant blood loss, incontinence, impotence, and prolonged convalescence. Advances in the understanding of pelvic neuromuscular anatomy by pioneers such as Patrick Walsh have resulted in a marked reduction in morbidity and mortality following radical retropubic prostatectomy (RRP) [3, 4]. Currently, with improvements in technique focusing on the preservation of potency and continence, reported quality of life scores in men undergoing surgery for low-grade prostate cancers are comparable to those receiving less invasive treatment modalities (external beam radiation, brachytherapy) [5] or watchful waiting [6].

As nerve-sparing RRP has become the gold standard extirpative intervention for clinically localized prostate cancer, recent efforts have shifted toward development of a minimally invasive operative approach to provide a faster recovery and decrease postoperative discomfort. Schuessler et al. [7] described the first laparoscopic radical prostatectomy (LRP) in 1997 but concluded that although the procedure was technically feasible, the laparoscopic approach offered no advantage over open surgery with regard to tumor removal, continence, potency, length of stay, convalescence, or cosmetic result due to prolonged operative times. Despite initial discouraging results, with dedicated effort Vallencien and Guilloneau were able to refine and standardize the laparoscopic technique in the late 1990s and the procedure subsequently gained popularity among urologists in both the Unites States and Europe [8]. In addition to the conventional advantages of minimally invasive surgery including reduced blood loss and quicker convalescence, in experienced hands, short-term and intermediate quality of life and oncologic outcomes are comparable to that of open RRP [9]. Limitations to laparoscopy including two-dimensional visualization, limited range of movement, and poor ergonomics due to the use of rigid instruments have resulted in a steep learning curve, most notably with intracorporeal suturing of the vesicourethral anastomosis. As a result, the majority of LRP procedures are still performed at centers of excellence with extensive laparoscopic experience.

M.C. Smaldone (✉)
Department of Surgical Oncology, Fox Chase Cancer Center, 333 Cottman Avenue, Philadelphia, PA 19111, USA
e-mail: smaldonemc@gmail.com

M.C. Ost (ed.), *Robotic and Laparoscopic Reconstructive Surgery in Children and Adults*, Current Clinical Urology, DOI 10.1007/978-1-60327-914-7_18, © Springer Science+Business Media, LLC 2011

Initially described by Abbou et al. in 2000 [10], the robotic-assisted laparoscopic prostatectomy(RALP) has been popularized by Menon's group at the Vattikuti Institute with the intention of decreasing the steep learning curve of the LRP and maximizing the advantages of a minimally invasive approach [11]. Advantages of the da Vinci robotic platform (Intuitive Surgical, Sunnyvale, CA, USA) include enhanced stereoscopic visualization offering true depth-of-field vision and enhanced dexterity (EndoWrist™ technology) allowing the ability to perform precise suturing for reconstruction, while the chief deterrents are increased cost and lack of tactile feedback. There is considerable debate regarding optimal oncologic and functional outcomes following prostatectomy and to date there have been no randomized, prospective trials comparing the three techniques. However, due to increased access and a more rapid learning curve, the robotic platform for RALP has been quickly embraced by the urologic community. With more than 70,000 procedures performed in 2008 alone, it was estimated that more than 75% of prostatectomies in the United States will be performed with robotic assistance in 2009 (personal communication, Intuitive). In this chapter, we review basic techniques with a focus on challenging anatomy and discuss current oncologic and functional outcomes following RALP.

Operative Considerations

Indications and Contraindications

In our practice, we encourage a minimally invasive approach to prostatectomy in men with suspected low-risk or organ-confined disease based on prostate-specific antigen (PSA) <10 ng/dl, Gleason score $\leq$7, and digital rectal examination ($\leq$cT2 disease) and no evidence of metastasis [12]. Although not an absolute contraindication, patients with evidence of locally advanced disease have a significant risk of disease progression and it is imperative that negative margins be obtained. In patients with intermediate- to high-risk prostate cancer, the decision regarding an open or a robotic approach is made on an individualized basis after consideration of patient age, co-morbidity, and anatomy. The literature suggests that patients with clinical evidence of nodal or metastatic disease do not benefit from prostatectomy [13]. Currently, this is our only disease-specific contraindication to open or minimally invasive prostatectomy in patients without clinical evidence of obstruction.

Co-morbid contraindications include significant cardiopulmonary compromise, peritonitis, ascites, and uncorrected bleeding diatheses. A history of stroke or cerebral aneurysm is a relative contraindication to robotic prostatectomy due to a prolonged duration in a steep Trendelenburg position. There are currently no absolute anatomic contraindications to a robotic-assisted approach. Although port placement and pelvic dissection can be more challenging in obese men or patients that have had prior abdominal surgery, successful outcomes have been reported for patients with a body mass index (BMI) >30, previous abdominal surgeries, enlarged prostate size (>60 g), a pronounced median lobe, and a previous history of prostate surgery, and have become incorporated into routine practice. High-volume surgeons have reported feasibility outcomes performing RALP in patients who have undergone prior neoadjuvant hormonal therapy, pelvic radiation, brachytherapy, and solid organ transplantation [14–16]. Although an open RRP is the preferred approach under these circumstances for the majority of urologists, encouraging results using the robotic platform have been achieved in select patients by minimally invasive surgeons with extensive experience.

Preoperative Preparation

As per the current AUA Best Practice Statement on Urologic Surgery Antibiotic Prophylaxis, a single intravenous dose of a first- or a second-generation cephalosporin is given within 1 h prior to skin incision to provide coverage for skin and urinary tract pathogens [17]. Alternative agents include an aminoglycoside plus metronidazole or clindamycin, and coverage is terminated in the immediate perioperative period. Prevention of deep vein thrombosis (DVT) is essential to perioperative care. Intermittent pneumatic compression devices or graduated compression stockings are mandatory during the surgery and perioperative stay until the patient is ambulatory, but DVT prophylaxis is generally not recommended in minor- or moderate-risk patients undergoing laparoscopic or robotic urologic surgery due to the risks of hemorrhage [18]. For patients with one or more high-risk factors, low-dose unfractionated heparin or low molecular weight heparin is recommended as per individual surgeon's preference. It is the opinion of the authors that DVT prophylaxis be administered for any robotic-assisted case in which the operative time is expected to be greater than 2 h in duration, particularly for institutions participating in residency training or early in the learning curve [19]. It is our practice to administer a single dose of low-dose unfractionated heparin preoperatively and in the immediate perioperative period. Bowel preparation with or without administration of an oral antibiotic for elective surgery is controversial [20] and is dependent on individual surgeon's preference. In our practice, we prescribe a clear liquid diet on the day before surgery and a gentle laxative (300 ml bottle of magnesium citrate) at noon on the day prior to surgery.

da Vinci Surgical System Components

The da Vinci Surgical System comprises the surgeon console, the vision tower, and the surgical patient cart. The control console consists of a three-dimensional video screen with one monitor for each eye, master handles that can be adjusted to transfer movement based on a motion scale (2:1, 3:1, 5:1), and foot controls which include control of the focus, clutch, camera, and electrocautery. The surgical patient cart consists of three or four individual devices that control the surgical instruments and the endoscope (0° or 30°) via input from the hand controls and foot pedals from the surgeon's control console (Fig. 18.1). A wide variety of 5- and 8-mm surgical instruments are available and are easily interchanged from the surgical arms by the assistants at the patient's bedside. The da Vinci S high-definition system includes a wider panoramic view as well as an integrated fourth arm for rapid deployment. The da Vinci Si high-definition system adds higher resolution video, a reconfigured control panel, and the option for dual-surgeon consoles for training purposes.

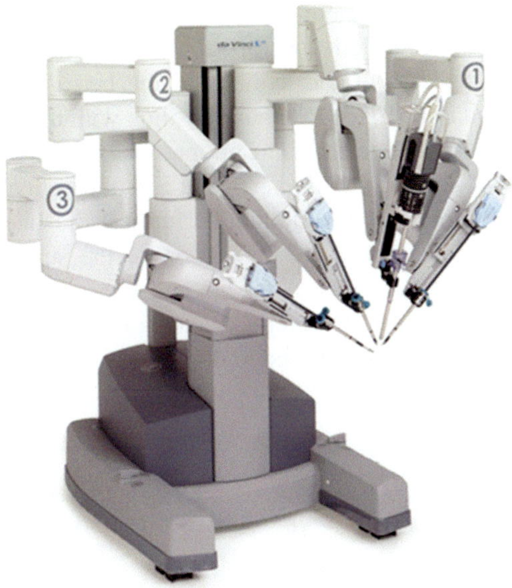

Fig. 18.1 *da Vinci* Si Patient Cart ©2009 Intuitive Surgical, Inc. (image reproduced with permission from Intuitive Surgical, Sunnyvale, CA, USA)

Patient Positioning

Proper patient positioning is essential prior to procedure initiation. Following informed consent, the patient is placed in the supine position with the legs in low lithotomy position. It is our preference to tuck the arms at the patient's sides, and pressure points (shoulders, legs, and arms) are padded with egg crate to prevent neuropraxic injury. The patient is secured to the operating table using cloth tape about the patient's chest at the level of the axilla, and the bed is fully tilted in full Trendelenburg position with the surgical and anesthesia team present to visually confirm that they are satisfied that the patient's position is secure and that no further adjustment is required prior to application of the surgical drapes (Fig. 18.2). After the abdomen and genitalia are sterilely prepped and draped, a 16-Fr Foley catheter is placed to drain the bladder.

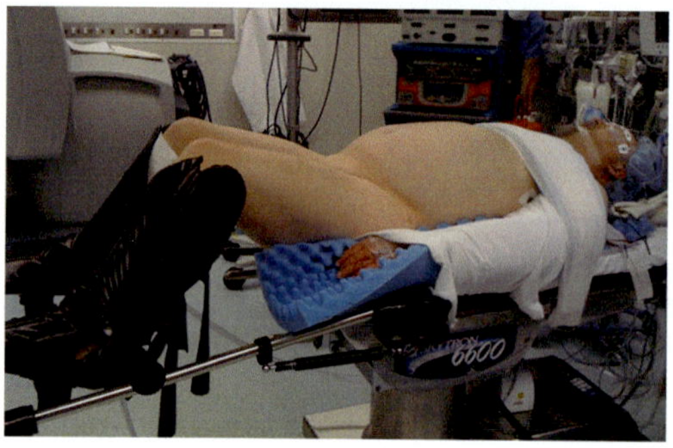

Fig. 18.2 The patient is placed in the supine position with the legs in low lithotomy position. It is our preference to tuck the arms at the patient's sides, and pressure points (shoulders, legs, and arms) are padded with egg crate to prevent neuropraxic injury

Port Placement

Port placement is critical to the ease of the procedure, and several variations as per individual surgeon's preference have been described for the transperitoneal approach. To obtain a pneumoperitoneum, with the patient in a supine position, a Veress needle is inserted into an upper quadrant at the anticipated site of the 5-mm assistant port. As an alternative, the Veress needle can be inserted at the umbilicus. If desired, the patient can be placed in a slight Trendelenburg position to allow the liver to fall in a cephalad position. After successful insufflation, access to the abdomen is obtained using a 12-mm VISIPORT^{TM} (US Surgical, Norwalk, CT, USA) blindly or under direct vision vertically in the midline 18–22 cm above the pubic symphysis, which in thin or non-obese patients is typically located in a supraumbilical position. In obese or tall men the camera port can be placed in an infraumbilical position. Alternatively the open Hassan technique can be utilized to enter the abdomen. A 0° endoscope is inserted and the abdomen and the pelvis are surveyed to ensure that there are no visceral injuries or significant adhesions. Three robotic ports and two assistant ports are then placed under direct vision. In our practice, two 8-mm robotic arm ports are placed 8 cm laterally from the midline (midclavicular line), at a distance of 15 cm from the superior edge of the midpoint of the pubic symphysis. The auxiliary (fourth arm) is placed approximately 2 cm superior and medial to the left anterior superior iliac spine (ASIS) and at least one handsbreadth from the left robotic port. A 12-mm assistant port is placed at the corresponding mirror-image position on the right. This port allows the assistant to pass sutures and the EndoCatch bag for specimen retrieval. A second 5-mm assistant port is placed in the right upper quadrant approximately two fingerbreadths below the costal margin at a point that bisects the camera port and the right robotic port. This is usually located at the site of Veress needle insertion and is primarily used for suction. Once the ports are in place (Fig. 18.3), the patient is placed in full Trendelenburg position and the robot is docked. Proper port placement is vital to maximize working space which can be limited in thin men with a narrow pelvis. Considerations include the need to place the ports high in the abdomen (at least one handsbreadth apart) to prevent contact between instruments. Similarly, it is necessary that the instruments reach the distal prostate and the pelvic floor to complete the critical parts of the operation, including ligation of the dorsal venous complex and urethrovesical anastomosis, which can be challenging in obese men. Communication between the primary surgeon at the console and the assistants at the bedside is essential to ensure rapid recognition of problems intraoperatively and a smooth transition between each step of the procedure.

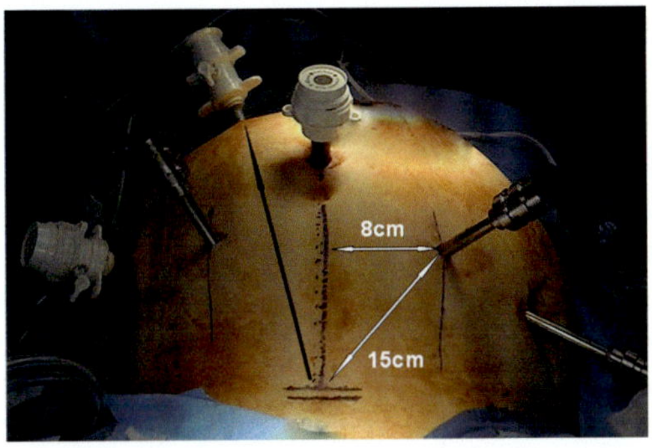

Fig. 18.3 Two 8-mm robotic ports are placed 8 cm laterally from the midline (midclavicular line), at a distance of 15 cm diagonally from the superior midpoint of the pubic symphysis. The auxiliary (fourth arm) is placed approximately 2 cm superior to the left anterior superior iliac spine approximately 8 cm from the left robotic port. A 12-mm assistant port is placed at the corresponding mirror-image position on the *right*. A second 5-mm assistant port is placed in the right upper quadrant approximately two fingerbreadths below the costal margin at a point that bisects the camera port and the right robotic port

Anesthesia Considerations

Pneumoperitoneum and alterations in patient positioning can result in several physiologic effects unique to laparoscopy. Hemodynamic shifts may not show clinically significant effects in healthy men but have been demonstrated to result in significant pathophysiologic changes in patients with preoperative cardiopulmonary disease [21]. Peritoneal insufflation pressures create a large gradient for CO_2 diffusion into the bloodstream resulting in hypercarbia. Carbon dioxide acts directly to inhibit the cardiovascular system, decreasing heart rate, cardiac contractility, and systemic vascular resistance while increasing pulmonary artery pressures, which can result in cardiac arrhythmias and respiratory acidosis [22].

Mechanical effects of increased intra-abdominal pressure from pneumoperitoneum may include reduced cardiac preload from compression of the great vessels as well as increased intrathoracic pressures which can result in decreased functional residual capacity and respiratory compliance. These effects can be magnified in obese patients or those placed in the pronounced Trendelenburg position for an extended duration [23]; in these cases, increasing the inspired O_2 concentration may be required to maintain oxygenation. Increased intra-abdominal pressures and its associated cardiovascular changes may also result in increased intracranial pressure, decreased visceral perfusion, and oliguria. A thorough pre-anesthesia assessment can assure that the patient is medically optimized in order to safely anticipate and tolerate these expected physiologic changes during laparoscopy.

Transperitoneal RALP Technique

Bladder Mobilization

After initial laparoscopic survey of the abdomen, the left colon is mobilized as needed using monopolar curved scissors without cautery. The parietal peritoneum overlying the bladder is taken down lateral to the medial umbilical ligaments from the urachus to the vas deferens bilaterally using a combination of blunt dissection and cautery. Using left-handed graspers, the right medial umbilical ligament is held on traction posteriorly, while the peritoneum is scored using monopolar cautery. The bladder is bluntly swept in a medial direction to help delineate the plane of dissection. On the left side, the assistant can use a laparoscopic grasper to hold traction on the left medial umbilical ligament. Dissection is continued into the pelvis until the pubic arches are visible. Once mobilized laterally, the urachus is transected using cautery and the bladder is "dropped" from the anterior abdominal wall at the midline. The extraperitoneal space is further developed by dissection anterior to the level of the pubic symphysis.

Exposure of the Prostatic Apex and Ligation of the Dorsal Venous Complex (DVC)

After the bladder is mobilized, the pre-prostatic fat is dissected using blunt dissection and monopolar cautery, exposing the endopelvic fascia and puboprostatic ligaments. The superficial dorsal vein is isolated and controlled with bipolar cautery. The endopelvic fascia is incised using scissors with or without cautery, and levator muscle fibers are gently teased laterally away from the prostatic base to apex until the edge of the dorsal vein is visualized. Mueller's ligament is carefully dissected free, sealed with bipolar cautery, and divided sharply. The puboprostatic ligaments are then placed on slight traction using posterior and cephalad pressure and divided with monopolar scissors. While in our practice, apical dissection is performed prior to ligation of the dorsal vein, some surgeons prefer to limit urethral dissection or division of the puboprostatic ligaments prior to placement of the dorsal vein stitch [24] with the belief that it may improve early continence results.

A 6-in. 0-Polysorb suture on a GS-21 needle (US Surgical, Norwalk, CT, USA) is used to control the DVC (Fig. 18.4). A sliding stitch is placed so that the tension can be adjusted prior to securing the knot. As per individual surgeon's preference, an additional stitch may be placed at the mid prostate; this can be used to decrease back bleeding when the DVC is divided or for prostatic manipulation during the posterior dissection.

Bladder Neck Transection

Once the DVC has been suture ligated, a 30° down lens may be placed to aid in the bladder neck dissection, depending on the patient's anatomy and individual surgeon's preference. Identifying the proper plane takes a degree of experience, but additional maneuvers such as manipulating the Foley catheter balloon or bimanual compression ("bladder neck pinch") can be utilized to identify the prostatovesical junction [25] (Fig. 18.5). Ideally, a shallow groove between the prostate and the horizontally orientated detrusor fibers can be distinguished, and in our experience, the prostatovesical junction is usually more clearly demarcated laterally rather than in the midline. Starting either medially or laterally, the bladder neck is incised using cautery. A lateral approach facilitates creation of a smaller bladder neck opening, minimizing the need for later reconstruction. Anecdotally, holding the monopolar scissors at a 90° angle to the tissue and using a sweeping motion with cautery facilitates separation of the tissue planes until the Foley catheter can be identified (Fig. 18.6). It is important to note that this should be essentially an avascular plane. Although there can be a degree of back bleeding from the prostate,

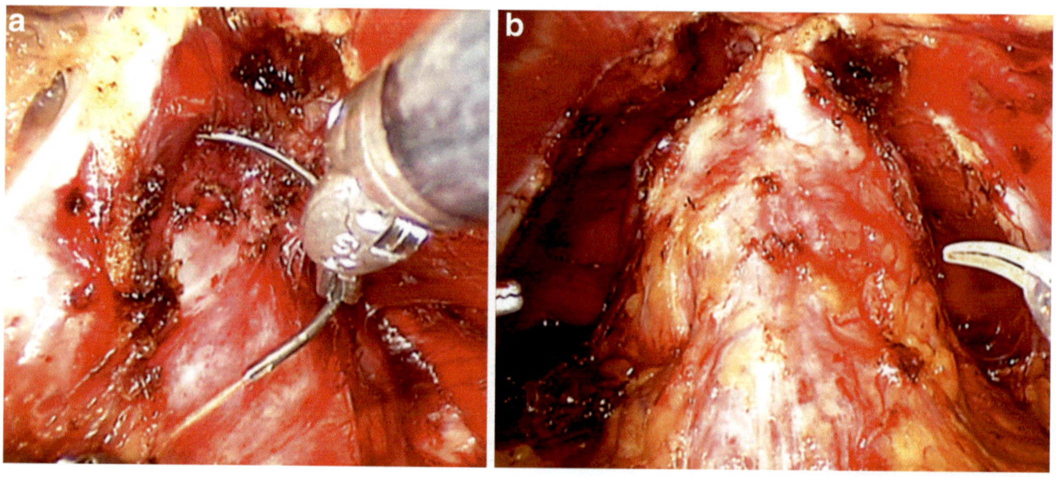

Fig. 18.4 After apical dissection is complete and the puboprostatic ligaments have been divided, a 0-Polysorb suture on a GS-21 needle is used to control the dorsal venous complex (**a**). A sliding stitch is placed so that tension can be adjusted prior to securing the knot (**b**)

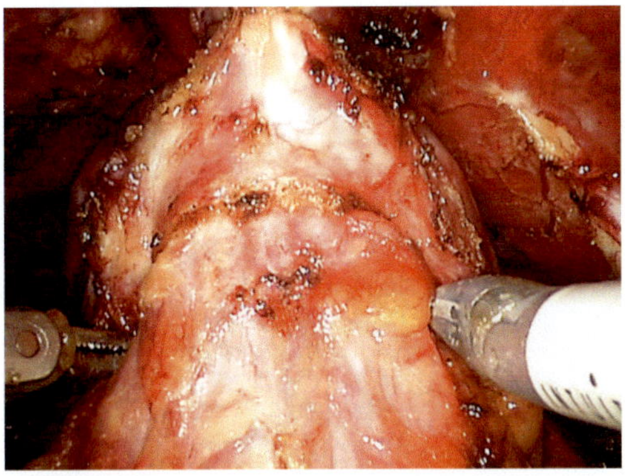

Fig. 18.5 Maneuvers such as manipulating the Foley catheter balloon or bimanual compression ("bladder neck pinch") can be utilized to identify the prostatovesical junction prior to bladder neck transection

pronounced bleeding should alert the surgeon to re-evaluate the surgical plane for inadvertent dissection within prostate tissue. The bedside assistant can intermittently provide traction on the catheter to seat the balloon at the bladder neck to help reassess the proper plane of dissection. When the anterior bladder neck has been divided exposing the catheter, the Foley balloon is deflated and the assistant retracts the catheter tip anteriorly toward the pubic symphysis, elevating the prostate and exposing the posterior bladder neck. We have found that exposure is improved by having the surgical technician pull the distal end of the catheter and placing a heavy clamp on the catheter close to the urethral meatus to maintain tension. The bladder neck is intermittently tented open with cephalad traction to allow for inspection of the ureteral orifices; in difficult cases, visualization can be facilitated by administering Indigo carmine dye. In patients with obscured anatomic planes this maneuver is also helpful to assess the orientation of the posterior bladder wall to facilitate dissection. The posterior bladder neck mucosa is then scored with the tips of the monopolar scissors and the detrusor muscle is divided. A separate layer of vertically orientated posterior bladder neck tissue must be incised before reaching Denonvilliers' fascia. This layer will later be utilized for reconstructing the posterior bladder neck.

Posterior Prostatic Dissection

Once the posterior bladder neck dissection is complete, the anterior layer of Denonvilliers' fascia can be visualized (Fig. 18.7a). This is sharply incised to expose the vasa deferentia and seminal vesicles. Each vas is carefully dissected as far distally as possible using controlled cautery and gentle sweeping motions to release the sheath and vessels. We have found that extended dissection to the level of the tip of the seminal vesicles aids in the subsequent seminal vesicle dissection. The vasa are transected using cautery and handed to the assistant for use as a handle for

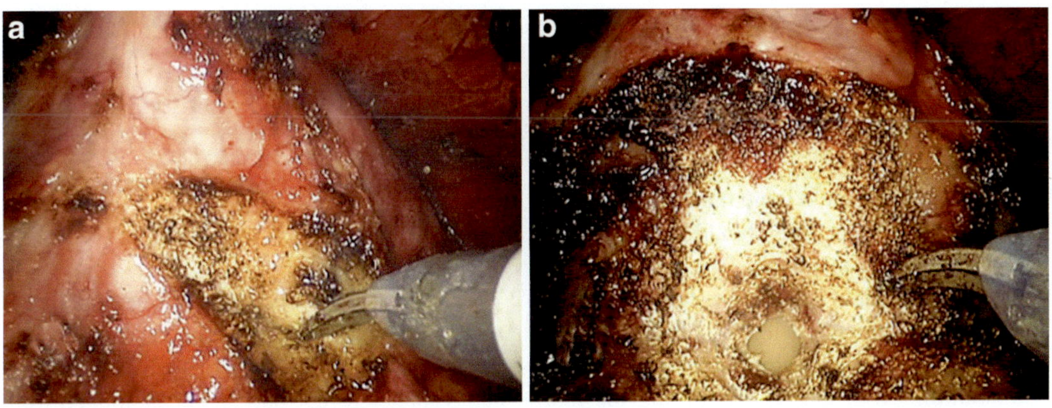

Fig. 18.6 Starting laterally (**a**), the bladder neck is incised with cautery using the monopolar scissors until the Foley catheter is identified (**b**)

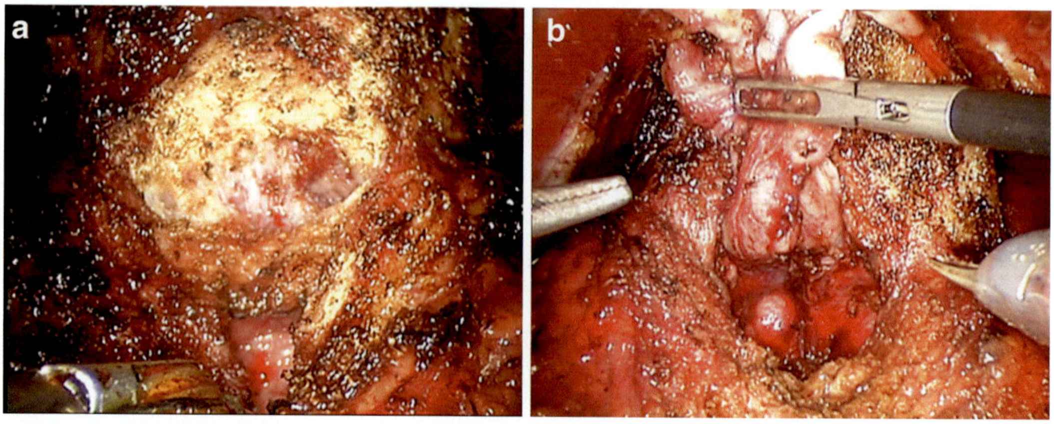

Fig. 18.7 Following dissection of the posterior bladder neck, the vas deferens and seminal vesicles are identified (**a**). Once dissected free, anterior retraction of the vasa and seminal vesicles exposes the surgical plane between the prostate and the rectum (**b**)

anterior traction. The seminal vesicles are then mobilized using a combination of blunt dissection and monopolar cautery, with attention paid to the deferential arteries which often lie in a posterior position. Care to avoid excessive use of cautery is essential, particularly near the tips of the seminal vesicles due to the close proximity of the neurovascular bundles. The seminal vesicles are then anteriorly retracted with the vasa to place the posterior layer of Denonvilliers' fascia on tension. Incision exposes the surgical plane between the prostate and the rectum which is developed bluntly (Fig. 18.7b). This plane can be difficult to identify in patients who have undergone multiple transrectal biopsies, saturation biopsy, and neoadjuvant hormonal therapy.

Management of Rectal Injury

Although uncommon in large minimally invasive prostatectomy series [26], should a rectal injury be identified intraoperatively, the prostatectomy should be completed and the prostate placed in a specimen entrapment device. The operative field should then be copiously irrigated with an antibiotic solution. After clearly identifying the margins of the rectal defect, if the edges appear viable with minimal fecal spillage, the rectotomy should be closed in two layers with absorbable suture and imbricated with a non-absorbable suture. In a patient with a history of pelvic radiation, a full-thickness cautery injury, significant fecal contamination, or a repair which cannot be completed without tension, a diverting colostomy is recommended [27]. Case reports have described further maneuvers to manipulate the rectal repair away from the urethrovesical anastomosis including tacking the rectum to the levator fibers on one side and placing an interposition omental flap that is secured posterior to the urethra [28]. In the case of primary closure of a rectal injury, it is our recommendation that a closed suction drain be placed away from the anastomosis, broad spectrum antibiotics be administered for at least 24 h, rectal dilation be performed, and the Foley catheter be left in place for a minimum of 14 days.

Retrovesical Dissection (Montsouris Technique)

The pure laparoscopic approach beginning with a retrovesical dissection of the vasa and seminal vesicles was initially described by Guillonneau and Vallancien [29] and has been applied to the robotic platform. With this technique, the bladder attachments to the anterior abdominal wall are initially preserved, and the vasa and seminal vesicles are targeted at the bottom of the peritoneal reflection at the base of the posterior bladder wall. The peritoneum is incised, and the rectum is retracted inferiorly by the assistant with the suction instrument. The vasa are identified, dissected free, and transected, exposing the seminal vesicles. The seminal vesicles are brought into the surgical field with traction, dissected free, and the tips are transected. Denonvilliers' fascia is then incised until pre-rectal fat is visualized, identifying a safe plane for posterior prostatic dissection, which is carried anteriorly to the rectourethralis muscle at the apex of the prostate. The bladder is subsequently dissected free from the abdominal wall to facilitate the apical prostatic dissection and division of the bladder neck, which proceeds using methods described above.

Neurovascular Bundle Dissection and Controlling the Lateral Pedicles

The decision to proceed with a nerve-sparing approach is multi-factorial and depends on each patient's tumor characteristics and baseline potency. Patients are counseled preoperatively that nerve sparing will not take precedence over cancer control and that the final decision will be made intraoperatively at the surgeon's discretion. However, nerve sparing is planned and carried out in the vast majority of cases of low- and intermediate-risk prostate cancer. It is our preference to perform nerve sparing in a retrograde manner prior to division of the prostatic pedicle, mimicking open techniques. The neurovascular bundle runs along the posterolateral aspect of the prostate and is enclosed by the periprostatic fascia medially, the levator layer of the periprostatic fascia laterally, and the anterior layer of Denonvilliers' fascia posteriorly [30]. It is our preference to perform a modified version of the "veil of Aphrodite" technique as described by Menon et al., including a high apical bundle release which has recently been incorporated into open techniques as well [31]. The plane between the prostatic fascia and the capsule of the prostate is entered using sharp dissection only, starting proximally where the prostatic fascia reflects off the lateral edge of the prostate and proceeding in an antegrade fashion toward the apex and the ipsilateral pubourethral ligament [32] (Fig. 18.8a). We then prefer to mobilize the neurovascular bundles away from the prostate in a retrograde fashion until the lateral prostatic pedicles are exposed.

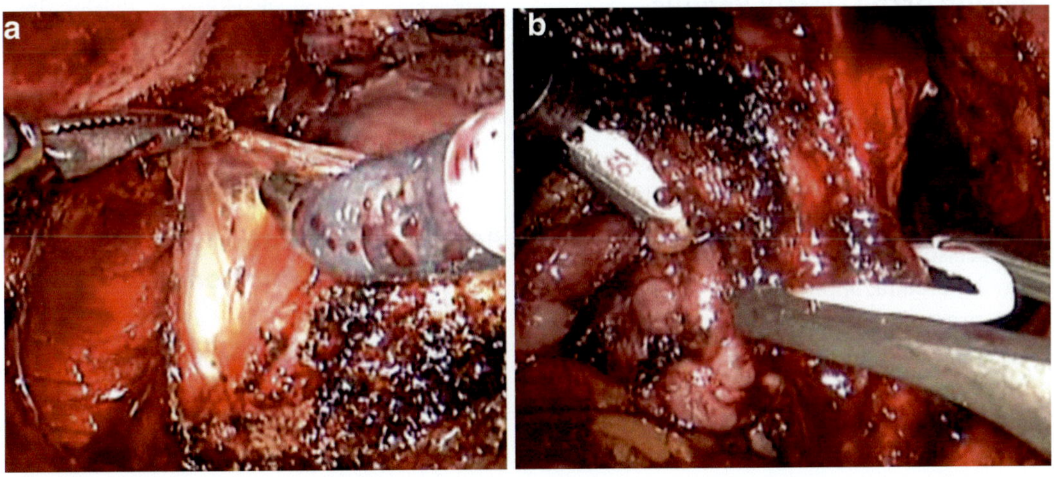

Fig. 18.8 To mobilize the neurovascular bundles, the plane between the prostatic fascia and the capsule of the prostate is entered near the apex using sharp dissection only. This plane is developed in a retrograde fashion back to the base of the prostate (**a**). The vascular pedicles are controlled using locking polymer clips and divided with scissors (**b**)

Using locking polymer clips, each pedicle is ligated and then divided sharply (Fig. 18.8b). The remaining posterior attachments are then cleared until the prostate has been mobilized to the level of the apex.

Modifications employed to improve nerve-sparing technique and improve potency outcomes have included preservation of all components of neurovascular tissue around the prostate, use of athermal scissors for the entire procedure, mobilization of the bundles away from the urethra apically to prevent damage during urethral transection, and anatomic reconstruction of the pelvic floor following urethrovesical anastomosis [33]. Additional novel efforts have focused on preservation of accessory pudendal branches [34], hypothermia to reduce traumatic inflammation [35], and hydrodissection to facilitate athermal bundle identification [36]. Prospective long-term data comparing these modifications are currently unavailable. We anticipate that future efforts will continue to capitalize on the increased understanding of pelvic neurovascular anatomy coupled with improved laparoscopic visualization in the pelvis to further improve nerve-sparing technique.

Division of the Dorsal Venous Complex and the Posterior Urethra

We traditionally use a 0° lens to incise the ligated DVC and complete our apical dissection. Once the nerve bundles and prostatic pedicles have been addressed, the DVC is incised sharply using scissors or monopolar cautery perpendicular to the urethra, approximately 5–10 mm distal to the prostatic apex to ensure an adequate urethral length and a negative margin. To facilitate this portion of the procedure, the assistant slides the lower jaw of a flat blunt grasper over the tip of the Foley catheter into the prostatic urethra and grasps the anterior lip of the base of the prostate (Fig. 18.9a). Cephalad and posterior traction can then be applied to the prostate to facilitate division of the DVC and the urethra (Fig. 18.9b). The Foley is then retracted to facilitate transaction of the posterior wall of the urethra and the rectourethralis muscle to free the prostate specimen (Fig. 18.9c). All attempts are made to minimize additional urethral fibromuscular skeletonization to aid in early return of continence. Some authors have suggested that cold incision of the DVC prior to suture ligation may result in decreased apical positive margin rates [37], but in our experience, early DVC ligation minimizes blood loss and improves intraoperative visualization without an appreciable adverse effect on apical margin status. Another alternative that has been described is the use of an endoscopic stapler to control the DVC, which is performed by the bedside assistant. However, in early investigations, no difference was shown with respect to blood loss, operative duration, or apical margin rates; as a result, this approach is performed sparingly at few centers [38].

Once mobilized, the surgical specimen is inspected while still in the abdomen. If there are concerns regarding capsular incision, extracapsular extension, or a grossly positive margin, additional specimens are sent for frozen section prior to completion of the urethrovesical anastomosis. We do not routinely send apical or bladder neck specimens for frozen section unless there is an increased clinical suspicion of tumor involvement. The surgical specimen is placed into a 10-mm EndoCatch™ bag (US Surgical, Norwalk, CT, USA) and moved into the upper abdomen for later retrieval.

Anatomic Restoration and the Urethrovesical Anastomosis

Technical modifications employed in RRP to help facilitate early return to continence that have been adapted by minimally invasive surgeons include sparing of the bladder neck [39], puboprostatic ligaments [40], puboprostatic collar [41], and posterior reconstruction of Denonvilliers' musculofascial plate [42]. Some authors advocate total anatomic restoration of the circumferential

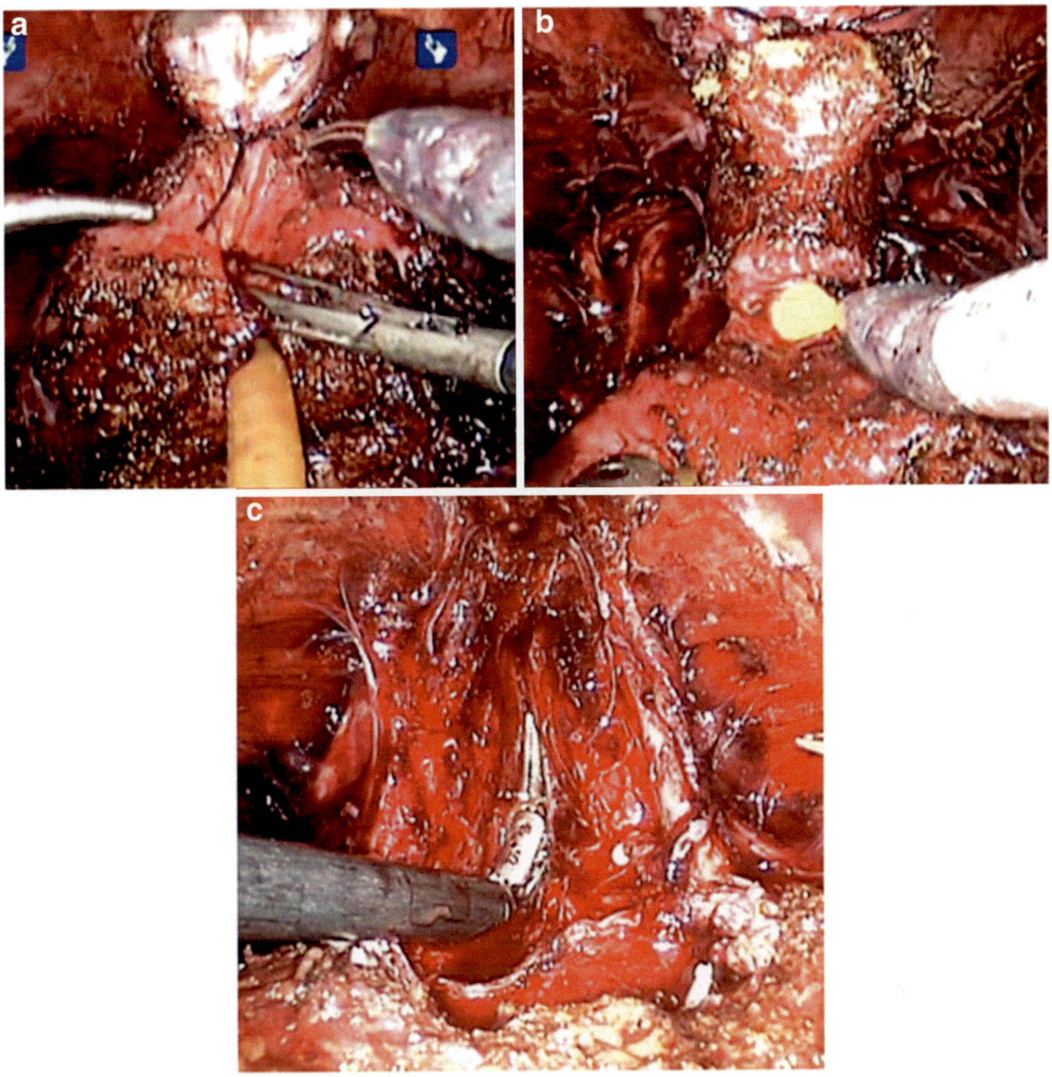

Fig. 18.9 Once the nerve bundles and prostatic pedicles have been addressed, the DVC is incised sharply using scissors or monopolar cautery. To facilitate this portion of the procedure, the assistant slides the lower jaw of a flat blunt grasper over the tip of the Foley catheter into the prostatic urethra and grasps the anterior lip of the base of the prostate (**a**). Once the urethra has been transected (**b**), the prostate specimen is placed into an entrapment bag, exposing the mobilized neurovascular bundles and the open bladder neck (**c**)

dynamic suspensory support system for the urethral sphincter complex. They believe that attenuating pelvic prolapse and downward pressure of the bladder on the healing anastomosis during micturition may relieve tension at the anastomosis, improve healing, and ultimately augment continence recovery [43].

It is our preference to spare the bladder neck during prostatic dissection and in our experience, reconstruction is rarely required prior to performing the urethrovesical anastomosis. If necessary, after completing the urethrovesical anastomosis, the remaining open bladder neck can be reconstructed with running or interrupted sutures incorporating full-thickness muscularis and bladder mucosa; this has been likened to a "reverse or anterior tennis racquet" technique [44]. We will often use a running 3-0 single-armed Monocryl suture on a RB-1 needle (Ethicon, Somerville, NJ, USA) with a Lapra-Ty (Ethicon, Somerville, NJ, USA) securing each end to reconstruct any remaining defect following completion of the anastomosis. In our practice, we still routinely divide the puboprostatic ligaments to facilitate exposure to the dorsal vein to assure adequate hemostasis, but we have recently amended our technique to minimize lateral and posterior apical dissection to preserve periurethral fibromuscular attachments to the pelvic floor. After the reports of encouraging short-term continence data, we have also incorporated posterior musculofascial reconstruction into our algorithm. Coined the "Rocco stitch," the cut edge of the distal Denonvilliers' plate and the cephalad Denonvilliers' musculofascial remnant posterior to the bladder neck is reapproximated in a running or an interrupted fashion in one or two layers [45, 46] (Fig. 18.10). This technique is thought to provide posterior support for the sphincteric mechanism and prevent caudal retraction of the urethra. As in bladder neck reconstruction, we utilize a running 3-0 Monocryl suture on an RB-1 needle (Ethicon Inc., Somerville, NJ, USA) with a Lapra-Ty (Ethicon Inc., Somerville, NJ, USA) securing each end. Perineal pressure by the bedside assistant helps to approximate the two edges. The tip of the Foley catheter is also brought in, grasped, and retracted anteriorly to identify and avoid incorporating the posterior urethral stump. Once these sutures are tied the bladder neck should lie close to the urethral stump. While the benefits to long-term postoperative continence remain undetermined, we have found that posterior musculofascial reconstruction takes tension off the anastomotic sutures helping to achieve a watertight urethrovesical anastomosis.

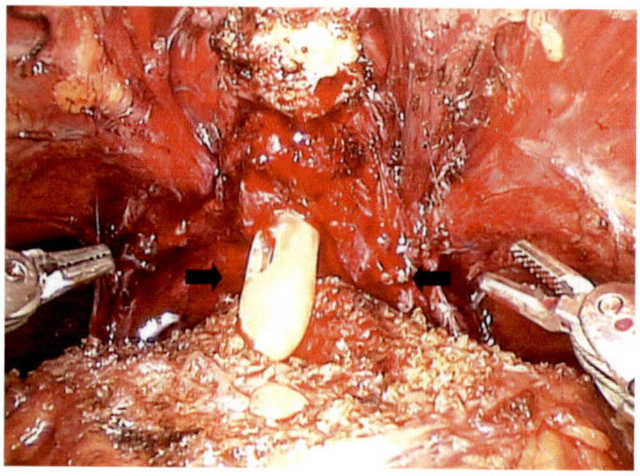

Fig. 18.10 The cut edge of the distal Denonvilliers' plate and the cephalad Denonvilliers' musculofascial remnant posterior to the bladder neck are reapproximated in a running fashion using a 3-0 Monocryl suture on an RB-1 needle with a Lapra-Ty securing each end. Posterior musculofascial reconstruction (*arrows*), coined the "Rocco stitch," provides posterior support for the sphincteric mechanism and takes tension off of the anastomotic sutures helping to achieve a watertight urethrovesical anastomosis

A single anastomotic suture is prepared by extracorporeally tying the tails of two 6.5-in. 3-0 Monocryl sutures to RB-1 needles (Ethicon, Somerville, NJ, USA) with one dyed and one undyed for identification purposes. For this portion of the procedure, we prefer to use the 0° endoscope and two large needle drivers. The urethrovesical mucosa-to-mucosa anastomosis is begun hemi-circumferentially starting with an outside-to-in throw of the dyed needle at 5 o'clock on the bladder neck, then passing the needle inside to out on the urethra (Fig. 18.11a). We follow the assistant's retracting urethral catheter to guide placement of the urethral sutures. After several throws to create adequate posterior reconstruction, the bladder is cinched down against the knot of the sutures lying on the posterior aspect of the bladder. The anastomosis is continued in a clockwise fashion to the 11 o'clock position (Fig. 18.11b), at which point the suture is temporarily tacked to the inside of the pubic arch on slight traction. Subsequently, the right-sided anastomosis is started using the undyed suture, passing it outside to in on the bladder and then inside to out on the urethra, starting from 5 o'clock and proceeding clockwise until the contralateral suture is reached. Of note, both sutures end on the outer aspect of the urethral side of the anastomosis. The new catheter is advanced into the bladder and the balloon is filled with 10–15 cm^3 of sterile water and pulled back to the bladder neck by the assistant to verify appropriate positioning. The two sutures are tied together and the integrity of the anastomosis is tested under direct vision by instilling 180 cm^3 of water or saline as per our routine. We no longer

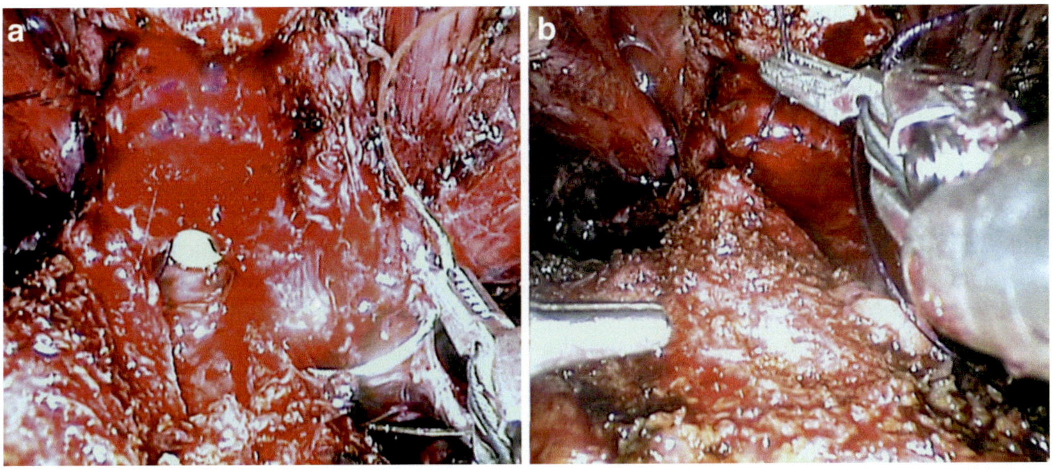

Fig. 18.11 Using a 0° endoscope and two large needle drivers, the urethrovesical anastomosis is performed using two 6.5-in. 3-0 Monocryl sutures on RB-1 needles (one dyed, one undyed) tied together extracorporeally (van Velthoven stitch). Using the dyed suture, the anastomosis is initiated with an outside-to-in throw at 5 o'clock on the bladder neck and then the needle is passed inside to out on the urethra in a clockwise manner until the 11 o'clock position is reached. The right-sided anastomosis is started using the undyed suture, passing it outside to in on the bladder and then inside to out on the urethra, starting from 5 o'clock and proceeding clockwise until the contralateral suture is reached. The two sutures are tied together and the integrity of the anastomosis is tested under direct vision

routinely leave closed suction drains in the vicinity of the anastomosis unless there is obvious fluid extravasation. Outcomes between interrupted and running urethrovesical anastomoses have been retrospectively compared in patients undergoing pure LRP [47], but it is the opinion of the authors that the robotic EndoWrist technology facilitates a watertight running anastomosis with decreased operative times and a shorter learning curve.

Lymph Node Dissection

The decision to perform a lymph node dissection at the time of prostatectomy is controversial and depends upon institutional protocol. We typically perform a node dissection in men with preoperative intermediate- to high-risk characteristics including palpable disease, PSA >10, and any Gleason score component of 4. As per surgeon's preference, the pelvic lymph node dissection can be performed any time after the bladder has been released from the anterior abdominal wall. In our practice, we most commonly perform the nodal dissection after the prostate specimen has been placed in an entrapment bag and prior to the urethrovesical anastomosis. The tissue overlying the external iliac vein is incised and the lymphatic nodal package is retracted medially until the pelvic side wall is visualized. The dissection is begun at the lymph node of Cloquet in the femoral canal and proceeds proximally toward the bifurcation of the iliac vessels. The obturator nerve represents the inferior limit of dissection and along with the obturator vessels must be carefully preserved. The nodal package between the obturator nerve and the hypogastric vein is also removed. Visible lymphatic structures are clipped and divided; alternatively, monopolar cautery may be used to free the nodal packets. We typically place a large locking polymer clip just beyond Cloquet's node prior to transecting the node packet. A second large clip is placed on the right packet for pathologic identification, and then both nodal packets are placed into one 10-mm EndoCatch™ bag for specimen retrieval.

Extraperitoneal Technique

The extraperitoneal (EP) technique for RALP has been described [48] and is currently the preferred approach of some surgeons. With this approach, the space of Retzius is developed using a round balloon dilator (US Surgical, Norwalk, CT) and by the placement of an infraumbilical 12-mm balloon trocar. Using the camera, the peritoneum is swept away from the anterior abdominal muscle, allowing the placement of the additional trocars under direct vision. Unlike the transperitoneal (TP) approach, only a 0° camera is necessary for the EP approach due to the lower camera port placement. The other procedural steps are similar to those of TP RALP, with the exception that posterior prostatic dissection must be performed following division of the bladder neck. Theoretical advantages include minimal risk to intra-abdominal organs, less peritoneal irritation to decrease the risk of postoperative ileus, and containment of urine or blood in the extraperitoneal space allowing for tamponade [49].

However, working within the confines of such a narrow working space can limit the ability to perform a posterior dissection resulting in more challenging neurovascular bundle preservation and urethrovesical anastomosis. Also, mimicking the anatomic limitations of the open RRP, an EP approach has an increased risk of lymphocele and requires placement of a closed suction drain if lymph node dissection is performed, which is not our routine in TP RALP. Retrospective series comparing TP and EP pure laparoscopic procedures have reported shorter operative times, decreased co-morbidity, and earlier time to convalescence [50], but these benefits have not been consistently reproduced in robotic series [51, 52]. In our experience the limitations of working within a more narrow space outweigh the potential benefits of staying out of the peritoneal cavity, but with comparable outcomes, surgeon comfort and experience will be the most significant factors in choosing a preferred approach.

Managing the Difficult Bladder Neck

As technological advances progress and more definitive functional outcomes data are reported, an increasing number of challenging cases will be performed robotically. These include patients with a large median lobe, large prostatic adenoma, and a history of prior prostatic surgery. When approaching a difficult bladder neck, general principles include placing traction on the Foley catheter balloon or performing a "pinch test" to identify the bladder neck margin. Entering an avascular fat plane also indicates that the proper prostatovesical junction has been identified; if there is doubt, some authors recommend dissecting in the midline to avoid excessive bleeding or dividing the bladder neck more proximally. It is important to err on the bladder side when the bladder neck anatomy is in question to ensure negative surgical margins.

Challenging Prostate Anatomy

A large median lobe can present several operative challenges during RALP. We do not routinely perform cystoscopy in the operating room on the day of scheduled RALP. If a large median lobe is seen at the time of transrectal ultrasound-guided prostate biopsy or suspected based on severe lower urinary tract symptoms, a cystoscopy may be electively performed in the office as part of preoperative planning. Intraoperatively, a large median lobe is suspected if the Foley catheter balloon deviates to one side when placed on traction. Fear of the potential for ureteral injury during the bladder neck resection can result in inadequate resection and positive margins at the posterior aspect and base of the prostate. An additional maneuver to increase bladder neck exposure and deliver the median lobe into the operative field is to perform a midline anterior cystotomy. We find that in most cases, retraction of the median lobe anteriorly using the left robotic instrument is adequate (Fig. 18.12a). Once the mucosa has been incised, care must be taken to stay out of the enucleation plane and continue through the posterior bladder neck (Fig. 18.12b). Prior dissection of the vasa and seminal vesicles may be helpful in such cases. If there is a history of previous prostatic surgery (TURP), anatomic landmarks are less evident due to postoperative scarring, and it may be necessary to take the bladder neck margin

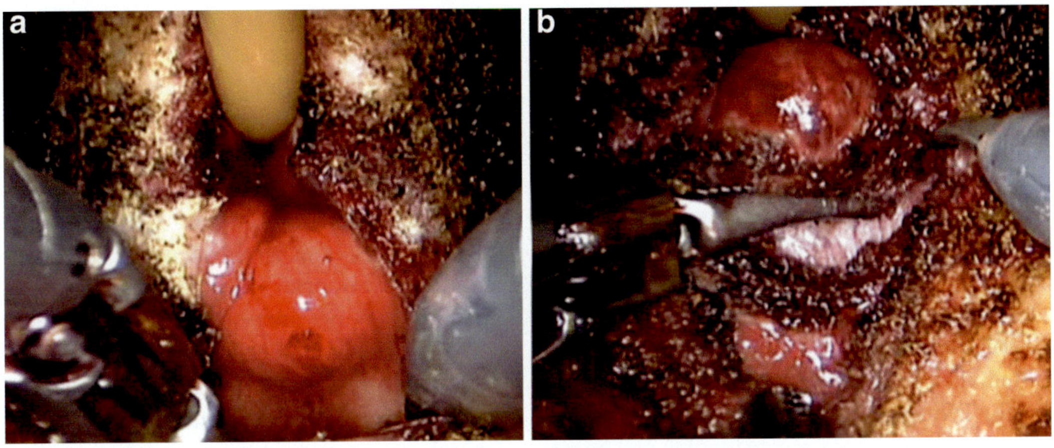

Fig. 18.12 In cases of a median lobe, retraction anteriorly using the left robotic instrument is often adequate to avoid ureteral injury during the bladder neck resection (**a**). Once the mucosa has been incised, care must be taken to stay out of the enucleation plane and continue through the posterior bladder neck (**b**)

even more proximally to ensure that a uniform negative margin is achieved.

Bladder Neck Reconstruction

The described maneuvers to resect adequate tissue to ensure a negative margin can result in a large bladder defect with the ureteral orifices close to the bladder neck (Fig. 18.13). Intraoperative administration of indigo carmine dye can be useful to identify the ureteral orifices to avoid iatrogenic injury, including local trauma during resection or subsequent obstruction during the urethrovesical anastomosis. It is important to continually inspect the bladder neck to identify the ureteral orifices as dissection proceeds. Once the cystotomy has been created, in rare cases, ureteral catheters or double-J ureteral stents can be placed intracorporeally without requiring cystoscopic access [53]. In complex cases it is our practice to place 5-Fr pediatric feeding tubes into the distal ureters and secure the ends with a single locking polymer clip for the duration of the repair. These are removed just prior to completion of the anterior portion of the urethrovesical anastomosis. If a large defect has been created, the bladder neck can be reconstructed using various techniques, including placement of interrupted vicryl sutures from the 2–4 o'clock and the 8–10 o'clock positions to narrow the diameter of the bladder neck to match the urethral diameter ("fish mouth") [54]. Our preference is to mobilize the bladder and perform posterior musculofascial reconstruction to both align and take tension off the urethrovesical anastomosis. When the anastomosis is complete, if further bladder neck reconstruction is required, the cystotomy

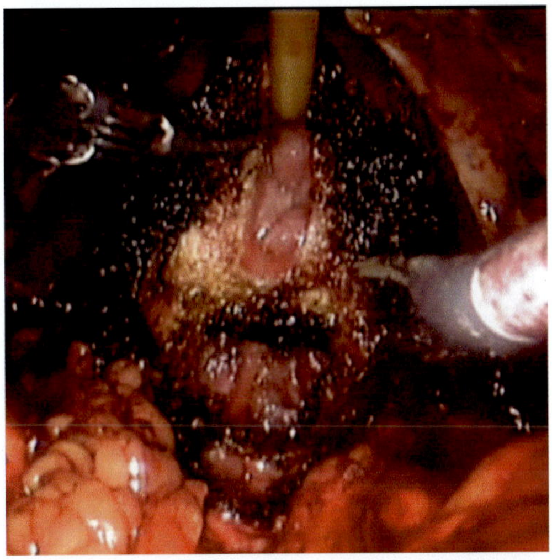

Fig. 18.13 Following prostate surgery, such as transurethral resection of the prostate, resecting adequate tissue to ensure a negative margin can result in a large bladder defect with the ureteral orifices close to the bladder neck. Consistent inspection of the bladder neck, intraoperative administration of indigo carmine dye, or placement of ureteral catheters can be useful to identify the ureteral orifices to avoid iatrogenic injury

can be closed with running or interrupted sutures in a reverse "tennis racquet" fashion. In all cases, it is recommended to fully test the anastomosis and to leave a closed suction drain if there is fluid extravasation or if an extensive bladder neck repair was undertaken. If the ureteral orifices are in close proximity to the urethrovesical anastomosis, some authors recommend leaving a stent or a ureteral catheter in place until the time of catheter removal to prevent postoperative obstruction [53].

Initial case series have demonstrated that minimally invasive prostatectomy techniques with complex bladder neck reconstruction can be performed in patients with significant gland size [55], median lobe [56], or previous prostate surgery [57]. Meeks et al. [58] reviewed 29 patients with a median lobe undergoing RALP and reported increases in operative times, estimated blood loss, and hospital stay, but no differences with regard to positive margins, postoperative complications, or continence at 6 months. Groups with more extensive experience have reported no significant differences in operative parameters, margin rates, or postoperative continence when comparing men with and without a large median lobe undergoing RALP [54]. Martin et al. [15] reported their experience performing RALP in patients with a history of prostate surgery (including simple prostatectomy, transurethral resection or photovaporization of the prostate, and open bladder neck reconstruction) and reported no significant differences with respect to operative parameters, complication rates, or margin status compared to normal controls. Currently long-term data are limited with regard to postoperative continence or the incidence of bladder neck contracture in patients that have undergone extensive bladder neck reconstruction. Outcomes in this select cohort of patients will surely be a focus of interest in future studies.

Management of Ureteral Injury

Reports of ureteral transection during open or minimally invasive prostatectomy are exceedingly rare [59], but patients with anatomic variations such as duplicated systems or ectopic insertion are at increased risk. Increased clinical suspicion for ureteral injury is necessary during dissection of the seminal vesicles or prostatovesical junction, particularly in patients with challenging anatomy that can distort distinguishing landmarks. If an iatrogenic injury is identified intraoperatively, open series have shown that distal ureteral injuries are better treated with ureteral reimplantation rather than primary ureteral repair [60]. After resection of the distal devitalized ureteral segment and spatulation, there have been several case reports describing robotic-assisted extravesical reimplantation using a running or an interrupted suture over a double JJ stent [61, 62] (Fig. 18.14). A closed suction drain should be left in the vicinity of the anastomosis and a cystogram should be performed prior to catheter removal. Postoperatively, an unrecognized injury to an ureteral orifice can present with decreased urine output, increased drain output, flank pain, an elevated serum creatinine from systemic urine reabsorption, or partial outflow obstruction from transient edema at the bladder

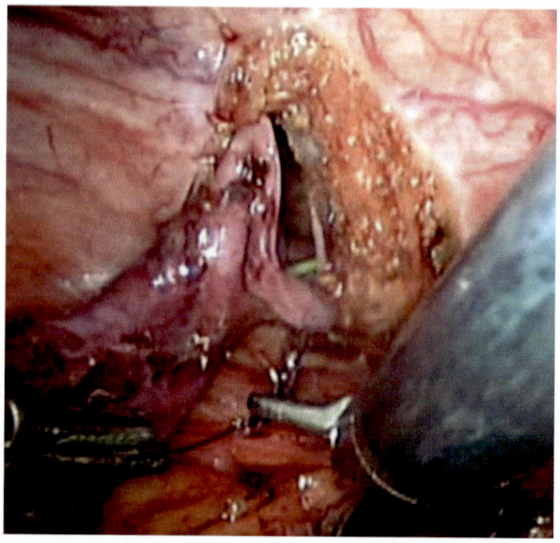

Fig. 18.14 If an iatrogenic ureteral injury is identified intraoperatively, after resection of the distal devitalized ureteral segment and spatulation, an extravesical reimplant can be performed using a running or an interrupted suture over a double JJ stent. A closed suction drain should be left in the vicinity of the anastomosis and a cystogram should be performed prior to catheter removal

neck [63]. A renal ultrasound can be performed to diagnose obstruction in the perioperative period; if detected, placement of a percutaneous nephrostomy drain and a subsequent staged repair is required to avoid disrupting a fresh anastomosis with a retrograde approach.

Oncologic Outcomes

Margin status is an important independent predictor of disease recurrence after radical prostatectomy and has been used as a surrogate for treatment efficacy [64]. While clinical and pathologic cancer characteristics are clearly associated with risk of a positive margin, it has been demonstrated that as a surgeon's experience increases, cancer control after radical prostatectomy improves. In a cohort of more than 7,700 patients undergoing RRP at four institutions over a 16-year period, Vickers et al. [65] reported a significant improvement in positive margin rates when stratified by number of cases performed (42%, <50 cases versus 11%, >1,000 cases). Although the learning curve for RALP is accelerated for surgeons already experienced with RRP (an estimated 12–100 cases) [66], these data are not trivial, and positive margin rates as high as 45% have been reported in early series [67]. As market forces have guided the adoption and application of new technology, a growing number of patients have been exposed to the learning curve with the potential for inferior oncologic outcomes.

As in open RRP, the apex of the prostate is at particular risk for positive margin due to poor definition of the prostate capsule, avoidance of the dorsal vein suture, and attempts to maximize urethral length [68, 69]. Maneuvers described to reduce apical margin rates include defatting the prostate over the endopelvic fascia, dividing the puboprostatic ligaments, cold incision of the DVC, and use of intraoperative frozen sections [37, 70]. Posterior positive margins due to errors in creating the plane of dissection between Denonvilliers' fascia and the rectum or tumor extension beyond the capsule and lateral margins due to overzealous nerve sparing can be avoided by carefully identifying anatomic planes and meticulous hemostasis [69]. An anterior bladder neck margin occurs when the boundary between the detrusor and the prostate is poorly defined and recent data have shown that bladder neck margin rates significantly decrease with cumulative surgical volume [71].

There is also speculation that an increased capsular incision rate, particularly during posterolateral neurovascular bundle mobilization early in the learning curve, may artificially inflate positive margin and extracapsular extension rates in RALP specimens [72]. Use of fine instruments and lack of haptic feedback may contribute to the iatrogenic capsular penetration in this patient population. While isolated capsular incision into tumor with otherwise organ-confined disease has been associated with an increased rate of disease recurrence in RRP specimens [73, 74], it remains unclear if an iatrogenic capsular incision into benign prostate tissue during nerve sparing has any significant impact on long-term prognosis.

In large series of surgeons with appropriate RALP experience, positive margin rates as low as 9.4–13% [11, 75] have been reported. In fact, a recent meta-analysis of 13 studies (3,039 patients) revealed no significant differences in overall risk or incidence of positive surgical margin comparing LRP and RALP with open RRP [76]. Surgeons with extensive experience with both open RRP and RALP have commented that the improved visualization, instrument precision, and reduced blood loss inherent to the robotic platform provide the opportunity to perform a better cancer operation compared to open techniques [77].

Unfortunately, prospective clinical trial data have failed to keep pace with the rapid dissemination of robotic technology into clinical practice. Currently it is unclear whether RALP is superior, equivalent, or inferior to open techniques with regard to cancer control. Until such data are available, decisions regarding surgical technique to afford optimal oncologic outcome will be determined by individual surgeon's experience and patient's preference.

Functional Outcomes

Comparing minimally invasive and open RRP, no significant differences have been shown with regard to incontinence or potency at 1 year [76]. However, the published literature must be carefully interpreted, as the majority of available studies are retrospective single-institution cohorts utilizing non-validated quality-of-life (QOL) instruments. In a recent analysis, Burnett et al. concluded that clinical studies reporting erectile function outcomes after localized prostate cancer treatment demonstrate poorly interpretable and inconsistent methods of assessment as well as widely disparate rates of erectile dysfunction [78]. Similarly, although the current consensus is that return to continence is more rapid following RALP [79], lack of a standard postprostatectomy incontinence (PPI) definition or validated measurement instrument has made comparison between differing techniques or institutional experiences challenging.

In the largest retrospective series to date, Baddani et al. reported an 82% potency rate in men with normal preoperative erections (SHIM>22) compared to 77% of men with mild preoperative erectile dysfunction, with >40% of men requiring phosphodiesterase-5 inhibitor (PDE5) therapy. Overall, 93% of men achieved urinary control at 1 year, defined as wearing ≤1 pad per day, and 82% had absence of any urinary leakage even on stress maneuvers [11]. Although these results are certainly encouraging, development and uniform distribution of validated QOL instruments is mandatory to discern differences between open and minimally invasive techniques.

Continence

Although no standardized definition of PPI exists, long-term continence data for men undergoing RALP have been reported. In one series, reported continence rates, defined as wearing ≤1 pad per day, were as high as 95% at 3 months [66]. Similar to RRP and LRP, continence rates tend to increase throughout the follow-up period, and at 12 months, continence rates as high as 84–98% have been reported [80, 81]. Although comparative data are limited, RALP appears to result in earlier return to continence compared to RRP [79] and LRP [82].

A mechanism to explain improved continence rates following RALP has not been fully delineated, but key factors appear to be minimal disturbance to the urethra and surrounding musculature and a tension-free urethrovesical anastomosis. Suggested technical modifications to improve continence include preservation of urethral length and varying degrees of anterior and posterior reconstruction. Tewari et al. [83] described a technique for preserving the puboprostatic collar and reported 95% continence rates at 4 weeks following catheter removal. Likewise, Patel et al. [75] reported excellent continence results utilizing a suspension suture between the urethra and the pubic symphysis. More recently, Rocco et al. [42] reported excellent short-term continence rates with restoration of the posterior aspect of the rhabdosphincter. In general, most robotic surgeons now employ one or a combination of modifications including preservation of the puboprostatic ligaments, suspension of the urethra and ligaments to the posterior pubis, and reconstruction of the posterior striated sphincter. Prospective evaluation of continence with standardized data collection techniques is needed to determine if there is any true benefit to these modifications.

Potency

Despite refinement of nerve-sparing technique to minimize local trauma and thermal injury, sexual outcomes remain widely variable following radical prostatectomy, and recent data have emerged demonstrating that clinically significant improvement in potency can occur beyond 2 years following RRP [84]. Factors influencing outcomes include differences in preoperative characteristics, patient age, baseline erectile function, surgeon's experience, surgical technique, and sparing of neurovascular structures [85]. Single-institution data using validated

QOL instruments have recently become available and report 90% potency at 2 years post-RALP; however, only 46% of patients returned to baseline function. Further, there were no significant differences between unilateral and bilateral nerve-sparing procedures. These data indicate that there is still considerable room for modification and improvement in nerve-sparing techniques [86].

The "veil of Aphrodite" (antegrade high fascial release) technique developed by Menon et al. and cautery-free dissection have been widely accepted and incorporated into clinical practice to minimize neurapraxia and traction injury during dissection of the neurovascular bundles [24]. It is important to note that the initial series incorporating these modifications did not report a significant increase in positive apical margin rates despite preservation of the prostatic fascia [87, 88]. Despite advances in the understanding of pelvic neurovascular anatomy, the contribution of accessory pudendal arterial branches and nervous tissue adjacent to the seminal vesicles to potency is purely speculative at this point and clinical outcomes data are lacking [89]. It remains to be seen if more experimental techniques including regional hypothermia and hydrodissection will translate into clinically significant improvement of potency outcomes. As with continence, prospective data collection with standardized validated QOL instruments is needed to determine whether improved visualization and preservation of neurovascular anatomy with the robotic platform provides any advantage with respect to long-term potency outcomes compared to conventional RRP or LP.

Bladder Neck Contracture

While bladder neck contracture (BNC) has been reported to occur in 6–15% of men undergoing open RRP [90], a significantly decreased incidence has been reported in men undergoing minimally invasive prostatectomy [91]. While follow-up is extremely limited, the reported incidence of BNC in large series of patients undergoing RALP is currently 0–2% [91–93]. The sequence of events contributing to stricture of the urethrovesical anastomosis is unclear, but potential technical and clinical factors implicated include urinary leakage, previous prostate surgery (TURP), operative technique, indwelling catheter duration, type of anastomotic suture, excessive luminal narrowing, failure of anastomotic approximation, excessive blood loss/pelvic hematoma, and anastomotic tension or ischemia [94].

Although controversial, it has been postulated that bladder neck "stomatization" during RRP (tennis racquet reconfiguration and eversion of the bladder neck mucosa), and not urinary leakage, may result in increased tissue ischemia and fibrosis resulting in increased contracture rates [91, 92]. While the optimal urethrovesical closure involves creating a watertight, tension-free anastomosis with mucosal apposition and correct realignment of the urethra, mucosal eversion may not in itself be necessary to produce a watertight anastomosis [95]. Whether bladder neck reconfiguration/mucosal eversion exacerbated by anastomotic defects and urinary extravasation plays a role in the development of BNC has not been established. However, it has become increasingly evident that these factors can be avoided using the robotic platform, and it will be interesting to see if these technical adjustments will translate into a reduced rate of BNC following RALP with long-term follow-up.

Conclusions

Compared to RRP, RALP offers the same advantages of minimally invasive surgery as LRP, including enhanced visualization, decreased bleeding and transfusion rates, shorter hospital stay, and faster recovery [79, 96, 97]. Early pathological outcomes are comparable to RRP and LRP with acceptable positive margin rates; however, long-term cancer control results are still maturing. With 1- and 2-year follow-up data available, continence and potency results appear equivalent to RRP and LRP, and with further technical modifications, RALP may ultimately prove to be superior. As market forces continue to drive the adoption and utilization of robotic technology, cost remains a matter of debate at the present time. For surgeons experienced with open RRP techniques, the learning curve of robotic prostatectomy is overcome more quickly compared to LRP, and with increasing experience, challenging anatomy and previous prostate surgery are no longer contraindications for a robotic-assisted approach.

Critical Operative Steps

1. Proper port placement is essential to maximize working space, prevent contact between instruments, and complete the critical portions of the operation, including ligation of the dorsal venous complex and urethrovesical anastomosis.
2. During apical dissection and ligation of the dorsal venous complex, minimizing dissection of periurethral attachments and puboprostatic ligaments may improve early return of continence.
3. Maneuvers such as manipulating the Foley catheter balloon or bimanual compression ("bladder neck pinch") can be utilized to identify the prostatovesical junction and facilitate bladder neck transection with negative margins in an avascular plane.
4. With anterior retraction of the vasa deferentia and seminal vesicles, posterior prostatic dissection should be performed by incising Denonvilliers' fascia and developing the plane between the prostate and the anterior rectum until the apex of the prostate is reached. This ensures sufficient tissue coverage over both the prostate specimen and the rectum and ensures adequate exposure for obtaining control of the lateral vascular pedicles.
5. For neurovascular bundle mobilization, the plane between the prostatic fascia and the capsule of the prostate is entered using sharp dissection only and the neurovascular bundles are dissected free in either an antegrade or a retrograde manner.
6. Posterior reconstruction of Denonvilliers' musculofascial plate ("Rocco stitch") and perineal pressure facilitate performance of a running watertight urethrovesical anastomosis, which in contemporary practice rarely requires placement of a closed suction drain.
7. Bladder neck reconstruction is rarely required prior to performing the urethrovesical anastomosis, but if necessary, the remaining open bladder neck can be reconstructed with running or interrupted sutures in a "reverse tennis racquet technique."

Critical Instruments and Supplies

1. Detailed pathologic and clinical staging information as well as baseline sexual health characteristics to guide decisions regarding nerve sparing.
2. Reliable preoperative transrectal ultrasound information to document prostate size and anatomic characteristics such as the presence of a median lobe to guide operative dissection.
3. Reliable bedside assistants and experienced operating room staff are essential to ensure smooth transitions between procedural steps.
4. *da Vinci robotic platform* (Intuitive Surgical, Sunnyvale, CA, USA)—advantages include high-definition stereoscopic visualization and enhanced dexterity (EndoWrist™ technology), allowing the ability to perform precise suturing for reconstruction.
5. *Gyrus PlasmaKinetic (PK) Bipolar Grasper* (Gyrus ACMI, Southborough, MA, USA)—Electrosurgical device utilizing high-powered pulsed bipolar energy that is designed to operate at temperatures that allow effective tissue dissection but result in minimal collateral damage and adherence to tissue.
6. *MicroFrance Johann Forceps* (Surgical Instrument Group Holdings, Ltd., Croydon, England)—5-mm rigid grasping instrument with a 20-mm fenestrated jaw provides reliable atraumatic retraction by the bedside assistant during prostatic dissection.

7. *Lapra-Ty Clip* (Ethicon Inc., Somerville, NJ, USA)—Polydioxanone suture clips that are useful as a substitute for knot tying during running suture for bladder neck and musculofascial reconstruction. The use during the urethrovesical anastomosis is avoided as per surgeon's preference due to the risks of clip migration and stone formation.
8. *Weck Hem-o-lok® Ligation System* (Teleflex Medical, Research Triangle Park, NC, USA)—Flexible non-absorbable polymer locking clips that can be utilized by the surgical assistant through a 12-mm port during ligation of the lateral prostate vascular pedicles.

References

1. Benjamin JA. Hugh Hampton Young 1870–1945. Science. 26 Oct 1945;102(2652):416–7.
2. Miller JA, Staunton MD. The birth of retropubic prostatectomy – Millin. J R Soc Med. Aug 1989;82(8):494–5.
3. Reiner WG, Walsh PC. An anatomical approach to the surgical management of the dorsal vein and Santorini's plexus during radical retropubic surgery. J Urol. Feb 1979;121(2):198–200.
4. Lepor H, Gregerman M, Crosby R, Mostofi FK, Walsh PC. Precise localization of the autonomic nerves from the pelvic plexus to the corpora cavernosa: a detailed anatomical study of the adult male pelvis. J Urol. Feb 1985;133(2):207–12.
5. Litwin MS, Gore JL, Kwan L, et al. Quality of life after surgery, external beam irradiation, or brachytherapy for early-stage prostate cancer. Cancer. 1 Jun 2007;109(11):2239–47.
6. Steineck G, Helgesen F, Adolfsson J, et al. Quality of life after radical prostatectomy or watchful waiting. N Engl J Med. 12 Sep 2002;347(11):790–6.
7. Schuessler WW, Schulam PG, Clayman RV, Kavoussi LR. Laparoscopic radical prostatectomy: initial short-term experience. Urology. Dec 1997;50(6):854–7.
8. Guillonneau B, Vallancien G. Laparoscopic radical prostatectomy: the Montsouris experience. J Urol. Feb 2000;163(2):418–22.
9. Rassweiler J, Seemann O, Schulze M, Teber D, Hatzinger M, Frede T. Laparoscopic versus open radical prostatectomy: a comparative study at a single institution. J Urol. May 2003;169(5):1689–93.
10. Abbou CC, Hoznek A, Salomon L, et al. Remote laparoscopic radical prostatectomy carried out with a robot report of a case. Prog Urol. Sep 2000;10(4):520–3.
11. Badani KK, Kaul S, Menon M. Evolution of robotic radical prostatectomy: assessment after 2766 procedures. Cancer. 1 Nov 2007;110(9):1951–8.
12. D'Amico AV, Whittington R, Malkowicz SB, et al. Biochemical outcome after radical prostatectomy or external beam radiation therapy for patients with clinically localized prostate carcinoma in the prostate specific antigen era. Cancer. 15 Jul 2002;95(2):281–6.
13. Daneshmand S, Quek ML, Stein JP, et al. Prognosis of patients with lymph node positive prostate cancer following radical prostatectomy: long-term results. J Urol. Dec 2004;172(6 Pt 1):2252–5.
14. Kaouk JH, Hafron J, Goel R, Haber GP, Jones JS. Robotic salvage retropubic prostatectomy after radiation/brachytherapy: initial results. BJU Int. Jul 2008;102(1):93–6.
15. Martin AD, Desai PJ, Nunez RN, et al. Does a history of previous surgery or radiation to the prostate affect outcomes of robot-assisted radical prostatectomy? BJU Int. Dec 2008;103(12):1696–8.
16. Jhaveri JK, Tan GY, Scherr DS, Tewari AK. Robot-assisted laparoscopic radical prostatectomy in the renal allograft transplant recipient. J Endourol. Nov 2008;22(11):2475–9.
17. Wolf JS, Jr., Bennett CJ, Dmochowski RR, Hollenbeck BK, Pearle MS, Schaeffer AJ. Best practice policy statement on urologic surgery antimicrobial prophylaxis. J Urol. Apr 2008;179(4):1379–90.
18. Forrest JB, Clemens JQ, Finamore P, et al. AUA best practice statement for the prevention of deep vein thrombosis in patients undergoing urologic surgery. J Urol. Mar 2009;181(3):1170–7.
19. Tsao AK, Smaldone MC, Averch TD, Jackman SV. Robot-assisted laparoscopic prostatectomy: the first 100 patients—improving patient safety and outcomes. J Endourol. Mar 2009;23(3):481–4.
20. Guenaga KK, Matos D, Wille-Jorgensen P. Mechanical bowel preparation for elective colorectal surgery. Cochrane Database Syst Rev. 2009; Issue 1. Art. No.: CD001544. DOI: 10.1002/14651858.CD001544.pub3
21. Girardis M, Da Broi U, Antonutto G, Pasetto A. The effect of laparoscopic cholecystectomy on cardiovascular function and pulmonary gas exchange. Anesth Analg. Jul 1996;83(1):134–40.
22. Hardacre JM, Talamini MA. Pulmonary and hemodynamic changes during laparoscopy – are they important? Surgery Mar 2000;127(3):241–4.
23. Phong SV, Koh LK. Anaesthesia for robotic-assisted radical prostatectomy: considerations for laparoscopy in the Trendelenburg position. Anaesth Intens Care. Apr 2007;35(2):281–5.
24. Menon M, Shrivastava A, Kaul S, et al. Vattikuti Institute prostatectomy: contemporary technique and analysis of results. Eur Urol. Mar 2007;51(3):648–57; discussion 648–57.

25. Tewari AK, Rao SR. Anatomical foundations and surgical manoeuvres for precise identification of the prostatovesical junction during robotic radical prostatectomy. BJU Int. Oct 2006;98(4):833–7.
26. Guillonneau B, Gupta R, El Fettouh H, Cathelineau X, Baumert H, Vallancien G. Laparoscopic [correction of laproscopic] management of rectal injury during laparoscopic [correction of laproscopic] radical prostatectomy. J Urol. May 2003;169(5): 1694–6.
27. Shekarriz B, Upadhyay J, Wood DP. Intraoperative, perioperative, and long-term complications of radical prostatectomy. Urol Clin North Am. Aug 2001;28(3):639–53.
28. Yee DS, Ornstein DK. Repair of rectal injury during robotic-assisted laparoscopic prostatectomy. Urology. Aug 2008;72(2):428–31.
29. Guillonneau B, Vallancien G. Laparoscopic radical prostatectomy: the Montsouris technique. J Urol. Jun 2000;163(6):1643–9.
30. Costello AJ, Brooks M, Cole OJ. Anatomical studies of the neurovascular bundle and cavernosal nerves. BJU Int. Nov 2004;94(7):1071–6.
31. Nielsen ME, Schaeffer EM, Marschke P, Walsh PC. High anterior release of the levator fascia improves sexual function following open radical retropubic prostatectomy. J Urol. Dec 2008;180(6):2557–64; discussion 2564.
32. Kaul S, Savera A, Badani K, Fumo M, Bhandari A, Menon M. Functional outcomes and oncological efficacy of Vattikuti Institute prostatectomy with veil of Aphrodite nerve-sparing: an analysis of 154 consecutive patients. BJU Int. Mar 2006;97(3): 467–72.
33. Martinez-Salamanca JI, Ramanathan R, Rao S, et al. Second prize: pelvic neuroanatomy and innovative approaches to minimize nerve damage and maximize cancer control in patients undergoing robot-assisted radical prostatectomy. J Endourol. Jun 2008;22(6):1137–46.
34. Rogers CG, Trock BP, Walsh PC. Preservation of accessory pudendal arteries during radical retropubic prostatectomy: surgical technique and results. Urology. Jul 2004;64(1):148–51.
35. Finley DS, Osann K, Skarecky D, Ahlering TE. Hypothermic nerve-sparing radical prostatectomy: rationale, feasibility, and effect on early continence. Urology. Apr 2009;73(4):691–6.
36. Guru KA, Perlmutter AE, Butt ZM, Peabody JO. Hydrodissection for preservation of neurovascular bundle during robot-assisted radical prostatectomy. Can J Urol. Apr 2008;15(2):4000–3.
37. Guru KA, Perlmutter AE, Sheldon MJ, et al. Apical margins after robot-assisted radical prostatectomy: does technique matter? J Endourol. Jan 2009;23(1):123–7.
38. Nguyen MM, Turna B, Santos BR, et al. The use of an endoscopic stapler vs suture ligature for dorsal vein control in laparoscopic prostatectomy: operative outcomes. BJU Int. Feb 2008;101(4):463–6.
39. Deliveliotis C, Protogerou V, Alargof E, Varkarakis J. Radical prostatectomy: bladder neck preservation and puboprostatic ligament sparing – effects on continence and positive margins. Urology. Nov 2002;60(5):855–8.
40. Stolzenburg JU, Liatsikos EN, Rabenalt R, et al. Nerve sparing endoscopic extraperitoneal radical prostatectomy – effect of puboprostatic ligament preservation on early continence and positive margins. Eur Urol. Jan 2006;49(1):103–11; discussion 111–2.
41. Takenaka A, Tewari AK, Leung RA, et al. Preservation of the puboprostatic collar and puboperineoplasty for early recovery of urinary continence after robotic prostatectomy: anatomic basis and preliminary outcomes. Eur Urol. Feb 2007;51(2):433–40; discussion 440.
42. Rocco F, Carmignani L, Acquati P, et al. Restoration of posterior aspect of rhabdosphincter shortens continence time after radical retropubic prostatectomy. J Urol. Jun 2006;175(6):2201–6.
43. Tewari A, Jhaveri J, Rao S, et al. Total reconstruction of the vesico-urethral junction. BJU Int. Apr 2008;101(7):871–7.
44. Menon M, Hemal AK, Tewari A, Shrivastava A, Bhandari A. The technique of apical dissection of the prostate and urethrovesical anastomosis in robotic radical prostatectomy. BJU Int. Apr 2004;93(6): 715–9.
45. Nguyen MM, Kamoi K, Stein RJ, et al. Early continence outcomes of posterior musculofascial plate reconstruction during robotic and laparoscopic prostatectomy. BJU Int. May 2008;101(9):1135–9.
46. Coughlin G, Dangle PP, Patil NN, et al. Surgery illustrated – focus on details. Modified posterior reconstruction of the rhabdosphincter: application to robotic-assisted laparoscopic prostatectomy. BJU Int. Nov 2008;102(10):1482–5.
47. Teber D, Erdogru T, Cresswell J, Gozen AS, Frede T, Rassweiler JJ. Analysis of three different vesicourethral anastomotic techniques in laparoscopic radical prostatectomy. World J Urol. Dec 2008;26(6):617–22.
48. Gettman MT, Hoznek A, Salomon L, et al. Laparoscopic radical prostatectomy: description of the extraperitoneal approach using the da Vinci robotic system. J Urol. Aug 2003;170(2 Pt 1):416–9.
49. Joseph JV, Rosenbaum R, Madeb R, Erturk E, Patel HR. Robotic extraperitoneal radical prostatectomy: an alternative approach. J Urol. Mar 2006;175(3 Pt 1):945–50; discussion 951.
50. Brown JA, Rodin D, Lee B, Dahl DM. Transperitoneal versus extraperitoneal approach to laparoscopic radical prostatectomy: an assessment of 156 cases. Urology. Feb 2005;65(2):320–4.
51. Atug F, Castle EP, Woods M, Srivastav SK, Thomas R, Davis R. Transperitoneal versus extraperitoneal robotic-assisted radical prostatectomy: is one better than the other? Urology. Nov 2006;68(5): 1077–81.

52. Madi R, Daignault S, Wood DP. Extraperitoneal v intraperitoneal robotic prostatectomy: analysis of operative outcomes. J Endourol. Dec 2007;21(12):1553–7.
53. Rehman J, Chughtai B, Guru K, Shabsigh R, Samadi DB. Management of an enlarged median lobe with ureteral orifices at the margin of bladder neck during robotic-assisted laparoscopic prostatectomy. Can J Urol. Feb 2009;16(1):4490–4.
54. Jenkins LC, Nogueira M, Wilding GE, et al. Median lobe in robot-assisted radical prostatectomy: evaluation and management. Urology. May 2008;71(5):810–3.
55. El-Hakim A, Leung RA, Richstone L, Kim TS, Te AE, Tewari AK. Athermal robotic technique of prostatectomy in patients with large prostate glands (>75 g): technique and initial results. BJU Int. Jul 2006;98(1):47–9.
56. Sarle R, Tewari A, Hemal AK, Menon M. Robotic-assisted anatomic radical prostatectomy: technical difficulties due to a large median lobe. Urol Int. 2005;74(1):92–4.
57. Jaffe J, Stakhovsky O, Cathelineau X, Barret E, Vallancien G, Rozet F. Surgical outcomes for men undergoing laparoscopic radical prostatectomy after transurethral resection of the prostate. J Urol. Aug 2007;178(2):483–7; discussion 487.
58. Meeks JJ, Zhao L, Greco KA, Macejko A, Nadler RB. Impact of prostate median lobe anatomy on robotic-assisted laparoscopic prostatectomy. Urology. Feb 2009;73(2):323–7.
59. Vallancien G, Cathelineau X, Baumert H, Doublet JD, Guillonneau B. Complications of transperitoneal laparoscopic surgery in urology: review of 1,311 procedures at a single center. J Urol. Jul 2002;168(1):23–6.
60. Schraudenbach P, Bermejo CE. Management of the complications of radical prostatectomy. Curr Urol Rep. May 2007;8(3):197–202.
61. Dinlenc CZ, Gerber E, Wagner JR. Ureteral reimplantation during robot assisted laparoscopic radical prostatectomy. J Urol. Sep 2004;172(3):905.
62. Larson JA, Tomaszewski JJ, Smaldone MC, Jackman SV. Robotic assisted laparoscopic extravesical ureteroneocystostomy for management of adult ureteral duplication with upper pole prostatic urethral insertion. JSLS. 2009;13(3):458–61.
63. Elliott SP, McAninch JW. Ureteral injuries: external and iatrogenic. Urol Clin North Am. Feb 2006;33(1):55–66, vi.
64. Stephenson AJ, Scardino PT, Eastham JA, et al. Postoperative nomogram predicting the 10-year probability of prostate cancer recurrence after radical prostatectomy. J Clin Oncol. 1 Oct 2005;23(28):7005–12.
65. Vickers AJ, Bianco FJ, Serio AM, et al. The surgical learning curve for prostate cancer control after radical prostatectomy. J Natl Cancer Inst. 1 Aug 2007;99(15):1171–7.
66. Ahlering TE, Skarecky D, Lee D, Clayman RV. Successful transfer of open surgical skills to a laparoscopic environment using a robotic interface: initial experience with laparoscopic radical prostatectomy. J Urol. Nov 2003;170(5):1738–41.
67. Atug F, Castle EP, Srivastav SK, Burgess SV, Thomas R, Davis R. Positive surgical margins in robotic-assisted radical prostatectomy: impact of learning curve on oncologic outcomes. Eur Urol. May 2006;49(5):866–71; discussion 871–862.
68. Sofer M, Hamilton-Nelson KL, Civantos F, Soloway MS. Positive surgical margins after radical retropubic prostatectomy: the influence of site and number on progression. J Urol. Jun 2002;167(6): 2453–6.
69. Smith JA, Jr., Chan RC, Chang SS, et al. A comparison of the incidence and location of positive surgical margins in robotic assisted laparoscopic radical prostatectomy and open retropubic radical prostatectomy. J Urol. Dec 2007;178(6):2385–9; discussion 2389–90.
70. Ahlering TE, Eichel L, Edwards RA, Lee DI, Skarecky DW. Robotic radical prostatectomy: a technique to reduce pT2 positive margins. Urology. Dec 2004;64(6):1224–8.
71. Weizer AZ, Ye Z, Hollingsworth JM, et al. Adoption of new technology and healthcare quality: surgical margins after robotic prostatectomy. Urology. Jul 2007;70(1):96–100.
72. Patel VR, Shah S, Arend D. Histopathologic outcomes of robotic radical prostatectomy. Sc World J. 2006;6:2566–72.
73. Chuang AY, Nielsen ME, Hernandez DJ, Walsh PC, Epstein JI. The significance of positive surgical margin in areas of capsular incision in otherwise organ confined disease at radical prostatectomy. J Urol. Oct 2007;178(4 Pt 1):1306–10.
74. Shuford MD, Cookson MS, Chang SS, et al. Adverse prognostic significance of capsular incision with radical retropubic prostatectomy. J Urol. Jul 2004;172(1):119–23.
75. Patel VR, Thaly R, Shah K. Robotic radical prostatectomy: outcomes of 500 cases. BJU Int. May 2007;99(5):1109–12.
76. Parsons JK, Bennett JL. Outcomes of retropubic, laparoscopic, and robotic-assisted prostatectomy. Urology. Aug 2008;72(2):412–6.
77. Skarecky DW, Brenner M, Rajan S, et al. Zero positive surgical margins after radical prostatectomy: is the end in sight. Expert Rev Med Devices. Nov 2008;5(6):709–17.
78. Burnett AL, Aus G, Canby-Hagino ED, et al. Erectile function outcome reporting after clinically localized prostate cancer treatment. J Urol. Aug 2007;178(2):597–601.
79. Tewari A, Srivasatava A, Menon M. A prospective comparison of radical retropubic and robot-assisted prostatectomy: experience in one institution. BJU Int. Aug 2003;92(3):205–10.

80. Bentas W, Wolfram M, Jones J, Brautigam R, Kramer W, Binder J. Robotic technology and the translation of open radical prostatectomy to laparoscopy: the early Frankfurt experience with robotic radical prostatectomy and one year follow-up. Eur Urol. Aug 2003;44(2):175–81.
81. Patel VR, Tully AS, Holmes R, Lindsay J. Robotic radical prostatectomy in the community setting – the learning curve and beyond: initial 200 cases. J Urol. Jul 2005;174(1):269–72.
82. Hakimi AA, Blitstein J, Feder M, Shapiro E, Ghavamian R. Direct comparison of surgical and functional outcomes of robotic-assisted versus pure laparoscopic radical prostatectomy: single-surgeon experience. Urology. Jan 2009;73(1):119–23.
83. Tewari AK, Bigelow K, Rao S, et al. Anatomic restoration technique of continence mechanism and preservation of puboprostatic collar: a novel modification to achieve early urinary continence in men undergoing robotic prostatectomy. Urology. Apr 2007;69(4):726–31.
84. Glickman L, Godoy G, Lepor H. Changes in continence and erectile function between 2 and 4 years after radical prostatectomy. J Urol. Feb 2009;181(2):731–5.
85. Walsh PC, Marschke P, Ricker D, Burnett AL. Patient-reported urinary continence and sexual function after anatomic radical prostatectomy. Urology. Jan 2000;55(1):58–61.
86. Rodriguez E, Jr, Finley DS, Skarecky D, Ahlering TE. Single institution 2-year patient reported validated sexual function outcomes after nerve sparing robot assisted radical prostatectomy. J Urol. Jan 2009;181(1):259–63.
87. Menon M, Kaul S, Bhandari A, Shrivastava A, Tewari A, Hemal A. Potency following robotic radical prostatectomy: a questionnaire based analysis of outcomes after conventional nerve sparing and prostatic fascia sparing techniques. J Urol. Dec 2005;174(6):2291–6, discussion 2296.
88. Ahlering TE, Eichel L, Chou D, Skarecky DW. Feasibility study for robotic radical prostatectomy cautery-free neurovascular bundle preservation. Urology. May 2005;65(5):994–7.
89. Mulhall JP, Secin FP, Guillonneau B. Artery sparing radical prostatectomy – myth or reality? J Urol Mar 2008;179(3):827–31.
90. Borboroglu PG, Sands JP, Roberts JL, Amling CL. Risk factors for vesicourethral anastomotic stricture after radical prostatectomy. Urology. Jul 2000;56(1):96–100.
91. Msezane LP, Reynolds WS, Gofrit ON, Shalhav AL, Zagaja GP, Zorn KC. Bladder neck contracture after robot-assisted laparoscopic radical prostatectomy: evaluation of incidence and risk factors and impact on urinary function. J Endourol. Jan 2008;22(1): 97–104.
92. Webb DR, Sethi K, Gee K. An analysis of the causes of bladder neck contracture after open and robot-assisted laparoscopic radical prostatectomy. BJU Int. Apr 2009;103(7):957–63.
93. El-Hakim A, Leung RA, Tewari A. Robotic prostatectomy: a pooled analysis of published literature. Expert Rev Anticancer Ther. Jan 2006;6(1):11–20.
94. Park R, Martin S, Goldberg JD, Lepor H. Anastomotic strictures following radical prostatectomy: insights into incidence, effectiveness of intervention, effect on continence, and factors predisposing to occurrence. Urology. Apr 2000;57(4):742–6.
95. van Velthoven RF, Ahlering TE, Peltier A, Skarecky DW, Clayman RV. Technique for laparoscopic running urethrovesical anastomosis: the single knot method. Urology. Apr 2003;61(4):699–702.
96. Herrmann TR, Rabenalt R, Stolzenburg JU, et al. Oncological and functional results of open, robot-assisted and laparoscopic radical prostatectomy: does surgical approach and surgical experience matter? World J Urol. Apr 2007;25(2):149–60.
97. Krambeck AE, DiMarco DS, Rangel LJ, et al. Radical prostatectomy for prostatic adenocarcinoma: a matched comparison of open retropubic and robot-assisted techniques. BJU Int. Feb 2009;103(4): 448–53.

Part VIII
NOTES and LESS—Future Directions in MIS Reconstructive Surgery

Chapter 19

The Role of NOTES and LESS in Minimally Invasive Reconstructive Urological Surgery

Mark D. Sawyer and Lee Ponsky

This chapter contains a video segment which can be found at the URL: http://www.springerimages.com/ost

Introduction

Natural orifice translumenal endoscopic surgery (NOTES^{TM}) and laparoendoscopic single-site surgery (LESS) are exciting new developments in the evolution of minimally invasive surgery with potential application to urologic reconstructive surgery. Both represent a natural progression of laparoscopic surgery with ever fewer and smaller incisions and each shares common challenges. NOTES^{TM} as a concept offers the potential for surgery without any transcutaneous abdominal incisions. LESS appears to offer a natural intermediate step toward a NOTES^{TM} approach and may prove more practical for many applications. LESS may be described as a laparoscopic procedure with a single cutaneous incision through which multiple trocars or ports are placed. The advantages of either approach relative to standard laparoscopy will need to be established. There are rapid technological advances that are propelling both approaches forward, making an exhaustive description of the techniques and equipment unfeasible. Each approach will ultimately need to demonstrate advantages and will require sufficient acceptance in the surgical community to be commercially viable for industry.

L. Ponsky (✉)
Division of Orologic Oncology, Department of Urology, Center of Urologic Oncology and Minimally Invasive Therapies, University Hospitals Case Medical Center, Cleveland, OH, USA
e-mail: lee.ponsky@uhhospitals.org

Potential Benefits of NOTES^{TM} and LESS

An obvious benefit of LESS is potential for improved cosmesis with fewer and possibly smaller scars, even a nearly invisible scar if performed at the umbilicus. Theoretically, there may be reduced pain as well. Potential benefits of NOTES^{TM} (in addition to cosmesis) could include reduced surgical site infections; reduced incidence of hernias at incision sites; reduction of adhesions (which could in turn reduce incidence of small bowel obstructions); reduced pain; and the possibility of performing procedures without anesthesia, even outside the operating room [1, 2]. Finally, it could be beneficial in certain patient populations, such as morbidly obese individuals, for whom internal organs might be more easily reached translumenally than via a transabdominal approach [1].

Technical Challenges of NOTES^{TM} and LESS

A surgical principle of traditional laparoscopy is a requirement for triangulation of instruments and the scope. As typically practiced, both LESS and NOTES^{TM} (unless using a multiple orifice approach) face challenges of coaxial instrumentation. With coaxial instrumentation, the scope and instruments are in the same

M.C. Ost (ed.), *Robotic and Laparoscopic Reconstructive Surgery in Children and Adults*, Current Clinical Urology, DOI 10.1007/978-1-60327-914-7_19, © Springer Science+Business Media, LLC 2011

working plane, which can limit perspective. Urologists are already familiar with this situation in the setting of transurethral surgery and endourology procedures of the upper urinary tract. However, these typically do not involve more than a single working instrument, as may be required for many NOTES™ and LESS procedures. Strategies for overcoming coaxial limitations are detailed later and include articulating instruments, novel platforms, and port devices, magnetic instruments [3], and potentially intracorporeal robotic platforms or "microrobots" [4].

Because of the similarities to traditional laparoscopy, we begin our discussion with LESS.

Laparoendoscopic Single-Site Surgery (LESS)

Nomenclature

Nomenclature for laparoscopy involving a single incision has been a source of both confusion and controversy. Terms and acronyms used in the literature have included SPA ("single-port access"), SILS ("single-incision laparoscopic surgery"), SAS ("single-access surgery"), OPUS ("one-port umbilical surgery"), and numerous others. Some have contended that the umbilicus represents an "embryonic natural orifice" and have proposed the term E-NOTES™ (with the "E" designating "embryonic") [5]. In an effort to reduce the confusion, there has been a desire to unify behind a single term that can be used across disciplines. The term "LESS" (laparoscopic endoscopic single-site surgery) was proposed by an interdisciplinary group of surgeons that formed a new organization called LESSCAR (Laparoendoscopic Single Site Consortium for Assessment and Research), which was modeled after NOSCAR™, a group that promotes research into NOTES™. The Urology NOTES™ & LESS Working Group of the Endourological Society in turn adopted "LESS" as the preferred description for laparoscopic surgery involving only a single transabdominal incision for publications in the field of Urology. This term can be amended with various modifiers, e.g., "U-LESS" for LESS using an umbilical incision. Finally, they clarified that "whether the surgery is performed via a single incision with multiple ports, a multi-channel port, or several small incisions grouped in one location, these procedures should probably be considered equivalent and included in LESS" [5].

Development of LESS

The first laparoscopic cases were diagnostic procedures, beginning with the initial report for peritoneoscopy in the canine by Georg Kelling in 1901 [6]. As such, these required only a single incision. However, the concept of single-incision laparoscopy implies therapeutic interventions, rather than simply diagnostic peritoneoscopy. Until relatively recently, most therapeutic procedures have required insertion of separate instruments through additional incisions in order to obtain triangulation. A notable exception is the description of laparoscopic female sterilization by Wheeless, who reported thousands of cases of bilateral partial salpingectomy using a single small incision beginning in 1969 [7]. Subsequent procedures described include hysterectomy (1991), appendectomy (1992), cholecystectomy (1997), ovarian cyst removal (2001), salpingectomy for ectopic pregnancy (2005), peritoneal dialysis catheter placement (2005), and Meckel's diverticulectomy (2007) [8].

Although Sanchez de Badajoz can be credited with the initial single-access hand-assisted laparoscopic nephrectomies in 2006 [9], the first reported purely laparoscopic single-access therapeutic procedures in urology were by Rane et al. in 2007 with a description of pyeloplasty, orchiopexy, orchiectomy, ureterolithotomy, and simple nephrectomy using an ASC Tri-Port device (Applied Surgical Concepts, Wicklow, Ireland) [10]. Subsequent LESS procedures using single-access combination ports in humans have included radical prostatectomy [11], simple prostatectomy with a transvesical access [12], varicocelectomy [13], pyeloplasty [14], adrenalectomy [15], renal cryoablation

[16], sacrocolpopexy [17], and wedge kidney biopsy [17]. A series of U-LESS donor nephrectomies was reported by Gill et al. [18]. Desai et al. [19] reported a LESS technique for bilateral Anderson–Hynes pyeloplasties (two patients), ileal ureter, and ureteroneocystostomy with psoas hitch, each using a single umbilical incision (between 1.5 and 3 cm). Finally, Raman et al. reported a series of 11 LESS nephrectomies in a case–control study comparing this approach to standard laparoscopic nephrectomy. Of note, in this study there were no significant differences in operative time, complications, change in post-operative hemoglobin, requirements for pain medications, or hospital stay. However, a lower intraoperative blood loss (20 ml vs. 100 ml) was reported in the LESS group [20].

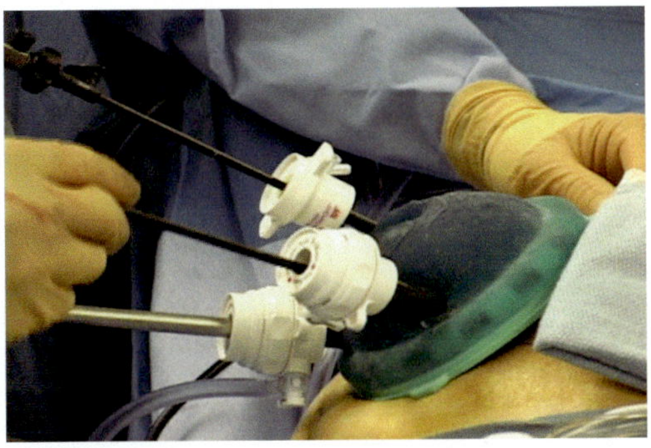

Fig. 19.1 GelPort™ with standard trocars and instruments, used for a LESS nephrectomy

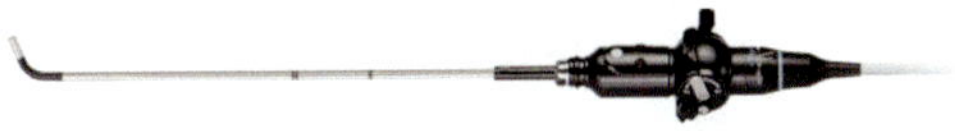

Fig. 19.2 Deflectable tip of 5-mm laparoscopic camera. Image courtesy of Olympus™

Equipment for LESS

Scope Innovations for LESS

Initial LESS procedures primarily used existing laparoscopic and endoscopic equipment. As noted, Sanchez de Badajoz [9] performed single-trocar hand-assisted nephrectomies, albeit with blind stapling of the hilum in 2006 in 74 patients. Raman et al. [21] described a LESS nephrectomy using three standard traditional laparoscopic trocars inserted adjacent to each other at the umbilicus. Ponsky et al. reported the initial use of a standard GelPort™ (Applied Medical, Rancho Santa Margarita, CA) with three trocars inserted through the gel port to perform a LESS radical nephrectomy with standard laparoscopic instruments (Fig. 19.1). This approach is well suited to patients with renal malignancy requiring intact specimen extraction [22].

The development of improved laparoscopic cameras, as well as articulating instruments, helps to overcome coaxial limitations and "sword fighting" of instruments [22]. Notable advances in laparoscopic scopes include reduced size and deflectable tips. The EndoEye™ (Olympus) (Fig. 19.2), for example, is a 5-mm scope that has a digital chip at the deflectable tip that allows for a wider field of view [15]. Examples of articulating instruments include grasping devices such as Autonomy™ Laparo-angle™ (Cambridge Endo, Framingham, MA) and RealHand™ (Novare Surgical Systems, Cupertino, CA) [23]. Cambridge Endo claims full articulation, seven degrees of freedom, and both rotatable tips and handles for their Autonomy™ series of instruments, which also include articulating scissors, hook cautery, and needle drivers.

The combination port device is a multiple instrument access port that typically will accommodate a scope and 2–3 additional instruments, and was specifically designed for LESS procedures. A growing number of reports are describing this type of access device, produced by several manufacturers, for a variety of procedures. Much of the initial published work used the ASC Triport™ (also referred to as the R-Port) (Figs. 19.3, 19.4, and 19.5) or the Uni-X™ Single Port Access (Pnavel Systems, Morganville, NJ). The AirSeal™ system (SurgiQuest, Orange, CT) also allows multiple instruments simultaneously through a single trocar.

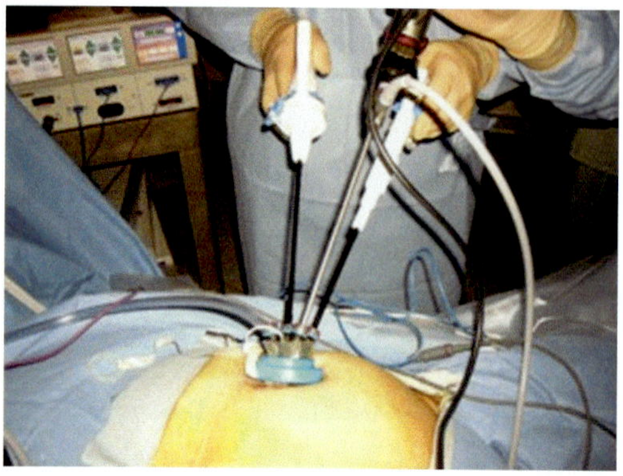

Fig. 19.3 Triport™ used in procedure at our institution

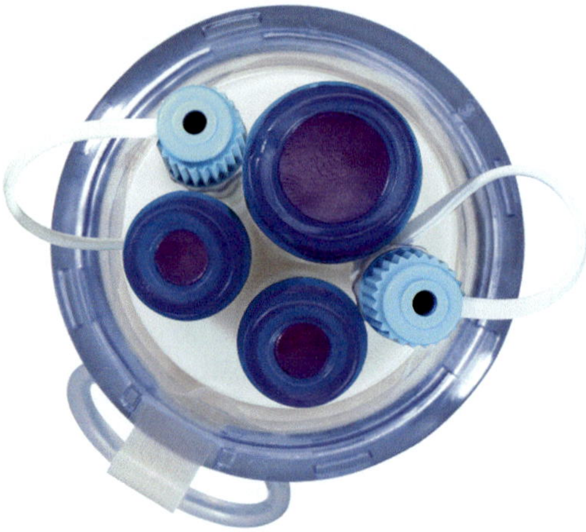

Fig. 19.4 QuadPort™ intended for LESS procedures (2.5–6.5 cm incisions). Image courtesy of Olympus™.

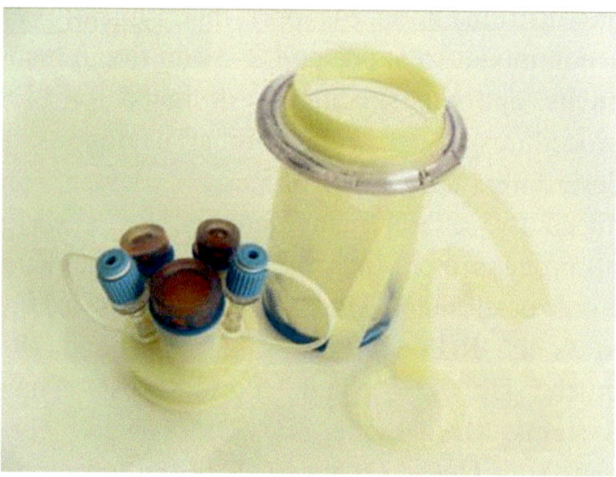

Fig. 19.5 TriPort™ intended for LESS procedures (as small as 1.5 cm). Image courtesy of Olympus™.

The da Vinci robotic platform (Intuitive Surgical, Sunnyvale, CA) has been adapted to LESS as well. Desai et al. [24] first described the use of the robot for transvesical radical prostatectomy in a cadaveric model. Subsequently, this group has performed robotic procedures using a gel port device to perform pyeloplasty, radical nephrectomy, and partial nephrectomy [25]. Newer generations of robots with flexible intracorporeal components could allow for more closely approximated instruments and smaller incisions.

Because of the overlap of some developing technologies for NOTES™ and LESS, discussion of future technologies such as intracorporeal devices will be deferred to later in this chapter.

Incisions for LESS

The "optimal" location of the single incision used for procedures is a current area of discussion, especially for cases requiring removal of a specimen. Previously described extraction sites that can be used for LESS radical nephrectomy include paramedian [22], umbilical [21] and Pfannenstiel [26] incisions, or a colpotomy [27].

The paramedian incision has been successfully used for LESS radical nephrectomy [22] and may be a reasonable transition access site for the novice to LESS. A notable disadvantage is a prominent scar compared to other extraction sites. Paramedian extraction sites may also have a higher risk of incisional hernias relative to umbilical and Pfannenstiel incisions [28].

As noted above, umbilical incisions for LESS have potential to be nearly scarless and may be particularly well suited to procedures such as pyeloplasties. The umbilical access is currently the best described access point for various procedures, including nephrectomies [18]. However, for extirpative procedures such as nephrectomies, a limitation is possible need to enlarge the incision to the detriment of the cosmetic result. In the case of donor nephrectomy, attempts to remove the kidney through too small of an incision at the umbilicus could potentially injure the kidney.

Our group has recently described a Pfannenstiel approach for both LESS radical nephrectomy and LESS nephroureterectomy which could be a reasonable alternative to the trans-umbilical technique. This approach offers excellent cosmesis even should the incision have to be extended for specimen removal, as it lies below the waistline typically covered by pubic hair. Other potential advantages may include reduced pain and possibly lower risk of incisional hernia [26].

Finally, Gill et al. [27] described the initial use of a colpotomy for removal of the kidney specimen during standard laparoscopic nephrectomies in 2002, a method that can easily be applied to LESS procedures. Transvaginal incisions will be discussed further in the section on NOTES™, but clearly use of this natural orifice would have the advantage of no cutaneous scars secondary to the extraction.

As a final comment, there is definitely a steep learning curve for LESS procedures. Experienced laparoscopists who would like to attempt LESS would be advised to plan from the onset of the case to convert to standard laparoscopy until comfortable with the new approach.

Natural Orifice Translumenal Endoscopic Surgery (NOTES™)

Natural orifices include the vagina, oral cavity, nares, urethra, and rectum. There is a long history of use of natural orifices for surgery. It should not be forgotten that the ancient Egyptians can be credited with the earliest use of a natural orifice access for cosmetic extraction of organs from cadavers, in this case transnasal removal of brain tissue. In the fifth century BC, the Ancient Greek scholar Herodotus described the Egyptian practice: "[T]he workmen, left alone in their place, embalm the body. If they do this in the most perfect way, they first draw out part of the brain through the nostrils with an iron hook, and inject certain drugs into the rest." [29]. Transsphenoidal surgery using access through the nares was then adapted early in the twentieth century for therapeutic procedures, although the approach gained popularity with the development of the endoscope [30]. Urologists have used the urethra for access to the bladder, ureters, or renal pelvis for well over a century. General surgeons and gastroenterologists have used both the oral cavity and the rectum for treatment of disorders of the alimentary tract. Gynecologists have likewise used the vagina for access to the uterus and for culdoscopy, as well as for vaginal hysterectomy.

Definition and Nomenclature

NOTES™ is defined by the Urology NOTES™ & LESS Working Group as a "surgical procedure that utilizes one or more patent natural orifices of the body with the intention to puncture a hollow viscera in order to enter an otherwise inaccessible body cavity." The term implies the use of endoscopic/laparoscopic equipment with insufflation of a cavity. By the new convention adopted by the urology working group, "NOTES™" without any prefix or modifier indicates no cutaneous incisions. This was to eliminate the term "pure NOTES™." According to this group, "the use of a transabdominal port should not be considered incompatible with NOTES™ but instead should be considered as part of the progression in the development of this technique." Therefore, the term "Hybrid NOTES™" is recommended for any procedure where more than 75% of the procedure is performed with instruments inserted through the natural orifice [31].

Development of NOTES™

The access of NOTES™ to the abdomen and the retroperitoneum has been described using incisions in the vagina, bladder, colon, and stomach. Gettman et al. [32] described perhaps the initial experience for translumenal surgery with a pure transvaginal nephrectomy using endoscopic equipment in a porcine model in 2002. The actual term NOTES™, and subsequent growth of interest for these procedures, followed the work of Kalloo et al. [33] with transgastric procedures beginning with peritoneoscopy and liver biopsy. The organization NOSCAR™ ("Natural Orifice Surgery Consortium for Assessment and Research") was established to promote research into this field and trademarked the term NOTES™. One of the significant contributions of this group was to attempt to anticipate the barriers to natural orifice surgery in a systematic manner in a 2006 White Paper. These challenges included access to the peritoneal cavity, closure of the access, maintenance of spatial position and orientation, anastomotic and suturing devices, and control of hemorrhage [34]. There has subsequently been an explosion of interest in this approach within various surgical specialties.

NOTES™ in Urology

Most of the work to date for NOTES™ procedures has been in the laboratory, although there is now an increasing experience with Hybrid NOTES™ procedures in humans. There is a growing experience of NOTES™ procedures in Urology using animal and cadaver models. NOTES™ nephrectomies have been reported in the porcine model using transvaginal access [32], combined transvaginal and transgastric access with transvaginal extraction [1], and combined transvesical and transgastric approaches (the latter without extraction) [35]. Both transurethral and transgastric partial cystectomies have been described by our group in a porcine model [36–38]. Transgastric partial nephrectomy was reported in abstract form in the porcine model using a thulium laser inserted through a gastroscope [39]. Transurethral radical prostatectomy including vesicourethral anastomosis was also described in a cadaver model [40].

In humans, urologic experience with NOTES™ has been limited to hybrid procedures and transitional procedures that do not fully qualify as NOTES™. Branco et al. [41] described a transvaginal nephrectomy for benign renal disease using two 5-mm transabdominal trocars in 2007. Allaf et al. recently reported a hybrid transvaginal donor nephrectomy with three transabdominal incisions (one at the umbilicus) in January 2009 [42]. Ribal Caparros et al. [43] published a report of a hybrid transvaginal nephrectomy for renal cell carcinoma in March 2009. This procedure involved two transabdominal ports (a 12- and a 5-mm port). These three reports could actually be considered precursors to hybrid NOTES™, as the instruments were primarily used through the transabdominal trocars and not through the orifice. Sotelo et al. [44] subsequently described a nephrectomy (also for renal malignancy) using multiport accesses both transvaginally and umbilically, which also represents a significant step toward hybrid NOTES™. Probably the closest to an actual transvaginal NOTES™ urologic procedure to date was the description by Kaouk et al. of a transvaginal hybrid NOTES™ radical nephrectomy, assisted by only a single transabdominal 5-mm trocar (for visualization and retraction). This group used a GelPort in the vagina for manipulation and visualization and most of the procedure was performed transvaginally [45]. This represents an important milestone toward the ultimate goal of an entirely transvaginal NOTES™ nephrectomy.

Transvesical peritoneoscopy using a transurethrally inserted ureteroscope has also been reported in a patient in conjunction with a radical prostatectomy procedure [46]. This represents the initial evaluation of transves ical scopes in humans as a precursor to transvesical NOTES™. We are not aware of any urologic applications of transgastric or transcolonic NOTES™ procedures in human patients to date.

Managing Coaxial Limitations

The lack of triangulation with single-access points has required strategies for compensating. For LESS, this has largely involved use of articulating instruments and cameras. NOTES™

procedures generally have even more limitations, given that the instruments must be small and sufficiently flexible to allow insertion through a scope. One method is a combined orifice approach. Described examples include combined transgastric and transvaginal nephrectomy [1] and combined transgastric and transvesical nephrectomy without extraction [35]. A combined approach carries a potential cost of increased morbidity, a larger team, and increased complexity of cases. An alternative is development of new platforms that will be more adaptable than conventional scopes.

Scopes and Equipment

Conventional Scopes

Early work in NOTES™ has principally relied on existing conventional endoscopic equipment, especially standard gastric endoscopes, although prototype scopes have been developed. Flexible scopes are required for access to the stomach and have significant advantages within the abdominal cavity, including ability to maneuver and even retroflex for procedures. However, this flexibility comes at significant cost including difficulties maintaining a given spatial position, easy disorientation (especially in retroflexion), poor force transmission (e.g., driving needles into tissue), and coaxial limitations. Additional factors to consider include scope sizes. For example, the size limit for transurethral access is probably less than 30 Fr. Size of the scope impacts the size of potential instruments, the number of simultaneous instruments, and the strength of illumination of the abdominal cavity. These limitations have already spurred industry to produce prototype scopes that address some of these issues.

New Scope and Platform Innovations for NOTES™

NeoGuide Systems (San Jose, CA) produces the NeoGuide Endoscopy System™ colonoscope which has 16 separate articulating segments each controlled by a computer. While intended for colonoscopy to allow smooth maneuverability around the flexures of the colon, this concept has promise for application to scopes used in NOTES™ procedures [47].

A proposed solution is to have a flexible scope that can lock into a fixed configuration. USGI Medical has produced the Cobra™ and ShapeLock™ prototypes and Olympus has described an "M" Scope that has ability to lock configurations [48, 49].

A more radical development has been novel platforms. A frequently described prototype platform is the Olympus R-Scope™ (Fig. 19.6), which has elevators at the tips which move in both vertical and horizontal planes and has two articulating sections. The USGI Transport™ (Fig. 19.7) is an FDA-approved platform with two 6-mm and two 4-mm channels that can lock even in a retroflexed position with independent maneuverability of the scope's tip. It also has ability to meter insufflation pressure (Fig. 19.8). Other concepts include multiple armed devices such as USGI's Cobra™ (with three arms that can move independently) [48]; Olympus' EndoSamurai (see Fig. 19.9); and Hansen Medical's ViaCath™ (Mountain View, CA) prototype which has attached robotic arms that can articulate [49]. The platforms created to date are primarily applicable to transgastric and transvaginal procedures, given their overall size.

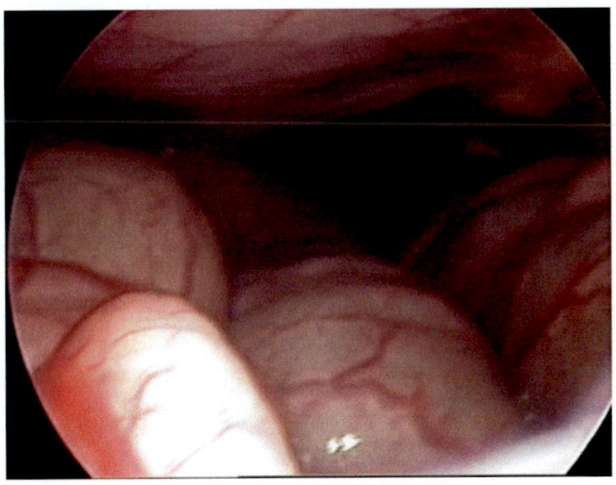

Fig. 19.6 Transvesical peritoneoscopy with rigid cystoscope in porcine model (illumination from cystoscope)

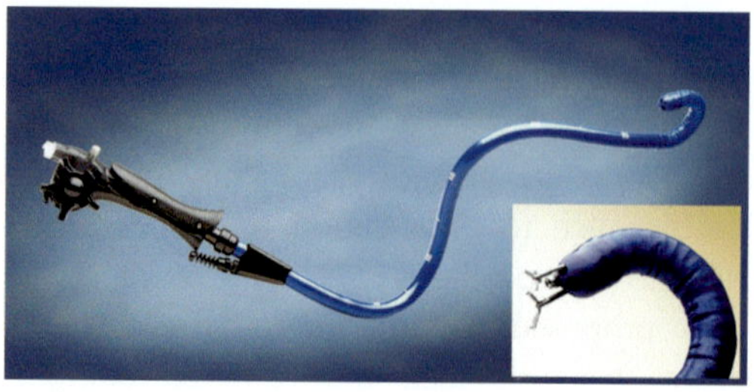

Fig. 19.7 Transport™ system. Images courtesy of USGI Medical™

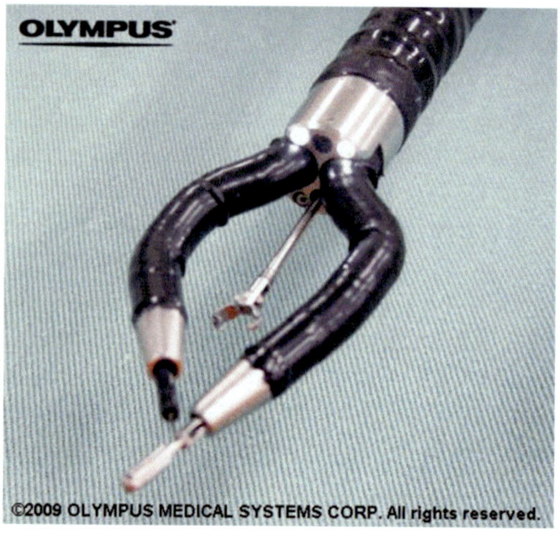

Fig. 19.8 The EndoSamurai™ prototype. Images courtesy of Olympus. ©2009 Olympus Medical Systems Corp. All rights reserved

Accesses

Transvaginal

The field of gynecology has been using a transvaginal approach for open surgery for many years. This orifice is very promising as a conduit for insertion of endoscopic instruments and cameras, given the relative ease of access. The original laboratory report of transvaginal nephrectomy by Gettman described the use of either a flexible cystoscope or a 5-mm laparoscope for visualization. An advantage of the vagina for extirpative procedures is potential for using the colpotomy for specimen extraction, e.g., the kidney [27]. The colpotomy is typically closed easily under direct vision with little morbidity or discomfort [50]. Indeed, the vast majority of initial clinical reports have used a hybrid transvaginal NOTES™ approach (including hybrid transvaginal NOTES™ cholecystectomy) [50]. An obvious disadvantage is its limited applicability to 50% of the population [51]. There also remain concerns about dyspareunia and leakage and patient positioning would need to be optimized.

Transgastric

Kalloo et al. [33] used a transgastric approach in their initial porcine studies that popularized the technique. Reddy and Rao described the

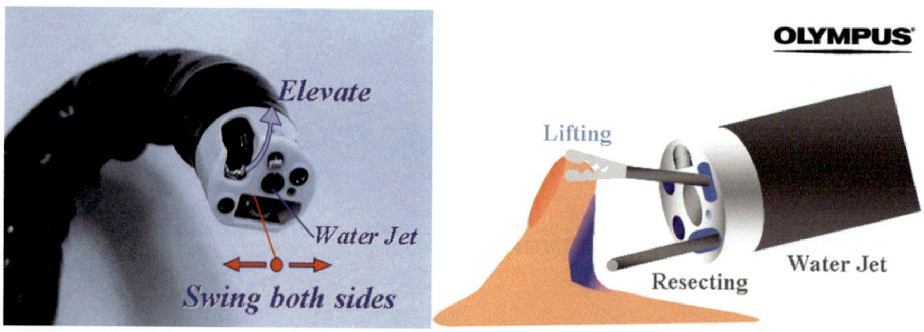

Fig. 19.9 Olympus R-Scope™ prototype. Images courtesy of Olympus. ©2009 Olympus Medical Systems Corp. All rights reserved

use of a transgastric approach for appendectomy in patients, although their work remains unpublished [34]. While there is significant interest in this approach, there remain significant questions of safe access and closure, especially given difficulties in sterilizing the stomach. This remains one of the most significant challenges for adapting transgastric surgery to humans. There have been various experimental closure devices used, including endoscopic clips and novel tissue approximation devices.

Transvesical

A significant advantage of a transvesical access is the relative sterility of urine, but the relatively small size of the orifice has limited investigations to date [46]. Early descriptions of transvesical access have included use of a ureteroscope through a 5.5-mm transvesical port in a porcine model by Lima et al. Use of such a small scope does not necessarily require closure in their experience [52]. Gettman and Blute [46] described transvesical peritoneoscopy in a patient using a ureteroscope. Our group has used both pediatric gastroscopes and rigid cystoscopes in the laboratory for transvesical peritoneoscopy in the porcine model, using the insufflation channel to maintain pneumoperitoneum [53]. An advantage is ability to use standard endoscopic equipment in the two working channels. A significant constraint for transvesical use is the relatively short length of current rigid scopes. On the other hand, other scopes either are too large to accommodate the urethra (e.g., standard gastric endoscopes); may have inadequate channel size for effective instrumentation; or have insufficient number of channels (e.g., pediatric gastroscopes and ureteroscopes) [54, 55]. Finally, safe and reliable closure of a vesicotomy will need to be established for larger bladder defects. Historically, this has required an open surgical treatment intervention in the setting of bladder perforations. A reliable endoscopic alternative method for repairing the vesicotomy would be necessary. Several such suggestions have been advocated. Lima's group described intravesical endoscopically applied sutures in the porcine model [56]. Our group has described use of standard endoscopic clips for closure also in a chronic porcine model [38, 55]. To urologists, this access site holds particular interest raising questions of the role urologists should have in transvesical approaches for non-urologic procedures and subsequent management of any complications.

Transcolonic/Transenteric

A transcolonic access has a potential advantage of size for scopes with the rectum tolerating reasonably large instruments. However, this access could be one of the most potentially controversial, given the high bacterial load of the colon and potential for infection with introduction of fecal matter into the peritoneum. A reliable method for thorough cleansing of the bowel contents would seem obligatory. Animal studies to date have included transcolonic cholecystectomy, ventral hernia repair, and distal pancreatectomy [57].

Pneumoperitoneum

Pneumoperitoneum can be established relatively easily with gastric endoscopes or even ureteroscopes [52]. However, conventional scopes have limited ability to regulate pressures, and the working channel of smaller scopes can limit gas flow and insufflation. Reasonable approaches to address this include using a transabdominal insufflation needle or a novel platform that includes a pressure regulation device.

Endoscopic Instruments

NOTES™ procedures will require optimization of equipment to allow retraction, cutting, retrieval of specimens, tissue approximation, and closure of access defects. Endoscopic devices necessarily must be smaller than standard laparoscopic instruments and typically must also have flexibility to fit within a scope. Articulating endoscopic instruments could also be advantageous.

Our group has used primarily needle knife electrocautery and wire snare electrocautery for intracorporeal incisions of tissue, with relatively little success with existing flexible endoscopic scissors. Manipulation of tissues can be effected with various grasping devices such as endoscopic forceps. Additionally, endoscopic loop devices can be used to hold tissues for excision, such as bladder specimens, and even to seal defects, such as the bladder (Fig. 19.10) [38].

Retrieval devices that can safely hold a specimen are also necessary instruments for many procedures. Various devices that are currently used for endoscopic procedures (e.g., to entrap polyps and foreign bodies of the GI tract) have been adapted to NOTES™. These include the Roth Net™ (US Endoscopy, Mentor, OH) and the Nakao SpiderNet™ retrieval device (ConMed Endoscopic Technologies, Utica, NY) [49, 58].

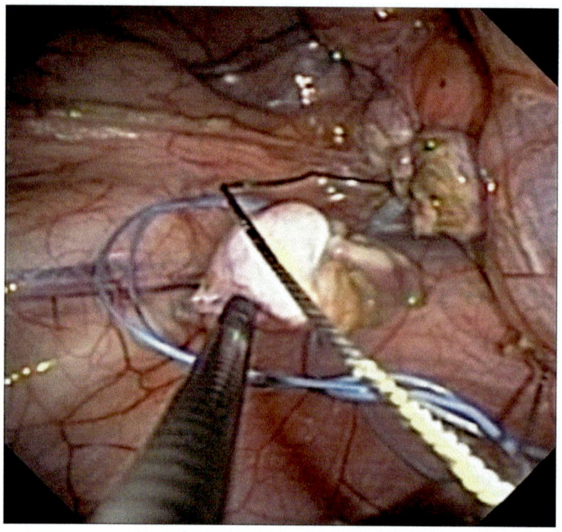

Fig. 19.10 Transgastric partial cystectomy: endoscopic loops seal both bladder specimen and remaining bladder in porcine model

Approximation of tissue is an extremely important concern for reconstructive procedures. This issue is of paramount importance for NOTES™ to be viable, given the need to close the visceral access in most cases. An early prototype described frequently in the literature is the Eagle Claw™ (Olympus, Tokyo, Japan). An experimental flexible-shafted stapling device for NOTES™ procedures is the iNOLC™ (intelligent Natural Orifice Linear Cutter, Power Medical Interventions, Langhorne, PA). Endoscopic clips have been described for both closure of gastrotomies and full-thickness bladder defects [53, 59]. Some more sophisticated clips have the ability to rotate and to open and close multiple times, e.g., the Resolution™ clip (Boston Scientific, Natick, MA). Other endoscopic suture devices include the T-tag™ system (Ethicon), g-Prox™ device (USGI Medical, San Clemente, CA) (Fig. 19.11), the T-tag™ system, and Tissue Approximation System, or TAS™, (Ethicon), the NDO Surgical Plicator™ (NDO, Mansfield, MA), and Endo Stitch™ (Covidien, Mansfield, MA) [49, 59, 60].

Internalized Instrumentation (NOTES™ and LESS)

Until recently, laparoscopic and endoscopic instruments have required continuity with an external part. A new paradigm is the use of independent internalized instruments. Two concepts

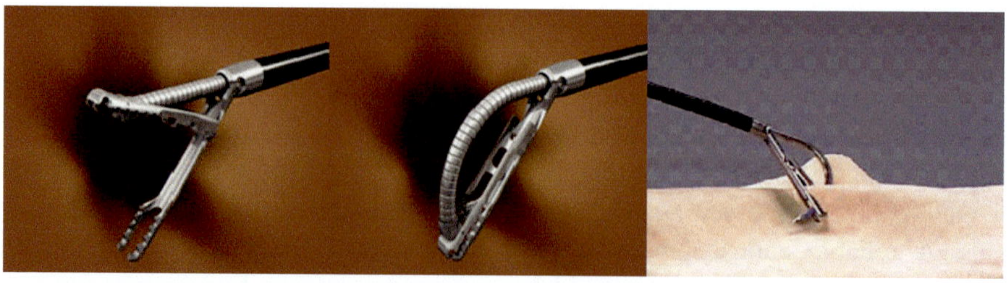

Fig. 19.11 The g-Prox™ tissue applicator. Images courtesy of USGI Medical™

deserve particular mention, namely magnetic instruments and miniature internalized robots or "microrobots."

Magnetic Instrumentation

Cadeddu et al. have described a novel and exciting use of magnetic instrumentation. Their "magnetic anchoring and guidance system" (MAGS) allows internalized instruments to be introduced through a single incision and then controlled extracorporeally with use of an external electromagnetic coupling device. Devices that have been used include graspers, cautery instruments, and a camera. This system was first successfully implemented for laboratory transvaginal NOTES™ nephrectomy and cholecystectomy and for LESS nephrectomy. Subsequently, there has been a successful clinical report of a LESS nephrectomy using a magnetically anchored camera. A challenge with these devices is the distance of the internal device from the external coupler, which would be potentially problematic for obese patients [3, 51, 61–63]. Nevertheless, this is a promising technology and has already been used clinically for a LESS nephrectomy [63].

Miniature Intracorporeal Robotics

Two prototype miniature robotic cameras were used to aid laparoscopic prostatectomy in a canine model. These are both remotely controlled and able to be inserted through a 15-mm incision. One prototype has a crawler function that gives the camera intracorporeal mobility. The other is stationary but has pan and tilt functionality that permits a 360° view of the abdomen but is relatively bulky (approximately 8 cm × 3 cm). The camera provides additional reference points to the surgeon. These prototypes do have significant limitations including size, inability to self-clean the lens, tethering of the device to external power, and need for a separate assistant to drive the camera [4]. Rentschler et al. used miniature robots for transgastric NOTES™ peritoneoscopy procedures. This group has suggested potential for use of "a family of robots working together inside the gastric and abdominal cavities after their insertion through the esophagus" [64]. In addition to camera functions, robots have also been developed that include illumination and retraction abilities. However, currently wireless robots have a battery life less than 1 h [65]. Further work will likely address some of the current limitations of these devices and potentially expand the repertoire of robotic tasks.

Conclusions

LESS and NOTES™ are intriguing approaches to surgery that may each represent a paradigm shift in operative management. Given the rapid pace of innovation to date, we anticipate further developments of instruments and devices. Of paramount importance in evaluating the role of these approaches is the need to critically assess these new technologies and ensure at least equivalency of these techniques for patient safety, including respect for established oncologic principles (when relevant), patient comfort, and efficacy.

References

1. Isariyawongse JP, McGee MF, Rosen MJ, Cherullo EE, Ponsky LE. Pure Natural Orifice Transluminal Endoscopic Surgery (NOTES) nephrectomy using standard laparoscopic instruments in the porcine model. J Endourol. Apr 17 2008;22(5):1087–91.
2. Marks JM, Ponsky JL, Pearl JP, McGee MF. PEG "rescue": a practical NOTES technique. Surg Endosc. May 2007;21(5):816–9.
3. Zeltser IS, Bergs R, Fernandez R, Baker L, Eberhart R, Cadeddu JA. Single trocar laparoscopic nephrectomy using magnetic anchoring and guidance system in the porcine model. J Urol. Jul 2007;178(1):288–91.
4. Joseph JV, Oleynikov D, Rentschler M, Dumpert J, Patel HR. Microrobot assisted laparoscopic urological surgery in a canine model. J Urol. Nov 2008;180(5):2202–5.

5. Box G, Averch T, Cadeddu J, et al. Nomenclature of natural orifice translumenal endoscopic surgery (NOTES) and laparoendoscopic single-site surgery (LESS) procedures in urology. J Endourol. Nov 2008;22(11):2575–81.
6. Kelling G. Ueber die Besichtigung der Speiseröhre und des Magens mit biegsamen Instrumenten. Vol 73. Leipzig: Verlag F.W.C. Vogel; 1902.
7. Wheeless CR Jr, Thompson BH. Laparoscopic sterilization. Review of 3600 cases. Obstet Gynecol. Nov 1973;42(5):751–8.
8. Canes D, Desai MM, Aron M, et al. Transumbilical single-port surgery: evolution and current status. Eur Urol. Nov 2008;54(5):1020–9.
9. Sanchez de Badajoz E, Jimenez Garrido A. Single trocar laparoscopic nephrectomy. Arch Esp Urol. Sep 2006;59(7):719–24.
10. Rané A, Rao P, Rao P. Single-port-access nephrectomy and other laparoscopic urologic procedures using a novel laparoscopic port (R-Port). Urology. Aug 2008;72(2):260–3.
11. Kaouk JH, Goel RK, Haber GP, Crouzet S, Desai MM, Gill IS. Single-port laparoscopic radical prostatectomy. Urology. Dec 2008;72(6):1190–3.
12. Desai MM, Aron M, Canes D, et al. Single-port transvesical simple prostatectomy: initial clinical report. Urology. Nov 2008;72(5):960–5.
13. Kaouk JH, Palmer JS. Single-port laparoscopic surgery: initial experience in children for varicocelectomy. BJU Int. Jul 2008;102(1):97–9.
14. Desai MM, Rao PP, Aron M, et al. Scarless single port transumbilical nephrectomy and pyeloplasty: first clinical report. BJU Int. Jan 2008;101(1):83–8.
15. Castellucci SA, Curcillo PG, Ginsberg PC, Saba SC, Jaffe JS, Harmon JD. Single port access adrenalectomy. J Endourol. Aug 2008;22(8):1573–6.
16. Goel RK, Kaouk JH. Single port access renal cryoablation (SPARC): a new approach. Eur Urol. Jun 2008;53(6):1204–9.
17. Kaouk JH, Haber GP, Goel RK, et al. Single-port laparoscopic surgery in urology: initial experience. Urology. Jan 2008;71(1):3–6.
18. Gill IS, Canes D, Aron M, et al. Single port transumbilical (E-NOTES) donor nephrectomy. J Urol. Aug 2008;180(2):637–41; discussion 641.
19. Desai MM, Stein R, Rao P, et al. Embryonic natural orifice transumbilical endoscopic surgery (E-NOTES) for advanced reconstruction: initial experience. Urology. Jan 2009;73(1):182–7.
20. Raman JD, Bagrodia A, Cadeddu JA. Single-incision, umbilical laparoscopic versus conventional laparoscopic nephrectomy: a comparison of perioperative outcomes and short-term measures of convalescence. Eur Urol. 13 Aug 2008;55(5): 1198–206.
21. Raman JD, Bensalah K, Bagrodia A, Stern JM, Cadeddu JA. Laboratory and clinical development of single keyhole umbilical nephrectomy. Urology. Dec 2007;70(6):1039–42.
22. Ponsky LE, Cherullo EE, Sawyer M, Hartke D. Single access site laparoscopic radical nephrectomy: initial clinical experience. J Endourol. Apr 2008; 22(4):663–6.
23. Kommu SS, Rane A. Devices for laparoendoscopic single-site surgery in urology. Expert Rev Med Devices. Jan 2009;6(1):95–103.
24. Desai MM, Aron M, Berger A, et al. Transvesical robotic radical prostatectomy. BJU Int. Dec 2008;102(11):1666–9.
25. Stein RJ, White WM, Goel RK, Irwin BH, Haber GP, Kaouk JH. Robotic laparoendoscopic single-site surgery using GelPort as the access platform. Eur Urol. Jan 2010;57(1):132–6. Epub 31 Mar 2009.
26. Ponsky LE, Steinway M, Lengu IJ, Hartke DM, Vourganti S, Cherullo EE. A Pfannenstiel single site nephrectomy and nephroureterectomy: a practical application of LESS surgery. Urology. Sep 2009;74(3):482–5.
27. Gill IS, Cherullo EE, Meraney AM, Borsuk F, Murphy DP, Falcone T. Vaginal extraction of the intact specimen following laparoscopic radical nephrectomy. J Urol. Jan 2002;167(1):238–41.
28. Bird VG, Au JK, Sandman Y, De Los Santos R, Ayyathurai R, Shields JM. Comparison of different extraction sites used during laparoscopic radical nephrectomy. J Urol. Apr 2009;181(4):1565–70.
29. Heroditus. The histories. Godley AD, translator. Cambridge, MA: Harvard University Press; 1920. Book 2, Ch 38. www.perseus.tufts.edu
30. Cappabianca P, de Divitiis E. Back to the Egyptians: neurosurgery via the nose. A five-thousand year history and the recent contribution of the endoscope. Neurosurg Rev. Jan 2007;30(1):1–7.
31. Box G, Averch T, Badlani G, Cadeddu J, Cherullo EE, Clayman R, Desai M, Frank I, Gettman M, Gill I, Gupta M, Haber GP, Kaouk J, Landman J, Lima E, Ponsky LE, Rane A, Sawyer MD, Humphreys M. Nomenclature of natural orifice translumenal endoscopic surgery (NOTES) and laparo-endoscopic single-site surgery (LESS) procedures in urology. J Endourol. Nov 2008;22(11):2575–8.
32. Gettman MT, Lotan Y, Napper CA, Cadeddu JA. Transvaginal laparoscopic nephrectomy: development and feasibility in the porcine model. Urology. Mar 2002;59(3):446–50.
33. Kalloo AN, Singh VK, Jagannath SB, et al. Flexible transgastric peritoneoscopy: a novel approach to diagnostic and therapeutic interventions in the peritoneal cavity. Gastrointest Endosc. Jul 2004;60(1):114–7.
34. Rattner D, Kalloo A. ASGE/SAGES working group on natural orifice translumenal endoscopic surgery. October 2005. Surg Endosc. Feb 2006;20(2): 329–33.
35. Lima E, Rolanda C, Pego JM, et al. Third-generation nephrectomy by natural orifice transluminal endoscopic surgery. J Urol. Dec 2007;178(6): 2648–54.

36. Sawyer MD, Cherullo EE, Ponsky LE Transurethral intravesical NOTES partial cystectomy: technical considerations in porcine model. Proceedings of the 23rd Meeting of Engineering and Urology Society, Orlando, FL; 2008.
37. Sawyer MD, Cherullo EE, Ponsky LE. Transgastric extravesical NOTES partial cystectomy: a novel pure NOTES approach in a porcine model. Proceedings of the 94th Congress of the American College of Surgeons, San Francisco, CA; 2008.
38. Sawyer MD, Cherullo EE, Elmunzer BJ, Schomisch S, Ponsky LE. Two methods of pure NOTES partial cystectomy: transurethral and transgastric approaches in a porcine model. Urology. Nov 2009;74(5):1049–53.
39. Lee BR, Boylu U, Oommen M, Fifer G, Thomas R, Joshi V. Natural orifice transluminal endoscopic surgery (NOTES) partial nephrectomy. J Urol. 2009;181(4):181.
40. Humphreys MR, Krambeck AE, Andrews PE, Castle EP, Lingeman JE. Natural orifice translumenal endoscopic surgical radical prostatectomy: proof of concept. J Endourol. Apr 2009;23(4):669–75.
41. Branco AW, Filho AJ, Kondo W, et al. Hybrid transvaginal nephrectomy. Eur Urol. 5 Nov 2007;53:1290–4.
42. Quasi-NOTES surgery used to remove donor kidney. Medical News, Surgery. 2009. http://www.medpagetoday.com/Surgery/General Surgery/12744.
43. Ribal Caparros MJ, Peri Cusi L, Molina Cabeza A, Garcia Larrosa A, Carmona F, Alcaraz Asensio A. First report on hybrid transvaginal nephrectomy for renal cancer. Actas Urol Esp. Mar 2009;33(3):280–3.
44. Sotelo R, de Andrade R, Fernandez G, et al. NOTES hybrid transvaginal radical nephrectomy for tumor: stepwise progression toward a first successful clinical case. Eur Urol. Jan 2010;57(1):138–44. Epub 22 Apr 2009.
45. Kaouk JH, White WM, Goel RK, et al. NOTES transvaginal nephrectomy: first human experience. Urology. Jul 2009;74(1):5–8.
46. Gettman MT, Blute ML. Transvesical peritoneoscopy: initial clinical evaluation of the bladder as a portal for natural orifice translumenal endoscopic surgery. Mayo Clin Proc. Jul 2007;82(7):843–5.
47. Eickhoff A, Jakobs R, Kamal A, Mermash S, Riemann JF, van Dam J. In vitro evaluation of forces exerted by a new computer-assisted colonoscope (the NeoGuide Endoscopy System). Endoscopy. Dec 2006; 38(12):1224–9.
48. Swanstrom LL, Khajanchee Y, Abbas MA. Natural orifice transluminal endoscopic surgery: the future of gastrointestinal surgery. Perm J. 2008;12(2):42–7.
49. Binmoeller KF. Endosurgery: what do we need? Gastrointest Endosc Clin N Am. Jul 2007;17(3): 617–34, ix.
50. Zorron R, Maggioni LC, Pombo L, Oliveira AL, Carvalho GL, Filgueiras M. NOTES transvaginal cholecystectomy: preliminary clinical application. Surg Endosc. Feb 2008;22(2):542–7.
51. Raman JD, Scott DJ, Cadeddu JA. Role of magnetic anchors during laparoendoscopic single site surgery and NOTES. J Endourol. May 2009;23(5):781–6.
52. Lima E, Rolanda C, Pego JM, et al. Transvesical endoscopic peritoneoscopy: a novel 5 mm port for intra-abdominal scarless surgery. J Urol. Aug 2006;176(2):802–5.
53. Sawyer MD, Cherullo EE, Ponsky LE Vesicotomy closure with novel use of endoscopic clips. Proceedings of the 23rd Meeting of Engineering and Urology Society, Orlando, FL; 2008.
54. Sawyer MD, Cherullo EE, Ponsky LE Visualization into the peritoneum: a urologic perspective on transvesical access including novel use of a rigid cystoscope. Proceedings of the 3rd International Conference on NOTES, San Francisco, CA; 2008.
55. Sawyer MD, Cherullo EE, Ponsky LE. Transvesical NOTES peritoneoscopy: initial experience with standard rigid cystoscope in a chronic porcine model. J Endourol. Nov 2008;22(Suppl 1):A188.
56. Lima E Endoscopic closure of transmural bladder wall perforations: the dawn of a new era in endourology. Proceedings of the 23rd Meeting of Engineering and Urology Society, Orlando, FL; 2008.
57. Shin EJ, Kalloo AN. Transcolonic NOTES: current experience and potential implications for urologic applications. J Endourol. May 2009;23(5):743–6.
58. Bounds BC. Endoscopic retrieval devices. Tech Gastrointest Endosc. 2006;8(1):16–21.
59. Swanstrom LL, Whiteford M, Khajanchee Y. Developing essential tools to enable transgastric surgery. Surg Endosc. Mar 2008;22(3):600–4.
60. McGee MF, Marks JM, Jin J, et al. Complete endoscopic closure of gastric defects using a full-thickness tissue plicating device. J Gastrointest Surg. Jan 2008;12(1):38–45.
61. Scott DJ, Tang SJ, Fernandez R, et al. Completely transvaginal NOTES cholecystectomy using magnetically anchored instruments. Surg Endosc. Dec 2007;21(12):2308–16.
62. Raman JD, Bergs RA, Fernandez R, et al. Complete transvaginal NOTES nephrectomy using magnetically anchored instrumentation. J Endourol. Mar 2009;23(3):367–71.
63. Cadeddu J, Fernandez R, Desai M, et al. Novel magnetically guided intra-abdominal camera to facilitate laparoendoscopic single-site surgery: initial human experience. Surg Endosc. Aug 2009;23(8): 1894–9.
64. Rentschler ME, Dumpert J, Platt SR, Farritor SM, Oleynikov D. Natural orifice surgery with an endoluminal mobile robot. Surg Endosc. Jul 2007;21(7):1212–5.
65. Canes D, Lehman AC, Farritor SM, Oleynikov D, Desai MM. The future of NOTES instrumentation: flexible robotics and in vivo minirobots. J Endourol. May 2009;23(5):787–92.

Part IX
Laparoscopy and Robotics in Incontinence and Pelvic Reconstructive Surgery

Chapter 20

Laparoscopy and Robotics in Stress Urinary Incontinence and Pelvic Reconstructive Surgery

Alvaro Lucioni and Kathleen C. Kobashi

This chapter contains a video segment which can be found at the URL: http://www.springerimages.com/ost

Introduction

The prevalence of pelvic floor disorders such as urinary incontinence and pelvic organ prolapse (POP) has seemingly increased over the last several decades. This increase could be attributed to longer life expectancy as well as the increased awareness of such disorders amongst health-care professional and patients. A recent epidemiological study found that the prevalence of at least one pelvic floor disorders among US women was 23.7% with the majority of them being affected by urinary incontinence [1]. Approximately 10% of women undergo surgery for treatment of urinary incontinence or POP. Thirty percent of these women will subsequently undergo one or more procedures after the first repair [2]. Proportionate to this increase in surgical management of pelvic floor disorders has been growth in the utilization of minimally invasive surgical treatments. Laparoscopic and robotic techniques allow surgeons to apply their open surgical skills in a minimally invasive fashion. Advantages of the laparoscopic and robotic approaches include improved visualization of the pelvis due to laparoscopic magnification and insufflation effects, shorter hospital stays, and decreased post-operative pain and recovery time. The purpose of this chapter is to review the surgical techniques and outcomes of laparoscopic and robotic surgeries for stress urinary incontinence, pelvic organ prolapse, and other pelvic reconstructive procedures such as vesicovaginal fistula repair and augmentation cystoplasty.

Stress Urinary Incontinence

The International Continence Society defines urinary incontinence as "the complaint of any involuntary loss of urine that is objectively demonstrable and a social or hygienic problem." Stress urinary incontinence (SUI) is described as "the involuntary loss of urine during coughing, sneezing, or physical exertion" [3] and is the most common type of urinary incontinence [3]. Despite the high prevalence of SUI, we do not have a complete understanding of the mechanisms that lead to urinary incontinence. Continence is believed to be maintained through a combination of factors including coaptation of the urethra, mechanical support of the bladder neck by the pelvic floor, a healthy submucosal vascular plexus, local hormonal balance, and an adequate neurologic reflex [4]. Various theories have been proposed to explain the development of SUI and attempts to mimic these theoretical mechanisms have been the basis of anti-incontinence procedures over the years. Creation of a suburethral hammock to reproduce the anatomic structural support of the urethra and procedures designed to restore the

A. Lucioni (✉)
The Continence Center at Virginia Mason Medical Center, Seattle, WA, USA
e-mail: alvaro.lucioni@vmmc.org

M.C. Ost (ed.), *Robotic and Laparoscopic Reconstructive Surgery in Children and Adults*, Current Clinical Urology, DOI 10.1007/978-1-60327-914-7_20, © Springer Science+Business Media, LLC 2011

retropubic position of the bladder neck to equalize pressure transmission between the bladder and the outlet have been successful techniques used to restore continence [5, 6, 7].

The Burch colposuspension which has fallen out of favor over the years has regained popularity with the increasing use of minimally invasive approaches, and review of the procedure and its outcomes is warranted.

Laparoscopic Burch Colposuspension

The open Burch colposuspension was introduced by Burch in 1961 [8]. By approximating the paravaginal fascia to Cooper's ligament, the procedure restores the bladder neck to its normal retropubic position. The laparoscopic Burch colposuspension utilizes the same surgical principles as the open approach.

Patient Evaluation

Patients should undergo a history and physical exam, including a thorough pelvic examination. Cystoscopy should be performed if there is any concern about any bladder or urethral pathology. In patients with a history of previous pelvic reconstructive surgery, the authors strongly recommend cystoscopic evaluation. Urodynamic evaluation should be performed to rule out any storage or voiding pathology particularly in patients with mixed urinary incontinence or patients who have undergone previous pelvic surgery.

Surgical Technique

Prior to surgery, some surgeons advocate the use of bowel preparation for ease in intraoperative bowel manipulation. After general anesthesia is induced, the patient is placed in a low lithotomy position with Trendelenburg as necessary. A Foley catheter is placed to drain the bladder. The procedure can be performed either extraperitoneally or intraperitoneally. The extraperitoneal approach has been associated with shorter operative times, fewer bladder injuries, and the ability to minimize the risk of post-operative pelvic adhesions [9, 10]. The extraperitoneal approach provides a shorter learning curve but does have a higher risk of CO_2 absorption leading to pneumomediastinum and pneumothorax [11, 12]; conversely the intraperitoneal approach provides a larger operating space and the ability to perform concomitant intraperitoneal surgery.

Three ports are placed: one periumbilical, one in the right, and one in the left lower quadrant just lateral to their respective epigastric vessels, approximately 3 cm medial and superior to the anterior–superior iliac spine. In the extraperitoneal approach, the space of Retzius is dissected using a balloon or a finger to aid with pneumodissection. The paravaginal fascia and Cooper's ligaments are then identified. Sutures are then used to approximate these two structures. Tensioning of the sutures is more difficult in the laparoscopic approach, given lack of tactile sensation. The number and type of sutures needed is debatable. The use of both absorbable and nonabsorbable sutures has been described. Persson and Wolner-Hanssen [13] advocated the use of two sutures on each side citing a higher success rate compared to using only one suture. Studies comparing suture placement versus mesh placement demonstrated higher success rates with suture [14]. Most authors advocate the use of cystoscopy after suture placement to rule out bladder injury.

Outcomes

Success rates for the laparoscopic approach range from 80 to 92%. A recent Cochrane review concluded that at 2 years postsurgery, there is no significant difference in outcomes between laparoscopic and open colposuspension [15]. However, most of the studies comparing both approaches are short term and thus durable long-term results comparing open versus laparoscopic approach are needed. The authors also commented that the newer vaginal sling procedures appear to offer greater benefits and objective outcomes in the

Table 20.1 Summary of recent studies evaluating efficacy of laparoscopic colposuspension

Author	Year	*N*(open/ laparoscopic)	Follow-up (months)	Subjective cure (%)	Objective cure (%)
Cheon et al. [53]	2003	43	12	86	86
		47		81	85
Ankardal et al. [54]	2004	98	12	89	92
		109		62	74
Kitchener et al. [55]	2006	147	24	55	70
		144		55	80
Carey et al. [56]	2006	104	44	70	NA
		96		58	

short term and thus the future utility of colposuspension is unclear. Table 20.1 summarizes the outcomes of the most recent studies comparing open versus laparoscopic Burch colposuspension.

Regarding complications, the overall rate is higher for laparoscopic Burch colposuspension compared to the open approach, with complication rates of 8–22% and 5–8%, respectively. The most common intraoperative complications include bladder, bowel, or vaginal injury, and ureteral kinking or injury. Reported peri-operative morbidities include urinary tract infection, pneumonia, transient urinary retention, and wound infection. Long-term complications include voiding dysfunction (urgency and urinary retention) and development of POP. Table 20.2 summarizes the complication rates of laparoscopic Burch colposuspension.

Robotic-Assisted Laparoscopic Colposuspension

With the success of the laparoscopic colposuspension, surgeons have started to use the robotic system to perform colposuspension. The shorter learning curve while using the robotic system has allowed surgeons to overcome the suturing difficulties in the laparoscopic procedure. A recent case report by Khan et al. [16] demonstrated the successful use of the robotic system to perform colposuspension in two patients. At 12-month follow-up, both patients were continent. Further evaluation in a larger cohort of patients is needed to evaluate the long-term efficacy of the robotic system for this operation.

Other Laparoscopic Procedures for SUI

Laparoscopy has also been used in the placement of vaginal slings. In this procedure, the space of Retzius is dissected laparoscopically and a midurethral dissection performed transvaginally. The sling material is passed from the vaginal incision to the retropubic space and secured laparoscopically to the Cooper's ligament. Phelps et al. [17] reported on their experience with this technique. They successfully performed a laparoscopic-assisted suburethral sling placement in 63 patients with overall satisfaction of 89%.

Table 20.2 Summary of complications of laparoscopic colposuspension

Author	*N*	Follow-up (months)	Bladder injury (%)	Bleeding (%)	UTI (%)	Urinary retention (%)	Urinary urgency (%)
Liu et al.	433	NA	1.8	NA	NA	3.5	3.2
Kitchener et al. [55]	144	24	2.8	0.7	5.7	NA	NA
Carey et al. [56]	96	44.4	5.2	1	NA	NA	63
Cooper et al. [11]	113	8.4	9.7	0.9	NA	NA	8.0

Pelvic Organ Prolapse

With a reported 37% prevalence of POP in the general population, treatment has increased significantly over the past several decades [18]. With aging, the prevalence of POP has been shown to increase to up to 65%. Traditional surgeries for POP repair with anterior and/or posterior wall plication, though initially successful, demonstrated suboptimal long-term results. In an effort to improve upon these suboptimal success rates, new techniques using a variety of synthetic and biological grafts have emerged, and there has been a dramatic increase in the number of surgical procedures performed by urologists and gynecologists for POP repair. With the advance of laparoscopic and robotic surgeries, many surgeons have utilized minimally invasive approaches to correct POP. Although laparoscopic and robotic-assisted procedures have been used for repair of anterior and posterior vaginal wall prolapse, these approaches have primarily been utilized for repair of apical defects.

The etiology of POP is complex and has been attributed to weakening of or damage to the connective tissues and innervation of the pelvis. A number of risk factors have been associated with the development of POP including obesity, parity, vaginal delivery, menopause, aging, genetic factors, trauma, musculoskeletal diseases, smoking, and prior surgery [19]. Parity and vaginal delivery are likely the most important risk factors. Tissue injury during vaginal delivery appears to be strongly related to ischemia; however mechanical forces may also contribute to the weakening of the connective tissue. Most of the damage during vaginal delivery likely occurs during the first delivery and subsequent deliveries may not necessarily worsen the damage already done [20]. Further, tissue remodeling is critical for tissue recovery following ischemic and mechanical injury. Patients with connective tissue disorders may be at a higher risk of developing prolapse because of ineffective or lack of tissue remodeling [21].

Patient Evaluation Prior to POP Repair

Similarly to patients undergoing surgery for SUI, POP patients should undergo a history and physical exam, including a thorough pelvic examination. Cystoscopy should be performed if concerned about any bladder or urethral pathology. Urodynamic evaluation should be performed to rule out any storage or voiding pathology particularly in patients with mixed urinary incontinence or patients who have undergone previous pelvic surgery. Urodynamic evaluation is also important to evaluate for occult SUI and determine the need for concomitant anti-incontinence procedure.

Brubaker et al. [22] reported on their outcomes in women undergoing sacrocolpopexy with or without Burch colposuspension and found that post-operatively, 23.8% of women in the Burch group compared to 44% in the non-Burch group had SUI ($p<0.001$). Based on this study, patients undergoing POP repair who have symptoms or urodynamic findings of SUI should be recommended to undergo a concomitant anti-incontinence procedure. However, the use of an anti-incontinence procedure in POP patients without evidence of SUI remains controversial. Anger et al. [23] recommends the use of a concomitant sling at the time of cystocele repair in women with grade III and IV cystoceles unless they have undergone a previous procedure for SUI. Ballert et al. [24] recently described that in women with high-grade POP without clinical or urodynamic SUI, the risk of intervention for de novo SUI after surgery was similar to the risk of intervention due to obstruction when a sling is placed. Thus, in patients without clinical history or urodynamic evidence of SUI, a thorough discussion of the risks of an anti-incontinence procedure versus the risk of developing SUI if an anti-incontinence procedure is not performed should be undertaken with the patient.

Radiologic evaluation with magnetic resonance imaging (MRI) in patient with POP has increased in recent years, particularly since the introduction of dynamic MRI technology. MRI may supplement information provided by physical examination and fluoroscopy by providing comprehensive and high-quality imaging of the entire pelvis, including pelvic support structures and organs. MRI has proven to be helpful in the evaluation of multi-compartment POP, particularly when one wants to determine the presence of an apical defect in patients with anterior and/or posterior compartment prolapse.

Laparoscopic and Robotics for Anterior and Posterior Vaginal Wall Prolapse

Laparoscopic Cystocele Repair

Transvaginal colporrhaphy, with or without synthetic or biograft, is the most common procedure used for cystocele repair. Unfortunately, failure rates of 10–70% have been reported [25–27]. Following the successful use of laparoscopic Burch colposuspension for SUI, pelvic surgeons began to apply laparoscopic skills and the surgical principles of the transvaginal approach to the repair of cystoceles.

Surgical Technique

Patient is placed in lithotomy position. Laparoscopic port placement is similar to that used during laparoscopic colposuspension. The bladder is mobilized, the space of Retzius developed, and the bladder neck, Cooper's ligament, and the lateral detachment of the endopelvic fascia from the arcus tendinious fasciae pelvis (ATFP) are identified. With insertion of a vaginal manipulator, the edges of the pubocervical fascia are identified and approximated to the ATFP with nonabsorbable sutures. These sutures should also incorporate vaginal tissue and the obturator internus and iliopectineal ligaments.

Outcomes

Behnia-Willison and colleagues [28] reported on their experience with laparoscopic cystocele repair in 212 patients (42 underwent concomitant hysteropexy or colpopexy and 47 underwent concomitant posterior repair). With a mean follow-up of 14.2 months, the objective cure rate, defined as POP-Q stage 0 or 1, was 76%. Eighteen of the 23 women with residual central defects subsequently underwent graft-reinforced anterior colporrhaphy.

Laparoscopic Rectocele Repair

The transvaginal approach remains the most common approach for repair of posterior compartment defects [29]. However, there are a few limited reports on the laparoscopic transabdominal approach for rectocele repair. Because of the approximate 10–41% risk of dyspareunia after rectocele repair, the authors recommend repairing rectoceles only in patients who are symptomatic (vaginal splinting and stool trapping).

Surgical Technique

Patient position and port placement is similar to that of laparoscopic Burch colposuspension. The rectovaginal space is then identified and carefully dissected to expose the rectovaginal septum. An EEA sizer may be used to identify and manipulate the vagina. The perineal body is then secured to the rectovaginal septum. The rectovaginal defect is closed with absorbable sutures, and, if needed, a levator ani plication is performed.

Outcomes

One study evaluating the efficacy of laparoscopic rectocele repair with polyglactin mesh in 20 patients reported that with 12-month follow-up, 16 of the patients had resolution of the symptoms

[30]. Another report by Thornton et al. compared the laparoscopic versus the transanal approach for rectocele repair. After 44-month follow-up, they noted a higher success rate with the transanal repair. Only 28% of the patients who underwent laparoscopic repair reported more than 50% symptom improvement.

Laparoscopic and Robotics for Repair of Apical Prolapse

Various procedures for apical prolapse repair have been described, including laparoscopic vaginal vault or uterine uterosacral ligament fixation, sacrocolpopexy, culdoplasty using the Moschcowitz and Halban procedures, and enterocele excision and closure. These techniques have been proven to be effective when performed in an open transabdominal fashion. Surgeons are now utilizing laparoscopy and robotics to perform these procedures in a minimally invasive fashion. The laparoscopic uterosacral fixation and sacrocolpopexy are the most commonly reported and thus will comprise the focus of the apical discussion.

Laparoscopic Uterosacral Ligament Fixation

Surgical Technique

During laparoscopic uterosacral ligament fixation the vaginal apex is approximated to the distal aspect of the uterosacral ligaments using nonabsorbable sutures. The rectovaginal fascia is then approximated to a more proximal aspect of the uterosacral ligaments. For the uterine suspension, a nonabsorbable suture is placed through the full thickness of the uterosacral ligament at the level of the ischial spine and then again at its insertion point into the lower uterine segment. Care must be taken to identify the ureter, usually located 1–1.5 cm lateral to the uterosacral ligament. Cystoscopy is performed at the end of the procedure to evaluate for bladder injury and for adequate urine efflux from both ureteral orifices.

Outcomes

Medina and Tacaks reported on their outcomes after laparoscopic uterosacral ligament fixation. They showed a significant improvement in the prolapse stage from an average POP-Q stage 2 to stage 0 at a follow-up of almost 16 months. No patients had symptomatic prolapse and no intraoperative complications were reported. Unfortunately, studies reporting outcomes using uterosacral ligament fixation have short follow-up and thus results must be interpreted with caution.

Laparoscopic and Robotic Sacrocolpopexy

Surgical Technique

After general anesthesia is obtained the patient is placed in dorsal lithotomy position. The patient's arms are tucked on both sides and adequately padded. The patient is then secured to the table and a metal cage is used to protect the patient's face. A Foley catheter is placed in the bladder. Pneumoperitoneum is obtained via open approach or Veress needle. For the laparoscopic approach an infraumbilical or a periumbilical port and two lower quadrant 10–12-mm ports are utilized (Fig. 20.1). One or two ancillary ports may be placed at the level of the umbilicus, lateral to the rectus muscle. If the robotic-assisted technique is used, then a 12-mm camera port is placed just above the umbilicus, and two 8-mm robotic arm ports are placed, 8 cm on either side of the midline and 17 cm from the symphysis pubis. Two assistant ports are placed: a 10-mm port 3 cm above the right anterior superior iliac spine and a right-sided, 5-mm port 8 cm lateral to the camera port (Fig. 20.2).

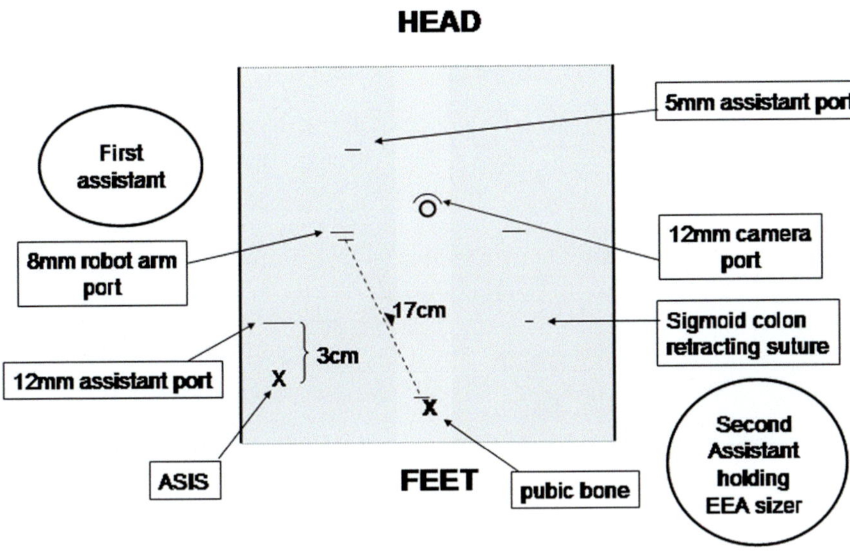

Fig. 20.1 Port placement for robotic-assisted laparoscopic sacrocolpopexy

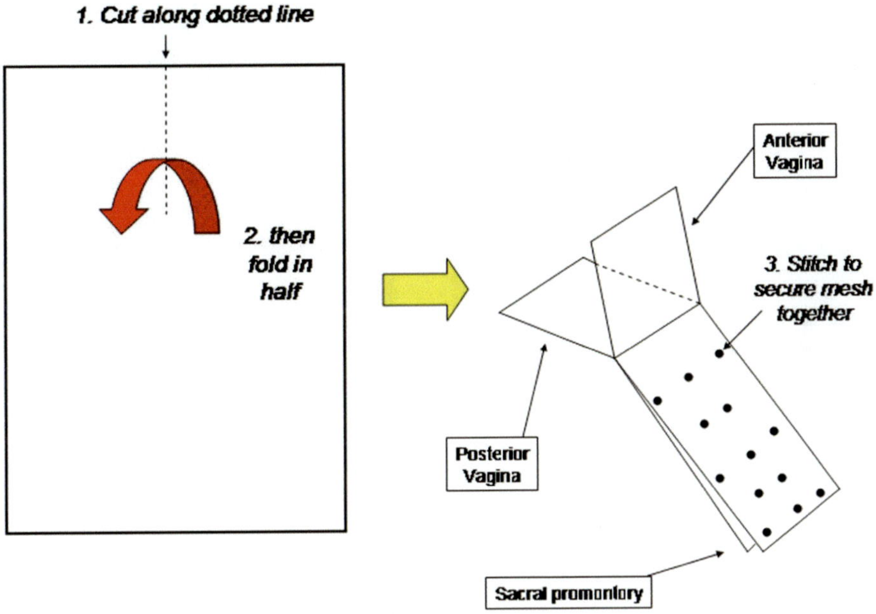

Fig. 20.2 Creation of Y-shaped mesh

After port placement, the patient is placed in steep Trendelenburg position to aid in visualization and bowel mobilization away from the surgical field. The sigmoid is retracted to the left with the use of an anchoring suture to the abdominal wall to provide excellent exposure of the posterior peritoneum and the vaginal apex. Using an EEA sizer or other vaginal obturator to facilitate the dissection, a peritoneal flap is dissected off the vaginal cuff (Fig. 20.3). Care is taken to avoid injury to the bladder. Saline can be instilled through the catheter to better

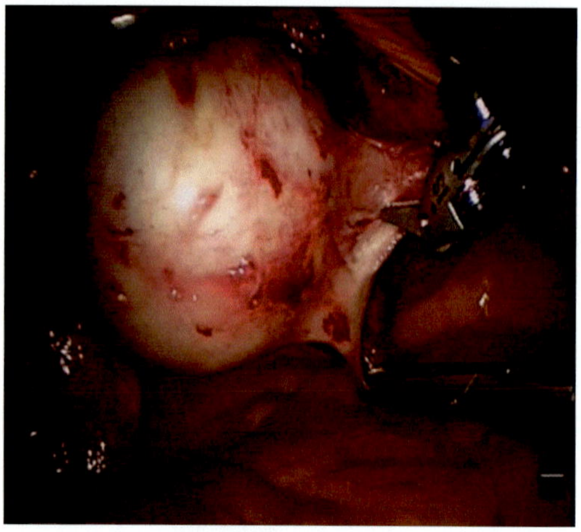

Fig. 20.3 Dissection of peritoneal flap at the vaginal cuff during robotic-assisted sacrocolpopexy

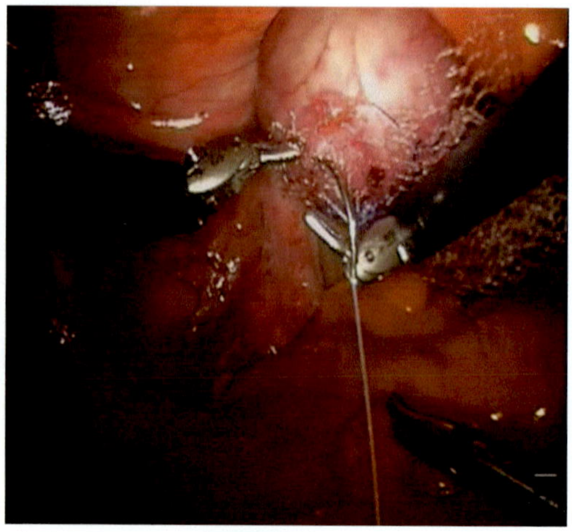

Fig. 20.5 Placement of anterior vaginal cuff sutures during robotic-assisted sacrocolpopexy

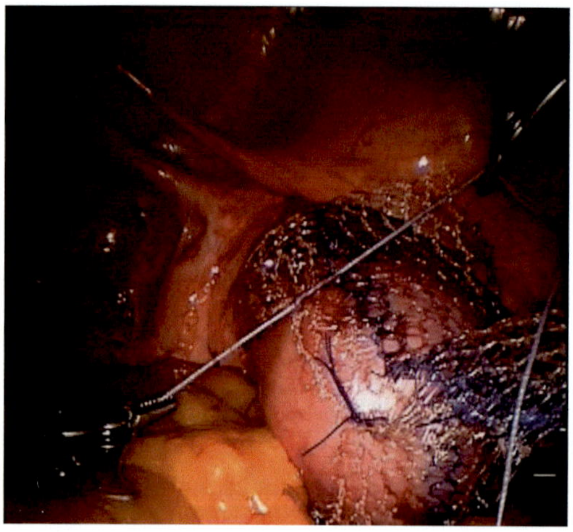

Fig. 20.4 Exposure of sacral periosteum ad pre-sacral ligaments during robotic-assisted sacrocolpopexy

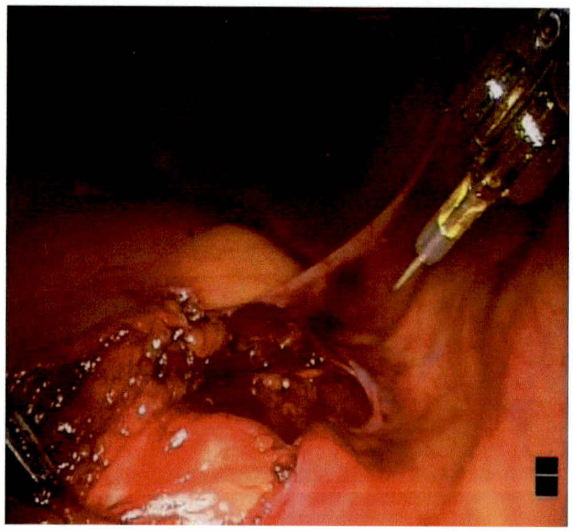

Fig. 20.6 Placement of posterior vaginal cuff sutures during robotic-assisted sacrocolpopexy

identify the bladder borders. The sacral promontory is then identified. The pre-sacral space and sacral periosteum are exposed with care taken to avoid injury to any pre-sacral veins (Fig. 20.4). The posterior peritoneum is then opened, connecting the vaginal peritoneal flap to the pre-sacral space. A Y-shaped synthetic mesh or a biologic graft is secured to the anterior and posterior aspects of the vaginal apex with full-thickness passes of nonabsorbable sutures (Figs. 20.2, 20.5, and 20.6). The base of the mesh or the graft is then secured to the pre-sacral ligaments and the periosteum with either two nonabsorbable sutures or with two bone anchors (Fig. 20.7). If bone anchors are used, an extra suprapubic port is placed just to the right of the midline for passage of the drill. The graft is secured with no tension. The mesh is retroperitonealized to minimize the risk of adhesions and bowel obstruction, although some studies have suggested that retroperitonealization of the mesh is unnecessary (Fig. 20.8) [31].

Hysterectomy can be performed concomitantly with the sacrocolpopexy. Earlier reports on

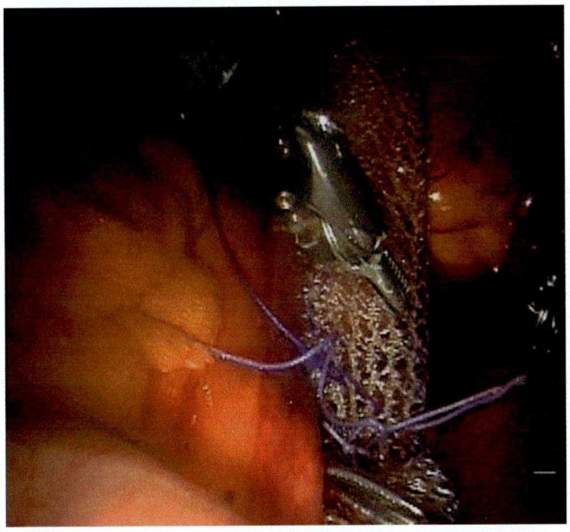

Fig. 20.7 Securing mesh to sacral promontory during robotic-assisted sacrocolpopexy

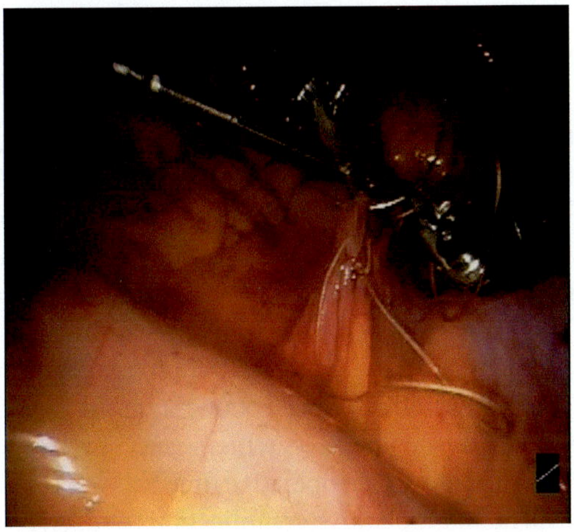

Fig. 20.8 Closure of posterior peritoneum over mesh material during robotic-assisted sacrocolpopexy

performing a hysterectomy at the time of sacrocolpopexy reported a high incidence of mesh extrusion. This higher extrusion rate has been attributed to surgical field contamination during vaginal opening at the time of complete hysterectomy. Given the higher incidence of mesh extrusion in this patient population, surgeons have reported on the use of a supracervical hysterectomy in select patients resulting in an extrusion rate of 0.8% [31]. Some authors stipulate that the cervix acts as a shock absorber that prevents mesh friction at the vaginal cuff and that preserving the cervix also helps maintain adequate blood supply to the vaginal apex [32].

Various mesh materials have been used for both open and laparoscopic sacrocolpopexy. The most commonly reported mesh materials include Mersilene (polyethylene terephthalate; Ethicon, Somerville, NJ), silicone-coated polyester (Cousin Biotech), and polypropylene (prolene; Ethicon, Somerville, NJ; Marlex, CR Bard, Cranston, RI). The ideal sling material should be one that is inert, pliable, nonantigenic, and nonallergenic, and that allows for tissue ingrowth avoiding infection. Biografts such as cadaveric fascia (Tutoplast; Coloplast, Minneapolis, MN) have also been used in sacrocolpopexy. Loffeld et al. [33] recently compared prolene mesh versus cadaveric fascia and reported a higher risk of intervention because of recurrent prolapse in the cadaveric fascia group (relative risk of 2.9). A prospective, randomized study evaluating the safety and efficacy of various mesh materials and biografts is needed.

Outcome

Ganatra et al. recently presented the results of a comprehensive review of laparoscopic sacrocolpopexy (Tables 20.3 and 20.4). This meta-analysis of greater than 1,000 patients revealed an overall satisfaction rate of 94.4% with a mean follow-up of 25 months [34]. The mean operative time was 158 min with a 2.7% conversion to open rate and a 1.6% early reoperation rate. The rate of recurrent prolapse after laparoscopic sacrocolpopexy was 6.2%, with 2.7% of patients presenting with mesh extrusion or erosion. The authors conclude that the laparoscopic sacrocolpopexy outcomes uphold the outcomes of the gold standard abdominal sacrocolpopexy but that longer prospective and randomized trials are needed to further evaluate the laparoscopic approach.

Since this meta-analysis, North et al. presented a prospective study evaluating laparoscopic sacrocolpopexy for management POP. At a minimum follow-up of 2 years, all 22

Table 20.3 Summary of recent studies evaluating the efficacy of laparoscopic sacrocolpopexy

Author	Year	*N*	Follow-up (months)	Subjective cure (%)	Objective cure (%)
Higgs et al. [57]	2005	140	66	79	92
Rozet et al. [58]	2005	363	15	96	96
Ross et al. [59]	2005	51	60	NA	93
Agarwala et al. [60]	2007	74	24	97	100
Rivoire et al. [61]	2007	131	34	98	89
Sarlos et al. [62]	2008	101	12	98	93

Table 20.4 Summary of complications of laparoscopic sacrocolpopexy

Author	*N*	Follow-up	Bladder injury (%)	Bowel injury (%)	Bleeding (%)	Mesh erosion (%)	Urinary dysfunction (%)	Fecal dysfunction (%)
Paraiso et al. [63]	56	14	11	2	0	4	NA	2
Higgs et al. [57]	140	66	1	1	3.6	8.7	17	17
Rozet et al. [58]	363	15	0	0	0	0.8	6	6
Ross et al. [59]	51	60	4	0	0	9	2	6
Agarwal et al. [60]	74	24	0	0	1	2.8	21	3
Rivoire et al. [61]	131	34	2	0	0	5.3	44	NA
Sarlos et al. [62]	101	12	4	1	1		34	19

women had stage 0 vault support (i.e., no visible prolapse) with one patient complaining of prolapse symptoms despite normal pelvic exam [35]. No patient complained of dyspareunia. In another recent study, Claerhout et al. [36] addressed the concern for the surgeon's learning curve when implementing the laparoscopic approach for sacrocolpopexy. Since 1996 they had performed 206 laparoscopic sacrocolpopexies. Seventeen percent of the cases were converted to an open procedure. Their major and minor complication rates were 4.4 and 12.6%, respectively. Their operation time declined significantly during the first 30 cases and remained steady at an average of 175 min after 90 cases. They concluded that adequate learning of the procedure occurred after 60 cases.

So far most preliminary reports of the robotic-assisted laparoscopic sacrocolpopexy have shown this procedure to be equally as successful as the laparoscopic approach [37–39]. Elliot et al. reported on the long-term results of robotic-assisted laparoscopic sacrocolpopexy in 30 patients with a mean follow-up of 24 months. Their mean operative time was 3.1 h. One patient was found to have dense adhesions between the bladder and the vagina necessitating conversion to an open procedure. All but one patient were discharged home on post-operative day one. At 1 year, 95% of patients had a successful repair without recurrent prolapse on pelvic exam. All patients reported satisfaction with the procedure. Two patients developed vaginal mesh extrusion. Another study by Kramer et al. [40] reported on 21 patients undergoing robotic-assisted laparoscopic sacrocolpopexy with a success rate of 95%. Their average operative time was 3 h 14 min with no intraoperative complications or open conversions. All but two patients were discharged on post-operative day 1. Thus far, robotic-assisted laparoscopic sacrocolpopexy has been proven to be a feasible and safe approach for surgical repair of POP. However, further study is needed to evaluate the long-term efficacy of the procedure.

Vesicovaginal Fistula

The most common cause of vesicovaginal fistula (VVF) in the developed world is iatrogenic during abdominal hysterectomy. They occur in approximately 1/1,800 hysterectomies and can present 1–6 weeks post-operatively [41]. Patients usually present complaining of continuous urinary incontinence; however, some patients may complain of SUI, urge incontinence, or vaginal drainage. VVF that results from operative injury can be successfully repaired in 75–97% of the cases. Most surgeons agree that the first attempt at VVF repair offers the patient the best opportunity for successful repair. VVF can be treated via a transabdominal or a transvaginal approach depending on location, size, and surgeon's preference. The transabdominal approach has been recommended in patients with upper tract involvement, proximity to ureteral orifice, multiple fistulas, or recurrent fistula [42]. With the advent of laparoscopy and robotic pelvic surgery, many surgeons are now using these minimally invasive techniques for VVF repair. The laparoscopic approach significantly reduces the access trauma of open surgery and provides magnified vision and less traumatic tissue handling [43].

Laparoscopic and Robotic VVF Repair

Patient Evaluation

After obtaining a history and performing a physical examination, including a thorough pelvic exam to attempt to identify the fistula tract, patients should undergo cystoscopy and upper tract evaluation. The latter could be obtained via computed tomography urogram or retrograde pyelogram. Often, patients may require an exam under anesthesia to perform a thorough pelvic exam, cystoscopy, and retrograde pyelogram. Upper tract evaluation is critical given that 10–15% of patients with VVF may have ureteral obstruction or ureterovaginal fistula [41]. The need for pre-operative urodynamic evaluation remains controversial. Most surgeons recommend urodynamic evaluation in patients with overactive bladder symptoms or when suspicious of intrinsic sphincter deficiency. The timing of VVF repair is also controversial. Traditionally surgeons recommended waiting 3–6 months after the initial injury; however most surgeons now state that VVF repair can be performed anytime after tissue edema and inflammation have resolved (4–6 weeks)[41].

Surgical Technique

The surgical technique has been previously described by Sotelo et al. [42]. After general anesthesia is obtained the patient is placed in the low lithotomy position. Cystoscopy is first performed to identify and catheterize the vesicovaginal fistula. If necessary both ureters can also be catheterized to facilitate ureteral identification intraabdominally. Pneumoperitoneum is the obtained and the laparoscopic ports are placed in a similar fashion to that of laparoscopic sacrocolpopexy.

The overall approach is similar to the open technique. The vagina is retracted posteriorly with use of an EEA sizer or a sponge retractor. The light from the cystoscope is identified in the proximity of the fistula tract. The posterior bladder wall is incised to the VVF tract using a harmonic scalpel. The incision is extended posteriorly and distally until the catheter marking the VVF tract and the vaginal retractor are fully exposed. The vaginal retractor is removed and a vaginal tampon is placed to prevent loss of pneumoperitoneum. The remaining borders of the fistulous tract are excised. The bladder is separated from the vagina. All necrotic or nonviable tissues are excised. The bladder is then closed in two layers in a running fashion using absorbable suture. The vaginal opening is then closed in one layer using absorbable suture. An anchoring suture is then placed distal to the fistulous tract. This will serve to anchor the omental interpositional flap. If omentum is not available, an epiploic appendix can be mobilized from the sigmoid colon. Watertight closure is then confirmed by filling the bladder with saline. A suprapubic catheter can then be placed if desired. A close drain system is also placed in the vicinity of the vaginal incision.

Bladder drainage is usually continued for 10–14 days or longer depending on the complexity of the repair. Most authors recommend the use of a cystogram to ensure fistula closure.

Robotic-assisted laparoscopic VVF repair is performed in a similar fashion. Port placement is the same as in robotic sacrocolpopexy. Instruments used include the da Vinci® long-tip grasper, hook, scissor, needle holder, and, if desired, the Maryland bipolar coagulating forceps.

Outcomes

The laparoscopic VVF repair was first described by Nezhat in 1994 [44]. One of the largest laparoscopic VVF repair experiences was reported by Sotelo et al. [42], with 15 patients and mean follow-up of 26.2 months. Their mean operative time was 170 min and an average post-operative hospital stay was 3 days. Only one patient had VVF recurrence. There were two operative complications: unrecognized epigastric artery injury necessitating exploration and enterotomy which was repaired laparoscopically.

Robotic-assisted laparoscopic VVF repaired was first described by Melamud et al. and then Sundaram et al. reported the first five-patient case series [43, 45]. In this series, all five patients underwent a successful repair. The mean operative time was 233 min and the mean hospital stay was 5 days. Hemal et al. recently reported on the use of robotics for recurrent supratrigonal VVF repair in seven patients. The average fistula size was 3 cm. Their mean operative time was 141 min. Mean hospital stay was 3 days. All seven patients had a successful repair with up to 12 month follow-up. With the increase in the use of laparoscopic and robotic techniques for pelvic surgery, surgeons are now tackling more complex cases such as recurrent VVF repairs. However, more long-term study is needed to prove the efficacy of these minimally invasive techniques.

Augmentation Cystoplasty

Augmentation cystoplasty has been successfully used to treat patients with low-volume, low-compliance bladders as well as patients with refractory overactive bladder [46, 47]. Given the complexity of the bowel handling (isolation and reconfiguration of the bowel segment and bowel anastomosis), most of the earlier reports of laparoscopic augmentation cystoplasty describe this portion of the procedure performed extracorporeally. With improvement in laparoscopic surgical technique, some surgeons are now performing the augmentation cystoplasty completely laparoscopically [48].

Patient Evaluation

History, physical exam, laboratory examination, cystoscopy, and urodynamic evaluation are used to identify adequate candidates for augmentation cystoplasty (AC). Indications for AC include poor bladder compliance, small bladder capacity, increased risk of upper tract injury (i.e., detrusor leak point pressure > 40 cmH_2O), and refractory overactive bladder. Contraindications include renal insufficiency, inflammatory bowel disease, short gut syndrome, and inability to perform clean intermittent catheterization. Patients should undergo mechanical bowel preparation prior to surgery.

Surgical Procedure

After general anesthesia is obtained, patients are positioned in low lithotomy and secured to the bed to allow for maximal Trendelenburg. Nasogastric tube and an 18-Fr Foley catheter are placed. Pneumoperitoneum is established via a Hasson technique or a Veress needle and a 12-mm port is placed at the midline or just to the left of the midline 18 cm cranially from the pubic bone [49]. Two 5-mm trocars are placed 15 cm from the pubic symphysis, approximately 1 handbreadth lateral on each side of the initial camera port. A left-sided 5-mm assistant port is placed approximately 8 cm lateral to our initial 5-mm left-sided trocar. The patient is then placed in steep Trendelenburg. The terminal ileum is identified by the presence of the ileocecal valve and appendix. The ileum is then tagged approximately 20–25 cm from the terminal ileum. A second silk suture is placed 20 cm proximal to the first suture. The space of

Retzius is then developed by dividing the obliterated umbilical ligaments and incising the anterior peritoneum lateral and superior to the urinary bladder. The peritoneum is then dissected away from the posterior aspect of the bladder. Next, the bowel segment is prepared in an extracorporeal fashion. The initial camera port incision is elongated 2 cm and the holding sutures are brought out of the incision, facilitating the desufflation and delivery of the previously selected bowel segment into the field. A 20-cm segment of the ileum is excluded from the bowel continuity using a gastrointestinal stapling device (US Surgical, Division of Tyco Healthcare, Princeton, NJ). The ileum is then brought back into continuity using either a standard hand-sewn two-layer side-to-side technique or stapled side-to-side technique. The small bowl mesentery defect is then closed. The isolated ileal segment is detubularized by opening it along the antimesenteric border. The patch is then reconfigured by folding it into a U-shaped fashion with the apex facing cranially, and the medial cut edges are brought into continuity with a running 2-0 Vicryl (Ethicon, Somerville, NJ) in a single full-thickness running suture line. It is critical to properly orient the ileal patch in order to avoid torsion of its mesentery. The anastomosis and detubularized patch are placed back into the abdomen. This incision is closed with interrupted suture leaving approximately a 1 cm opening at the cranial apex of the incision to reinsert our 12-mm port. Pneumoperitoneum is reestablished and the bowel segments are inspected for vascularization and proper orientation. The bladder is then bivalved and the 3 and 6 o'clock positions marked. The enterocystotomy is then performed maintaining correct orientation with the apex of the U aligning with the anterior portion of the cystotomy. Prior to completing the enterocystotomy, left-sided 5-mm assistant port is enlarged to allow placement of a 24-Fr malecot through a cystotomy in the anterior quadrant of the bladder. The malecot is secured to the bladder with purse-string 2-0 chromic suture. After the enterocystotomy is completed, a watertight closure is confirmed. A closed drain is placed over the space of Retzius.

If performing the procedure with robotic assistance, 7-mm da Vinci® trocars (Intuitive Surgical, Sunnyvale, CA) are placed at the same position as the 5-mm ports. A 12-mm assistant port is placed 1 handbreadth superior and 8 cm lateral to the initial 5-mm right-sided trocar. Instruments used include the da Vinci® long-tip grasper, hook, scissor, needle holder, and, if desired, the Maryland bipolar coagulating forceps.

Outcomes

The use of laparoscopic and robotic techniques for augmentation cystoplasty in adults is limited to case series. In 2000, Gill et al. reported on successful laparoscopic enterocystoplasty in three patients with a neurogenic bladder. One patient underwent an ileocystoplasty, another a sigmoid cystoplasty, and the third patient underwent a cystoplasty with cecum and proximal ascending colon and a continent, catheterizable ileal conduit with an umbilical stoma. Bowel exclusion and reanastomosis were performed extracorporeally, and the enterovesical anastomosis was performed laparoscopically in all three patients [50]. More recently, Noguera et al. reported on the successful use of a single-port augmentation cystoplasty in a 20-year-old female with neurogenic bladder [51]. One of the largest series of laparoscopic augmentation cystoplasty was reported by El-Feel et al. [52]. With a mean follow-up of 39 months, 23 patients underwent successful enterocystoplasty. Their estimated bladder volume increased from 111 to 788 ml, while the maximum detrusor pressure decreased from 92 to 15 cmH_2O. Though laparoscopic augmentation cystoplasty has been shown to be feasible and safe, study evaluating long-term outcomes is necessary.

Conclusions

With the increased use of laparoscopic and robotic techniques in pelvic floor surgery, more complex pelvic reconstructive procedures are being performed. Recent studies have demonstrated that laparoscopy and robotic-assisted surgery are safe and feasible for treatment of SUI,

POP, VVF, and AC. However, long-term studies are needed to properly assess and compare the efficacy of these minimally invasive techniques to the traditional open approach.

Acknowledgments Paul Kozlowski, MD, and David E. Rapp, MD, for their collaboration in the video preparation.

References

1. Nygaard I, Barber MD, Burgio KL, et al. Prevalence of symptomatic pelvic floor disorders in US women. JAMA. 17 Sep 2008;300(11):1311–6.
2. Olsen AL, Smith VJ, Bergstrom JO, Colling JC, Clark AL. Epidemiology of surgically managed pelvic organ prolapse and urinary incontinence. Obstet Gynecol. Apr 1997;89(4):501–6.
3. Luber KM. The definition, prevalence, and risk factors for stress urinary incontinence. Rev Urol. 2004;6(Suppl 3):S3–9.
4. Rapp DE, Kobashi KC. The evolution of midurethral slings. Nat Clin Pract Urol. Apr 2008;5(4):194–201.
5. DeLancey JO. Structural support of the urethra as it relates to stress urinary incontinence: the hammock hypothesis. Am J Obstet Gynecol. Jun 1994;170(6):1713–20; discussion 1720–3.
6. Petros PE, Ulmsten UI. An integral theory of female urinary incontinence. Experimental and clinical considerations. Acta Obstet Gynecol Scand Suppl. 1990;153:7–31.
7. Enhorning G. Simultaneous recording of intravesical and intra-urethral pressure. A study on urethral closure in normal and stress incontinent women. Acta Chir Scand Suppl. 1961;Suppl 276:1–68.
8. Burch JC. Cooper's ligament urethrovesical suspension for stress incontinence. Nine years' experience – results, complications, techniques. 1968. Am J Obstet Gynecol. Aug 2002;187(2):512; discussion 513.
9. Frankel G, Kantipong M. Sixteen-month experience with video-assisted extraperitoneal laparoscopic bladder neck suspension. J Endourol. Jun 1995;9(3):259–64.
10. Raboy A, Hakim LS, Ferzli G, Antario JM, Albert PS. Extraperitoneal endoscopic vesicourethral suspension. J Laparoendosc Surg. Oct 1993;3(5):505–8.
11. Cooper MJ, Cario G, Lam A, Carlton M. A review of results in a series of 113 laparoscopic colposuspensions. Aust N Z J Obstet Gynaecol. Feb 1996;36(1):44–8.
12. Wolf JS, Jr, Monk TG, McDougall EM, McClennan BL, Clayman RV. The extraperitoneal approach and subcutaneous emphysema are associated with greater absorption of carbon dioxide during laparoscopic renal surgery. J Urol. Sep 1995;154(3):959–63.
13. Persson J, Wolner-Hanssen P. Laparoscopic Burch colposuspension for stress urinary incontinence: a randomized comparison of one or two sutures on each side of the urethra. Obstet Gynecol. Jan 2000;95(1):151–5.
14. Zullo F, Palomba S, Russo T, et al. Laparoscopic colposuspension using sutures or prolene meshes: a 3-year follow-up. Eur J Obstet Gynecol Reprod Biol. 1 Dec 2004;117(2):201–3.
15. Dean NM, Ellis G, Wilson PD, Herbison GP. Laparoscopic colposuspension for urinary incontinence in women. Cochrane Database Syst Rev. 2006;3:CD002239.
16. Khan MS, Challacombe B, Rose K, Dasgupta P. Robotic colposuspension: two case reports. J Endourol. Sep 2007;21(9):1077–9.
17. Phelps JY, Lin L, Liu CY. Laparoscopic suburethral sling procedure. J Am Assoc Gynecol Laparosc. Nov 2003;10(4):496–500.
18. Bump RC, Mattiasson A, Bo K, et al. The standardization of terminology of female pelvic organ prolapse and pelvic floor dysfunction. Am J Obstet Gynecol. Jul 1996;175(1):10–7.
19. Schaffer JI, Wai CY, Boreham MK. Etiology of pelvic organ prolapse. Clin Obstet Gynecol. Sep 2005;48(3):639–47.
20. Sultan AH, Stanton SL. Preserving the pelvic floor and perineum during childbirth–elective caesarean section? Br J Obstet Gynaecol. Aug 1996;103(8):731–4.
21. Alperin M, Moalli PA. Remodeling of vaginal connective tissue in patients with prolapse. Curr Opin Obstet Gynecol. Oct 2006;18(5):544–50.
22. Brubaker L, Cundiff GW, Fine P, et al. Abdominal sacrocolpopexy with Burch colposuspension to reduce urinary stress incontinence. N Engl J Med. 13 Apr 2006;354(15):1557–66.
23. Anger JT, Raz S, Rodriguez LV. Severe cystocele: optimizing results. Curr Urol Rep. Sep 2007;8(5):394–8.
24. Ballert KN, Biggs GY, Isenalumhe A Jr, Rosenblum N, Nitti VW. Managing the urethra at transvaginal pelvic organ prolapse repair: a urodynamic approach. J Urol. Feb 2009;181(2):679–84.
25. Sand PK, Koduri S, Lobel RW, et al. Prospective randomized trial of polyglactin 910 mesh to prevent recurrence of cystoceles and rectoceles. Am J Obstet Gynecol. Jun 2001;184(7):1357–62; discussion 1362–4.
26. Weber AM, Walters MD, Piedmonte MR, Ballard LA. Anterior colporrhaphy: a randomized trial of three surgical techniques. Am J Obstet Gynecol. Dec 2001;185(6):1299–304; discussion 1304–6.
27. Maher C, Baessler K, Glazener CM, Adams EJ, Hagen S. Surgical management of pelvic organ prolapse in women: a short version Cochrane review. Neurourol Urodyn. 2008;27(1):3–12.
28. Behnia-Willison F, Seman EI, Cook JR, O'Shea RT, Keirse MJ. Laparoscopic paravaginal repair of

anterior compartment prolapse. J Minim Invasive Gynecol. Jul–Aug 2007;14(4):475–80.
29. Daneshgari F, Paraiso MF, Kaouk J, Govier FE, Kozlowski PM, Kobashi KC. Robotic and laparoscopic female pelvic floor reconstruction. BJU Int. Sep 2006;98(Suppl 1):62–8; discussion 69.
30. Cundiff GW, Fenner D. Evaluation and treatment of women with rectocele: focus on associated defecatory and sexual dysfunction. Obstet Gynecol. Dec 2004;104(6):1403–21.
31. Gadonneix P, Ercoli A, Salet-Lizee D, et al. Laparoscopic sacrocolpopexy with two separate meshes along the anterior and posterior vaginal walls for multicompartment pelvic organ prolapse. J Am Assoc Gynecol Laparosc. Feb 2004;11(1):29–35.
32. Gadonneix P, Ercoli A, Scambia G, Villet R. The use of laparoscopic sacrocolpopexy in the management of pelvic organ prolapse. Curr Opin Obstet Gynecol. Aug 2005;17(4):376–80.
33. Loffeld CJ, Thijs S, Mol BW, Bongers MY, Roovers JP. Laparoscopic sacrocolpopexy: a comparison of Prolene and Tutoplast mesh. Acta Obstet Gynecol Scand. 2009;88(7):826–30.
34. Ganatra AM, Rozet F, Sanchez-Salas R, et al. The current status of laparoscopic sacrocolpopexy: a review. Eur Urol. 4 Feb 2009;55(5):1103–5.
35. North C, Ali-Ross N, Smith A, Reid F. A prospective study of laparoscopic sacrocolpopexy for the management of pelvic organ prolapse. BJOG. 28 May 2009;116(9):1251–7.
36. Claerhout F, Roovers JP, Lewi P, Verguts J, De Ridder D, Deprest J. Implementation of laparoscopic sacrocolpopexy-a single centre's experience. Int Urogynecol J Pelvic Floor Dysfunct. 29 May 2009;20(9):1119–25.
37. Ayav A, Bresler L, Hubert J, Brunaud L, Boissel P. Robotic-assisted pelvic organ prolapse surgery. Surg Endosc. Sep 2005;19(9):1200–3.
38. Daneshgari F, Kefer JC, Moore C, Kaouk J. Robotic abdominal sacrocolpopexy/sacrouteropexy repair of advanced female pelvic organ prolaspe (POP): utilizing POP-quantification-based staging and outcomes. BJU Int. Oct 2007;100(4):875–9.
39. Elliott DS, Krambeck AE, Chow GK. Long-term results of robotic assisted laparoscopic sacrocolpopexy for the treatment of high grade vaginal vault prolapse. J Urol. Aug 2006;176(2):655–9.
40. Kramer BA, Whelan CM, Powell TM, Schwartz BF. Robot-assisted laparoscopic sacrocolpopexy as management for pelvic organ prolapse. J Endourol. Apr 2009;23(4):655–8.
41. Miller EA, Webster GD. Current management of vesicovaginal fistulae. Curr Opin Urol. Jul 2001;11(4):417–21.
42. Sotelo R, Mariano MB, Garcia-Segui A, et al. Laparoscopic repair of vesicovaginal fistula. J Urol. May 2005;173(5):1615–8.
43. Sundaram BM, Kalidasan G, Hemal AK. Robotic repair of vesicovaginal fistula: case series of five patients. Urology. May 2006;67(5):970–3.
44. Nezhat CH, Nezhat F, Nezhat C, Rottenberg H. Laparoscopic repair of a vesicovaginal fistula: a case report. Obstet Gynecol. May 1994;83(5 Pt 2): 899–901.
45. Melamud O, Eichel L, Turbow B, Shanberg A. Laparoscopic vesicovaginal fistula repair with robotic reconstruction. Urology. Jan 2005;65(1):163–6.
46. Hasan ST, Marshall C, Robson WA, Neal DE. Clinical outcome and quality of life following enterocystoplasty for idiopathic detrusor instability and neurogenic bladder dysfunction. Br J Urol. Nov 1995;76(5):551–7.
47. Mundy AR, Stephenson TP. "Clam" ileocystoplasty for the treatment of refractory urge incontinence. Br J Urol. Dec 1985;57(6):641–6.
48. Meng MV, Anwar HP, Elliott SP, Stoller ML. Pure laparoscopic enterocystoplasty. J Urol. Mar 2002;167(3):1386.
49. Hasson HM. A modified instrument and method for laparoscopy. Am J Obstet Gynecol. 15 Jul 1971;110(6):886–7.
50. Gill IS, Rackley RR, Meraney AM, Marcello PW, Sung GT. Laparoscopic enterocystoplasty. Urology. Feb 2000;55(2):178–81.
51. Noguera RJ, Astigueta JC, Carmona O, et al. Laparoscopic augmentation enterocystoplasty through a single trocar. Urology. Jun 2009;73(6):1371–4.
52. El-Feel A, Abdel-Hakim MA, Abouel-Fettouh H, Abdel-Hakim AM. Laparoscopic augmentation ileocystoplasty: results and outcome. Eur Urol. 7 Apr 2008;55(3):721–7.
53. Cheon WC, Mak JH, Liu JY. Prospective randomised controlled trial comparing laparoscopic and open colposuspension. Hong Kong Med J. Feb 2003;9(1):10–4.
54. Ankardal M, Ekerydh A, Crafoord K, Milsom I, Stjerndahl JH, Engh ME. A randomised trial comparing open Burch colposuspension using sutures with laparoscopic colposuspension using mesh and staples in women with stress urinary incontinence. BJOG. Sep 2004;111(9):974–81.
55. Kitchener HC, Dunn G, Lawton V, Reid F, Nelson L, Smith AR. Laparoscopic versus open colposuspension–results of a prospective randomised controlled trial. BJOG. Sep 2006;113(9): 1007–13.
56. Carey MP, Goh JT, Rosamilia A, et al. Laparoscopic versus open Burch colposuspension: a randomised controlled trial. BJOG. Sep 2006;113(9):999–1006.
57. Higgs PJ, Chua HL, Smith AR. Long term review of laparoscopic sacrocolpopexy. BJOG. Aug 2005;112(8):1134–8.
58. Rozet F, Mandron E, Arroyo C, et al. Laparoscopic sacral colpopexy approach for genito-urinary prolapse: experience with 363 cases. Eur Urol. Feb 2005;47(2):230–6.
59. Ross JW, Preston M. Laparoscopic sacrocolpopexy for severe vaginal vault prolapse: five-year

outcome. J Minim Invasive Gynecol. May–Jun 2005;12(3):221–6.
60. Agarwala N, Hasiak N, Shade M. Laparoscopic sacral colpopexy with Gynemesh as graft material–experience and results. J Minim Invasive Gynecol. Sep–Oct 2007;14(5):577–83.
61. Rivoire C, Botchorishvili R, Canis M, et al. Complete laparoscopic treatment of genital prolapse with meshes including vaginal promontofixation and anterior repair: a series of 138 patients. J Minim Invasive Gynecol. Nov–Dec 2007;14(6):712–8.
62. Sarlos D, Brandner S, Kots L, Gygax N, Schaer G. Laparoscopic sacrocolpopexy for uterine and post-hysterectomy prolapse: anatomical results, quality of life and perioperative outcome—a prospective study with 101 cases. Int Urogynecol J Pelvic Floor Dysfunct. Oct 2008;19(10):1415–22.
63. Paraiso MF, Walters MD, Rackley RR, Melek S, Hugney C. Laparoscopic and abdominal sacral colpopexies: a comparative cohort study. Am J Obstet Gynecol. May 2005;192(5):1752–8.

Subject Index

Note: Locators followed by 'f' and 't' refer to figures and tables respectively.

A

Accesses
 port placement, robot docking, 58–59
 retrocolic/transmesenteric, 114
 retroperitoneal, 32–34
 role of NOTES and LESS
  augmentation enterocystoplasty, 169
  endoscopic instruments, 269–270
  internalized instrumentation (NOTES^{TM} and LESS), 270–271
  pneumoperitoneum, 269
  transcolonic/transenteric, 269
  transgastric, 268–269
  transvaginal, 268
  transvesical, 269
Adult laparoscopic and robotic-assisted pyeloplasty, 85
 complications, 91
 contraindications, 85–86
 critical instruments and supplies, 91
 critical operative steps, 91
 indications, 85
 outcomes, 90–91
 postoperative care, 88
  Bilateral UPJO, 90
  body habitus, 90
  concomitant pyelolithotomy, 90
  crossing vessels, 89
  horseshoe kidney, 90
  secondary pyeloplasties, 89–90
  technical considerations, 88–89
 preoperative preparation and positioning, 86
 surgical technique, 87–88
Adult laparoscopic partial nephrectomy for renal cell carcinoma
 critical instruments and supplies, 51
 critical operative steps, 51
 epidemiology, 43
 indications, 43–45
 outcomes
  complications, 50–51
  positive margins, 49–50
  recurrence and survival, 50
  tumor spillage and port site metastasis, 50
 preoperative preparation, 45
 special considerations
  dissectors, 49
  hemostasis, 48–49
  Hilar control, 47–48
 technique, 45–47
Adult robotic-assisted partial nephrectomy for renal cell carcinoma, 55
 access, port placement, robot docking, 58–59
 bowel mobilization and Hilar dissection, 60–61
 conversions and complications, 67–68
 critical instruments and supplies, 69
 critical operative steps, 69
 Hilar control and tumor extirpation, 62–63
 indications and contraindications, 56
 patient preparation, 56–57
 postoperative course, 65
 renal mobilization, tumor identification, and exposure, 61–62
 renorrhaphy, specimen retrieval, and closure, 63–65
 results, 65–67
 robotic surgery for complex tumors, 67–68
 ureteral catheter placement and patient positioning, 57–58
Anastomosis, 147f
 completed, 147f
 preparations for, 222–223
 using a running suture, 113f
Anesthetic risk and pediatric laproscopy, 186
Anterior pedicle, division of, 157
Antireflux surgery, 185, 194
Apical prolapse, laparoscopic and robotics for repair of, 282
Asymptomatic *vs.* symptomatic, laparoscopic pyeloplasty, 97–98
Augmentation cystoplasty, 288–289
Augmentation enterocystoplasty
 access, 169
 bladder incision and cystoplasty, 171
 bowel anastomosis, 170

Current Clinical Urology, DOI 10.1007/978-1-60327-9147, © Springer Science+Business Media, LLC 2011

Augmentation enterocystoplasty (*cont.*)
detubularization, 171
isolation of bowel segment, 169–170

B

Bilateral intra-abdominal "peeping" testicles, 208f
Bilateral non-palpable testicles and laparoscopic orchiopexy, 211–213
Bilateral UPJO, 90
Bipolar cautery, 13
Bipolar electrosurgery with thin blades, 37f
Bipolar energy, 4–5
Bipolar forceps, 11–12
Bladder augmentation, 25, 167–168
Bladder cancer, 153–154
Bladder neck, managing difficult, 248
bladder neck reconstruction, 249–250
challenging prostate anatomy, 248–249
management of ureteral injury, 250–251
Bowel anastomosis, 170
Bowel graspers, 20f
Bowel mobilization and Hilar dissection, 60–61
Bowel segment, isolation of, 169–170
Bulldog clamping of renal Hilum, 63f

C

Clamp
laparoscopic bulldog, 47
Satinsky, 3–4
vascular, 9–10
Computerized tomography, 95
Concomitant pyelolithotomy, 90
Conduit, 21, 153, 160
Continent catheterizable stomas, 167–174
access, 172
appendicovesicostomy, 172
isolation and harvest of appendix, 172
Curved scissors, 20f
Cystectomy, benign indications for partial, 161t
Cystoplasty, bladder incision and, 171

D

Da Vinci instruments, 11t, 14t
Da Vinci surgical system, 10, 17–19, 55, 109, 237
components, 239
DeBakey forceps, 20f
Deflectable tip of 5-mm laparoscopic camera, 263f
Detubularization, 171
Diagnostic laparoscopy, 17, 58, 202–203
Dismembered pyeloplasty, 114f
Diuretic radionuclide renography, 96
Donor ureter transection, 146f
Dorsal venous complex (DVC)
controlling, 158f
division of, 157–158
exposure of prostatic apex and ligation of, 239–240

E

Ectopic ureter, 73, 126–127, 135
EndoSamurai™, 268f
Endoscopic surgery, 25, 29, 31, 36–38
EndoWrist®, 3, 10–11, 18–19, 236, 254
Extirpation of renal mass, 63f
Extraperitoneal technique, 247–248
Extravesical ureteral reimplantation
description of robotic-assisted extravesical technique, 189–190
positioning and port placement, 188
results, 190–191

F

Fowler–Stephens orchiopexy, 202, 204–205, 207–208, 210

G

GelPort™, 263f
G-Prox™, 270f
Grasper, 4, 11, 14
Grasping and blunt dissection, instrumentation for, 35

H

Hemostatic devices, 6f
Hilar control, 47–48
and tumor extirpation, 62–63
Hilar dissection, 60–61
"Hitch stitch," placement of, 146f

I

Incising and hemostasis, instrumentation for, 35–37
Inguinal canal, 201, 203, 206
Instrumentation during pediatric laparoscopic anastomoses and reconstruction, 29
critical instruments and supplies, 39
critical operative steps, 39
instrumentation for
aspiration and irrigation, 38
grasping and blunt dissection, 35
incising and hemostasis, 35–37
insufflation/insufflators, 30–31
suturing and tissue anastomosis, 37–38
trocars, 31–32
visualization, 29–30
primary access and port placement, 32–35
Instrumentation during pediatric robotic anastomoses and reconstruction, 17–18
Da Vinci surgical system, 18–19
instruments, 19–21
robotic-assisted laparoscopic bladder surgeries, 24–25
robotic-assisted laparoscopic pyeloplasty, 21–22
robotic-assisted laparoscopic renal surgery, 22–23
robotic-assisted laparoscopic ureteral reimplantation, 23–24
Instruments and supplies, critical
adult laparoscopic and robotic-assisted pyeloplasty, 91
adult laparoscopic partial nephrectomy for renal cell carcinoma, 51
adult robotic-assisted partial nephrectomy for renal cell carcinoma, 69

instrumentation during pediatric laparoscopic anastomoses and reconstruction, 39
laparoscopic anastomoses and bladder neck reconstruction, 233
laparoscopic ureteral reimplant surgery to correct reflux disease
extravesical reimplantation, 183
intravesical reimplantation, 183
laparoscopic ureteroureterostomy and correction of ureteral defects, 137
pediatric laparoscopic and robotic upper pole nephrectomy, 79
pediatric robotic pyeloplasty, 119
robotic anastomoses and bladder neck reconstruction, 254
robotic intravesical and extravesical reimplantation, 195
Insufflation/insufflators, instrumentation for, 30–31
Interrupted suture technique, 223–224
Intra-abdominal testicle, 203, 205, 207–209, 211, 213–214
Intravenous pyelogram, 95
Intravesical ureteral reimplantation
description of robotic-assisted intravesical technique, 192–193
positioning and port placement, 191–192
results, 193–194
Ipsilateral ureteroureterostomy
indications for, 126–127
principles of, 129

K

Kidney, 35, 38, 61–62
cancer, 55, 68
horseshoe, 90
Kocherization of duodenum, 61f

L

Laparoscopic anastomoses and bladder neck reconstruction, 221
critical instruments and supplies, 233
critical operative steps
interrupted suture, 232–233
preparation of anastomosis, 232
running suture, 233
discussion, 230–232
interrupted suture technique, 223–224
position of patient and surgeon, 221–222
preparations for anastomosis, 222–223
running suture technique, 224–225
single-knot method, 225–230
Laparoscopic and robotic instrumentation for urologic reconstructive surgery, 3
laparoscopy *vs.* robotics, 3–4
robotic instruments, 10–11
bipolar cautery, 13
clip appliers, 14
five-millimeter instruments, 14–15
graspers, 14
monopolar cautery, 11–12
scissors, 13
ultrasonic energy, 13
standard laparoscopic instrumentation
graspers and dissectors, 4
incision and hemostasis, 4–7
port-site closure, 10
retraction, 8–9
stapling/clipping, 8
suction/irrigation, 8
suturing, 7–8
vascular clamps, 9–10
Laparoscopic and robotic orchiopexy for impalpable undescended testicle
bilateral non-palpable testicles and laparoscopic orchiopexy, 211–213
complications, 213–214
laparoscopic management of non-palpable testicle
diagnostic laparoscopy, 202–203
laparoscopic orchiopexy, 203–204
laparoscopic orchiopexy, 201
diagnostic workup, 201–202
preoperative assessment, 201
timing of surgery, 202
laparoscopic technique for non-palpable testicle, 204–205
blind-ending testicular vessels, 206
cord structures entering internal ring, 206–207
intra-abdominal testis, 207–208
laparoscopy in management of high-palpable undescended testicle, 213
open surgical management of non-palpable testicle, 202
primary laparoscopic orchiopexy
closure and exiting abdomen, 210–211
creating neo-inguinal hiatus and testicular delivery into the scrotum, 210
establishing peritoneal pedicle flap, 208–210
gaining additional cord length and securing testicle, 210
second-stage fowler–Stephens, 211
Laparoscopic and robotics
for anterior and posterior vaginal wall prolapse
laparoscopic cystocele repair, 281
laparoscopic rectocele repair, 281–282
for repair of apical prolapse, 282
sacrocolpopexy, 282–286
Laparoscopic augmentation cystoplasty, 168, 288–289
Laparoscopic bladder augmentation and creation of continent-catheterizable stomas, 167
augmentation enterocystoplasty
access, 169
bladder incision and cystoplasty, 171
bowel anastomosis, 170
detubularization, 171
isolation of bowel segment, 169–170
contraindications, 168
creation of continent-catheterizable stoma, 171–172

Laparoscopic bladder augmentation (*cont.*)
access, 172
appendicovesicostomy, 172
isolation and harvest of appendix, 172
critical surgical instruments, 174
indications, 167–168
post-operative management, 173–174
surgical procedure, 168–169
surgical technique
pre-operative considerations, 168
Laparoscopic colposuspension, 279–279t, 281
Laparoscopic cystectomy, 153, 156
Laparoscopic cystocele repair, 281
Laparoscopic graspers, 4f
Laparoscopic instrumentation, standard
graspers and dissectors, 4
incision and hemostasis, 4–7
port-site closure, 10
retraction, 8–9
stapling/clipping, 8
suction/irrigation, 8
suturing, 7–8
vascular clamps, 9–10
Laparoscopic ipsilateral ureteroureterostomy
reports of, 135
steps in, 135–136
Laparoscopic management of non-palpable testicle
diagnostic laparoscopy, 202–203
laparoscopic orchiopexy, 203–204
Laparoscopic orchiopexy, 201, 204t
diagnostic workup, 201–202
preoperative assessment, 201
timing of surgery, 202
Laparoscopic partial nephrectomy for renal cell carcinoma (adults)
advantages and disadvantages, 75t
critical instruments and supplies, 51
critical operative steps, 51
epidemiology, 43
indications, 43–45
outcomes
complications, 50–51
positive margins, 49–50
recurrence and survival, 50
tumor spillage and port site metastasis, 50
preoperative preparation, 45
robotic-assisted partial nephrectomy *vs.*, 66t
special considerations
dissectors, 49
hemostasis, 48–49
Hilar control, 47–48
technique, 45–47
Laparoscopic pyeloplasty, pediatric, 93
asymptomatic *vs.* symptomatic, 97–98
critical instruments, 107
critical operative steps
for retroperitoneal-assisted laparoscopic pyeloplasty, 106–107
for retroperitoneal laparoscopic pyeloplasty, 106
for robotic-assisted retroperitoneal pyeloplasty, 107
for robotic-assisted transperitoneal pyeloplasty, 107
for transperitoneal laparoscopic pyeloplasty, 105–106
diagnostic assessment
computerized tomography, 95
diuretic radionuclide renography, 96
intravenous pyelogram, 95
pressure flow study, 96–97
ultrasonography, 94–95
voiding cystourethrogram, 96
etiology and presentation of ureteropelvic junction obstruction, 93–94
surgical management, 98
instruments in pediatric laparoscopy, 98–99
pre-operative assessment, 98
retroperitoneal approach, 101–103
robotic-assisted laparoscopic pyeloplasty, 103–104
robotic-assisted retroperitoneal approach, 104–105
robotic-assisted transperitoneal approach, 104
transperitoneal laparoscopic pyeloplasty, 99–101
Laparoscopic rectocele repair, 281–282
Laparoscopic renal surgery
retroperitoneal
patient positioning, 33f
port placement, 33f
transperitoneal
patient positioning, 34f
port placement, 34f
Laparoscopic sacrocolpopexy, 282, 285–286, 286t
Laparoscopic surgery, 25, 35–36, 130–131
Laparoscopic technique for non-palpable testicle, 204–205
blind-ending testicular vessels, 206
cord structures entering internal ring, 206–207
intra-abdominal testis, 207–208
Laparoscopic transureteroureterostomy
reports of, 136
steps in, 136–137
Laparoscopic treatment of VUR, surgical techniques for
intravesical procedures, 177–178
megaureter, 178–179
patient and surgeon position, 176–179
robotic-assisted ureteroneocystostomy, 179
Laparoscopic ultrasound of kidney and renal mass, 62f
Laparoscopic ureteral reimplantation procedures, outcomes of, 182t
Laparoscopic ureteral reimplant surgery to correct reflux disease, 175
critical instruments and supplies
extravesical reimplantation, 183
intravesical reimplantation, 183
critical operative steps
extravesical reimplantation, 181–183
intravesical reimplantation, 183

evolution, 175–176
outcomes and discussion
extravesical techniques, 179–180
intravesical techniques, 180–181
robotic surgery, 183
surgical techniques for laparoscopic treatment of VUR
intravesical procedures, 177–178
megaureter, 178–179
patient and surgeon position, 176–179
robotic-assisted ureteroneocystostomy, 179
Laparoscopic ureteral surgery, 130
Laparoscopic ureteroureterostomy and correction of ureteral defects, 125
critical instruments and supplies, 137
critical operative steps, 137
ipsilateral ureteroureterostomy
indications for, 126–127
principles of, 129
laparoscopic ipsilateral ureteroureterostomy
reports of, 135
steps in, 135–136
laparoscopic transureteroureterostomy
reports of, 136
steps in, 136–137
laparoscopic ureteral surgery, 130
laparoscopic ureteroureterostomy of single ureter to itself
reports of, 130–131
steps in, 131–134
traditional open surgical approach, principles of, 127
transureteroureterostomy, principles of, 129–130
ureteral surgery, indications for, 125
ureteroureterostomy of single ureter to itself
indications for, 125–126
principles of, 128–129
Laparoscopic ureteroureterostomy of single ureter to itself
reports of, 130–131
steps in, 131–134
Laparoscopic ureteroureterostomy of single ureter to itself, steps in, 131–134
Laparoscopic uterosacral ligament fixation, 282
Laparoscopic UU, indications for, 142t
Laparoscopy
in management of high-palpable undescended testicle, 213
robotics *vs.*, 3–4
in stress urinary incontinence and pelvic reconstructive surgery, 277–289
Laparoscopy and robotics in stress urinary incontinence and pelvic reconstructive surgery, 277
augmentation cystoplasty, 288–289
laparoscopic and robotic sacrocolpopexy, 282–286
laparoscopic and robotics for anterior and posterior vaginal wall prolapse
laparoscopic cystocele repair, 281
laparoscopic rectocele repair, 281–282
laparoscopic and robotics for repair of apical prolapse, 282
laparoscopic uterosacral ligament fixation, 282
pelvic organ prolapse, 280
patient evaluation prior to repair, 280–281
stress urinary incontinence, 277–278
laparoscopic burch colposuspension, 278–279
robotic-assisted laparoscopic colposuspension, 279
vesicovaginal fistula, 286–287
laparoscopic and robotic VVF repair, 287–288
LESS (Laparoendoscopic Single Site Surgery)
development of, 262–263
equipment for
incisions for, 264–265
scope innovations for, 263–264
nomenclature, 262
role in minimally invasive reconstructive urological surgery, 261–271
potential benefits of, 261
technical challenges of, 261–262
Lymph node dissection at aortic bifurcation, 158f

M

Maryland dissector, 20f
Minimally invasive reconstructive urological surgery, 261
LESS
development of, 262–263
equipment for, 263–264
incisions for, 264–265
nomenclature, 262
NOTES™, 265
development of, 265–266
managing coaxial limitations, 266–267
in urology, 266
potential benefits of NOTES™ and LESS, 261
scopes and equipment
conventional scope, 267
new scope and platform innovations for NOTES™, 267
technical challenges of NOTES™ and LESS, 261–262
Minimally invasive surgery, 17–18, 25, 86, 119, 235
Moieties, 73–79
Monopolar, 19, 23
cautery, 11–12
Monopolar cautery hook, 19f
Montsouris technique, *see* Retrovesical dissection (Montsouris technique)

N

Needle driver, 7, 11, 14, 21–21f, 22, 24, 187
Needle holder, 37f
Neobladder, orthotopic, 153, 156, 159–160
Nephrectomy, 3, 5, 43–51, 55–69, 73–79
Nephron sparing surgery, 50, 55, 67, 127
Non-dismembered pyeloplasty, 113f–115f
Non-palpable testicle, 201–204

NOTES and LESS in minimally invasive reconstructive urological surgery, role of, 261
  accesses
    endoscopic instruments, 269–270
    internalized instrumentation (NOTES™ and LESS), 270–271
    pneumoperitoneum, 269
    transcolonic/transenteric, 269
    transgastric, 268–269
    transvaginal, 268
    transvesical, 269
  LESS
    development of, 262–263
    equipment for, 263–264
    incisions for, 264–265
    nomenclature, 262
  NOTES™, 265
    development of, 265–266
    managing coaxial limitations, 266–267
    in urology, 266
  potential benefits of NOTES™ and LESS, 261
  scopes and equipment
    conventional scope, 267
    new scope and platform innovations for NOTES™, 267
  technical challenges of NOTES™ and LESS, 261–262
NOTES (Natural Orifice Translumenal Endoscopic Surgery), 25, 68
  role in minimally invasive reconstructive urological surgery, 261–271
    potential benefits of, 261
    technical challenges of, 261–262

O

Olympus R-Scope™, 268f
Open ipsilateral ureteroureterostomy, principles of, 129
Open surgical management of non-palpable testicle, 202
Open transureteroureterostomy, principles of, 129–130
Open ureteroureterostomy of single ureter to itself, principles of, 128–129
Operative steps, critical
  adult laparoscopic and robotic-assisted pyeloplasty, 91
  adult laparoscopic partial nephrectomy for renal cell carcinoma, 51
  adult robotic-assisted partial nephrectomy for renal cell carcinoma, 69
  instrumentation during pediatric laparoscopic anastomoses and reconstruction, 39
  laparoscopic anastomoses and bladder neck reconstruction
    interrupted suture, 232–233
    preparation of anastomosis, 232
    running suture, 233
  laparoscopic ureteral reimplant surgery to correct reflux disease
    extravesical reimplantation, 181–183
    intravesical reimplantation, 183
  laparoscopic ureteroureterostomy and correction of ureteral defects, 137
  pediatric laparoscopic and robotic upper pole nephrectomy, 79
  pediatric laparoscopic pyeloplasty
    for retroperitoneal-assisted laparoscopic pyeloplasty, 106–107
    for retroperitoneal laparoscopic pyeloplasty, 106
    for robotic-assisted retroperitoneal pyeloplasty, 107
    for robotic-assisted transperitoneal pyeloplasty, 107
  pediatric robotic pyeloplasty, 119
  robotic anastomoses and bladder neck reconstruction, 254
  robotic radical cystectomy and use of intestinal segments, 164
  robotic ureteral reimplant surgery to correct reflux disease, 194
Orchiectomy, 206–207, 262
Orchiopexy
  laparoscopic, 201, 203–204, 211–212
    diagnostic workup, 201–202
    preoperative assessment, 201
    timing of surgery, 202
  primary laparoscopic, 208–210
Outcomes, 90–91
  adult laparoscopic and robotic-assisted pyeloplasty, 90–91
  adult laparoscopic partial nephrectomy for renal cell carcinoma
    positive margins, 49–50
  augmentation cystoplasty, 289
  complications, 50–51
  continent cutaneous urinary diversion, 160–161
  laparoscopic and robotic VVF repair, 288
  laparoscopic burch colposuspension, 278–280
  laparoscopic cystocele repair, 281
  laparoscopic rectocele repair, 281–282
  of laparoscopic ureteral reimplantation, 182
  laparoscopic ureteral reimplant surgery, 179–180
  laparoscopic uterosacral ligament fixation, 282
  minimally invasive partial cystectomy, 163
  oncologic, 251
  positive margins, 49–50
  recurrence and survival, 50
  retroperitoneal approach, 102–103
  robotic anastomoses and bladder neck reconstruction, 252
  of robotic-assisted laparoscopic pyeloplasty, 89
  robotic-assisted retroperitoneal approach, 104–105
  transperitoneal laparoscopic pyeloplasty, 101
  tumor spillage and port site metastasis, 50

P

Partial cystectomy
  benign indications for, 161
  minimally invasive, 161
  transgastric, 270

Pediatric laparoscopic anastomoses and reconstruction, instrumentation during, 29
- aspiration and irrigation, 38
- critical instruments and supplies, 39
- critical operative steps, 39
- grasping and blunt dissection, 35
- incising and hemostasis, 35–37
- instrumentation for access
  - trocars, 31–32
- insufflation/insufflators, 30–31
- primary access and port placement, 32–35
- suturing and tissue anastomosis, 37–38
- visualization, 29–30

Pediatric laparoscopic and robotic upper pole nephrectomy, 73
- complications, 78–79
- critical instruments and supplies, 79
- critical operative steps, 79
- indications, 73
- preoperative evaluation, 73–75
- retroperitoneal prone and lateral, 78
- robotic-assisted transperitoneal approach, 75–78
- surgical approach, 75

Pediatric laparoscopic pyeloplasty, 93
- asymptomatic *vs.* symptomatic, 97–98
- critical instruments, 107
- critical operative steps
  - for retroperitoneal-assisted laparoscopic pyeloplasty, 106–107
  - for retroperitoneal laparoscopic pyeloplasty, 106
  - for robotic-assisted retroperitoneal pyeloplasty, 107
  - for robotic-assisted transperitoneal pyeloplasty, 107
  - for transperitoneal laparoscopic pyeloplasty, 105–106
- diagnostic assessment
  - computerized tomography, 95
  - diuretic radionuclide renography, 96
  - intravenous pyelogram, 95
  - pressure flow study, 96–97
  - ultrasonography, 94–95
  - voiding cystourethrogram, 96
- etiology and presentation of ureteropelvic junction obstruction, 93–94
- surgical management, 98
  - instruments in pediatric laparoscopy, 98–99
  - pre-operative assessment, 98
  - retroperitoneal approach, 101–103
  - robotic-assisted laparoscopic pyeloplasty, 103–104
  - robotic-assisted retroperitoneal approach, 104–105
  - robotic-assisted transperitoneal approach, 104
  - transperitoneal laparoscopic pyeloplasty, 99–101

Pediatric robotic anastomoses and reconstruction, instrumentation during, 17–18
- Da Vinci surgical system, 18–19
- instruments, 19–21
- robotic-assisted laparoscopic bladder surgeries, 24–25
- robotic-assisted laparoscopic pyeloplasty, 21–22
- robotic-assisted laparoscopic renal surgery, 22–23
- robotic-assisted laparoscopic ureteral reimplantation, 23–24

Pediatric robotic pyeloplasty, 109–110
- critical instruments and supplies, 119
- critical operative steps, 119
- diagnosis, 110
- indications, 110–111
- instruments and supplies, 111
- postoperative management and follow-up
  - intraoperative complications, 116–117
  - postoperative care and follow-up, 115–116
  - postoperative pain management, 115
- redo robotic pyeloplasty, 117–118
- retrocolic/transmesenteric access, 114
  - dismembered/non-dismembered robotic pyeloplasty, 114–115
- robotic procedures for recurrent UPJO, 117
- robotic ureterocalicostomy, 118–119
- surgical technique, 111–113
- transperitoneal/retroperitoneal approach, 113

Pediatric robotic urologic surgery, instruments, 25t

Pelvic lymph node dissection, 158

Pelvic organ prolapse, 277, 280
- patient evaluation prior to repair, 280–281

Port, placement, 32–35, 144–145, 156, 179, 187–189, 191–192, 238–239

Posterior bladder and prostatic pedicles, division of, 157

Pressure flow study, 96–97

Primary access and port placement, 32–35

Primary laparoscopic orchiopexy
- closure and exiting abdomen, 210–211
- creating neo-inguinal hiatus and testicular delivery into the scrotum, 210
- establishing peritoneal pedicle flap, 208–210
- gaining additional cord length and securing testicle, 210

Prostatectomy, 221–222, 230–232, 235–236, 247–248

Pyeloplasty, 8, 11, 21–22, 85–91, 93, 103–107, 109–119

Pyeloplasty, laparoscopic and robotic-assisted, 85
- complications, 91
- contraindications, 85–86
- critical instruments and supplies, 91
- critical operative steps, 91
- indications, 85
- outcomes, 90–91
- postoperative care, 88
  - Bilateral UPJO, 90
  - body habitus, 90
  - concomitant pyelolithotomy, 90
  - crossing vessels, 89
  - horseshoe kidney, 90
  - secondary pyeloplasties, 89–90
  - technical considerations, 88–89

Pyeloplasty, laparoscopic and robotic-assisted (*cont.*)
preoperative preparation and positioning, 86
surgical technique, 87–88

Q
QuadPort™, 264f

R
Radical cystectomy, 153–164
and anterior pelvic exenteration, 159
Reconstructive surgery, 3–15, 277–290
Reconstructive urology, 68
Rectocele, 281–282
Redo robotic pyeloplasty, 117–118
Reflux disease, 175–183
Reimplant surgery, 175–183
Renal mobilization, tumor identification, and exposure, 61–62
Renorrhaphy, completion of, 64f
Renorrhaphy, specimen retrieval, and closure, 63–65
Retractors, 9f
Retrocolic/transmesenteric access, 114
dismembered/non-dismembered robotic pyeloplasty, 114–115
Retroperitoneal access, 32–35, 101–104, 106–107, 113
Retroperitoneal heminephrectomy, 79f
Retroperitoneal laparoscopic pyeloplasty, 38f
Retrovesical dissection (Montsouris technique), 242–243
anatomic restoration and urethrovesical anastomosis, 244–247
division of dorsal venous complex and posterior urethra, 244
lymph node dissection, 247
neurovascular bundle dissection and controlling lateral pedicles, 243–244
Robotic anastomoses and bladder neck reconstruction, 235–236
critical instruments and supplies, 254
critical operative steps, 254
extraperitoneal technique, 247–248
functional outcomes, 252
bladder neck contracture, 253
continence, 252
potency, 252–253
managing difficult bladder neck, 248
bladder neck reconstruction, 249–250
challenging prostate anatomy, 248–249
management of ureteral injury, 250–251
oncologic outcomes, 251
operative considerations
anesthesia considerations, 239
Da Vinci surgical system components, 237
indications and contraindications, 236
patient positioning, 237–238
port placement, 238–239
preoperative preparation, 236–237
retrovesical dissection (Montsouris technique), 242–243
anatomic restoration and urethrovesical anastomosis, 244–247
division of dorsal venous complex and posterior urethra, 244
lymph node dissection, 247
neurovascular bundle dissection and controlling lateral pedicles, 243–244
transperitoneal RALP technique
bladder mobilization, 239
bladder neck transection, 240–241
exposure of prostatic apex and ligation of DVC, 239–240
management of rectal injury, 242
posterior prostatic dissection, 241–242
Robotic-assisted laparoscopic surgeries
bladder surgeries, 24–25
laparoscopic colposuspension, 279
laparoscopic pyeloplasty, 21–22, 103–105
outcomes, 89t
laparoscopic renal surgery, 22–23
laparoscopic sacrocolpopexy
port placement for, 283
laparoscopic ureteral reimplantation, 23–24
renal surgery, 22–23
Robotic-assisted laparoscopic ureterocalicostomy, 119f
Robotic-assisted partial nephrectomy, 57f–59f
operative results, 66t
vs. laparoscopic partial nephrectomy, 66t
Robotic-assisted partial nephrectomy for renal cell carcinoma (adults), 55
access, port placement, robot docking, 58–59
bowel mobilization and hilar dissection, 60–61
conversions and complications, 67
critical instruments and supplies, 69
critical operative steps, 68–69
hilar control and tumor extirpation, 62–63
indications and contraindications, 56
patient preparation, 56–57
postoperative course, 65
renal mobilization, tumor identification, and exposure, 61–62
renorrhaphy, specimen retrieval, and closure, 63–65
results, 65–67
robotic surgery for complex tumors, 67–68
ureteral catheter placement and patient positioning, 57–58
Robotic-assisted surgeries
advantages and disadvantages of, 56t
radical cystoprostatectomy, port placement for, 155f
robotic-assisted radical cystoprostatectomy, 153
robotic-assisted retroperitoneal pyeloplasty, 107
robotic-assisted sacrocolpopexy, 284–285
robotic-assisted transperitoneal approach, 75–78
robotic-assisted ureteroneocystostomy, 179
upper pole nephrectomy, 76f
Robotic instruments, 10–11, 12f
bipolar cautery, 13
clip appliers, 14
five-millimeter instruments, 14–15
graspers, 14
monopolar cautery, 11–12

scissors, 13
ultrasonic energy, 13
Robotic procedures for recurrent UPJO, 117
Robotic pyeloplasty, pediatric, 109–110
critical instruments and supplies, 119
critical operative steps, 119
diagnosis, 110
indications, 110–111
instruments and supplies, 111
postoperative management and follow-up
intraoperative complications, 116–117
postoperative care and follow-up, 115–116
postoperative pain management, 115
redo robotic pyeloplasty, 117–118
retrocolic/transmesenteric access, 114
dismembered/non-dismembered robotic pyeloplasty, 114–115
robotic procedures for recurrent UPJO, 117
robotic ureterocalicostomy, 118–119
surgical technique, 111–113
transperitoneal/retroperitoneal approach, 113
Robotic radical cystectomy and use of intestinal segments, 153
critical instruments, 164
critical operative steps, 163–164
robotic-assisted radical cystoprostatectomy, 153
anterior bladder release, 157
development of posterior plane, 157
division of anterior pedicle, 157
division of dorsal venous complex, 157–158
division of posterior bladder and prostatic pedicles, 157
extended pelvic lymph node dissection, 158
identification and transection of ureters, 156
indications and contraindications, 153–154
operating roomsetup, 154
patient preparation and positioning, 154–156
port placement, 156
radical cystectomy and anterior pelvic exenteration, 159
transposition of left ureter to right side, 158
urinary diversion
continent cutaneous urinary diversion, 160
cystoscopy, 162–163
minimally invasive partial cystectomy, 161–162
orthotopic neobladder, 159–160
positioning and trocar placement, 161–162
Robotic renal surgery, 68t
Robotics
laparoscopy *vs.*, 3–4
miniature intracorporeal, 271
in stress urinary incontinence and pelvic reconstructive surgery, 277–289
Robotic sacrocolpopexy, 282–286
Robotic surgery, 3, 183
for complex tumors, 67–68
Robotic ureteral reimplant surgery to correct reflux disease, 185
anesthetic risk and pediatric laproscopy, 186
critical instruments and supplies: robotic intravesical and extravesical reimplantation, 195
critical operative steps: intravesical reimplantation, 195
extravesical ureteral reimplantation
description of robotic-assisted extravesical technique, 187–190
positioning and port placement, 188
results, 190–192
indications for intervention, 186
intravesical ureteral reimplantation
description of robotic-assisted extravesical technique, 192–195
positioning and port placement, 191–193
results, 193
patient preparation and setup, 186–187
patient selection, 186
port placement and selection of instruments, 187
specifics of robotic approach, 187–189
Robotic ureterocalicostomy, 118–119
Robotic ureteroureterostomy and correction of ureteral defects, 141–142
approach and identification of ureteral obstruction, 145–147
operative considerations, 147
post-operative considerations, 148
surgical considerations, 147
indications, 142
surgical technique
patient positioning, 143–144
port placement, 144–145
pre-operative preparation, 143
Running suture technique, 224–225
single-knot method, 225–230

S

Scissors, 13
laparoscopic, 35–36
monopolar, 157
Second-stage fowler–Stephens, 211
Single-knot running vesicourethral anastomosis, 227–229t
Single site surgery, 261
Stress urinary incontinence, 277–278
laparoscopic burch colposuspension, 278–289
laproscopy and robotics, 277–289
robotic-assisted laparoscopic colposuspension, 279
Suture, 14, 20–21, 37, 64, 69, 133–134, 148, 172, 223–225, 232–233
placement of, 169
Suture technique
interrupted, 223–224
running, 224–225
single-knot method, 225–230
Suturing and tissue anastomosis, instrumentation for, 37–38
Suturing instruments, 7f

T

Traditional open surgical approach, 127
Transabdominal traction sutures, 170f
Transgastric partial cystectomy, 274
Transperitoneal, 24, 34–35, 46, 75–77, 99–101, 104–107, 113–114
Transperitoneal RALP technique
  bladder mobilization, 239
  bladder neck transection, 240–241
  exposure of prostatic apex and ligation of the dorsal venous complex (DVC), 239–240
  management of rectal injury, 242
  posterior prostatic dissection, 241–242
Transperitoneal/retroperitoneal approach, 113
Transport™, 268f
Transposition of left ureter to right side, 158
Transureteroureterostomy, 129–130
Transvesical peritoneoscopy, 267
Triport™, 264f
Trocars, 31–32
  placement of, 169
Tumors
  extirpation, 62–63
  robotic surgery for complex, 67–68

U

Ultrasonography, 94–95
Undescended testis, 148, 202
Ureteral catheter placement, 57–58
Ureteral defects, 125–137, 141–148
Ureteral injury, 252–253
Ureteral obstruction, 22, 65, 141–142, 145–147
Ureteral reimplantation, 24–25, 175–183, 185–195
Ureteral surgery, 125–126, 128, 130
  indications for, 125–126
  principles for, 128t
Ureter and renal hilum, identification, 61f
Ureterocalicostomy, 118f
Ureterocele, 73, 126–127, 129, 144, 146
Ureteropelvic junction obstruction (UPJO), 85–91, 93–107, 109–119
  access through mesentary, 100f
  CT scan appearance, 96f
  etiology and presentation of, 93–94
  exposure of, 100f
  intrinsic causes of, 94f
  Mag 3 Lasix scan drainage curve in setting of, 97f
  retrograde pyelogram, 86f
  typical appearance, 95f
Ureteropelvic junction, transection, 87f
Ureteroureterostomy of single ureter to itself
  indications for, 125–126
  principles of, 128–129
Ureters, identification and transection of, 156
Urinary diversion, 50, 117, 156, 158–161
  continent cutaneous urinary diversion, 160
  cystoscopy, 162–163
  minimally invasive partial cystectomy, 161–162
  orthotopic neobladder, 159–160
  positioning and trocar placement, 161–162
Urology, 18, 21, 25, 68, 141, 188, 263, 266

V

Vascular clamps, 10f
Vesicoureteral reflux, 22–24, 73, 96, 110, 126, 141, 175, 180, 185
Vesicourethral anastomosis, choreographed sequence of successive stitches
  in interrupted, 224t
  in running, 226t
    "single-knot," 226t
Vesicovaginal fistula, 182, 277, 286–287
  laparoscopic and robotic VVF repair, 287–288
Voiding cystourethrogram, 96

Y

Y-shaped mesh, 283f

MIX
Papier aus verantwortungsvollen Quellen
Paper from responsible sources
FSC® C105338

If you have any concerns about our products,
you can contact us on
ProductSafety@springernature.com

In case Publisher is established outside the EU,
the EU authorized representative is:
Springer Nature Customer Service Center GmbH
Europaplatz 3, 69115 Heidelberg, Germany

Printed by Libri Plureos GmbH
in Hamburg, Germany